Pulmonary Embolism

Eyal Herzog
Editor

Pulmonary Embolism

Springer

Editor
Eyal Herzog
Hadassah Medical Center
Jerusalem, Israel

ISBN 978-3-030-87089-8 ISBN 978-3-030-87090-4 (eBook)
https://doi.org/10.1007/978-3-030-87090-4

This Springer imprint is published by the registered company Springer Nature Switzerland AG
The registered company address is: Gewerbestrasse 11, 6330 Cham, Switzerland

Contents

Pathway for the Diagnosis and Management of Pulmonary Embolism

Eyal Herzog, Gabby Elbaz-Greener, David Planer, Tali Koren, Offer Amir, Janet Shapiro, and Yosef Kalish

1 Introduction

Venous Thromboembolism (VTE), the combined syndromes of deep vein thrombosis (DVT) and pulmonary embolism (PE), is currently the third most frequent acute cardiovascular syndrome globally behind myocardial infarction and stroke [1]. In the past decade we have seen a remarkable improvement in new diagnostic tools as well as novel therapeutic options to manage patients with VTE.

Multiple societies from around the globe have published guidelines for the management of VTE. The most recently updated document is the 2019 European Society of Cardiology (ESC) guidelines for the diagnosis and management of acute pulmonary embolism which was developed in collaboration with the European Respiratory Society (ERS) [2]. A major limitation of the currently published guidelines is its complexity.

To aid health care providers caring for patients with acute PE, our team developed a novel, comprehensive yet straightforward, pathway for the management of patients with PE, which we believe can be used in many health care systems around the globe [3].

The necessity to develop such a pathway at our institution was compelling, and typical of the need at many other large medical centres. It has become increasingly difficult for all health care providers to grasp all the subtleties in the management of VTE to rapidly, efficiently, and accurately implement clinical protocols. It should

E. Herzog (✉) · G. Elbaz-Greener · D. Planer · T. Koren · O. Amir
Department of Cardiology, Heart Institute, Hadassah Hebrew University Medical Center, Jerusalem, Israel

J. Shapiro
Department of Medicine, Mount Sinai Morningside, New York, NY, USA

Y. Kalish
Department of Hematology, Hadassah Hebrew University Medical Center, Jerusalem, Israel

E. Herzog (ed.), *Pulmonary Embolism*,
https://doi.org/10.1007/978-3-030-87090-4_1

be emphasized that this pathway is the opinion of our group and may differ somewhat from the published guidelines.

Our pathway for the diagnosis and management of pulmonary embolism is divided into three steps as demonstrated in Fig. 1:

Step 1: Diagnosis of PE (top third of pathway)
Step 2: Acute management of patients with PE (middle third of pathway)
Step 3: Recommendations for the chronic management of patients with PE (the bottom third of the pathway).

In each step we propose key questions that lead to "yes" and "no" answers which will further aid the health care providers to easily navigate the pathway.

The Pulmonary Embolism Response Team (PERT) is a multispecialty team involved in the decision-making for the individual patient. The ESC guidelines recommend establishment of a team of experts to convene for every case of intermediate or high risk pulmonary embolism. The composition of the team depends on the local resources and expertise. The PERT team brings together specialists from different disciplines including, but not limited to, cardiology, pulmonology, Emergency Medicine, hematology, vascular medicine, anaesthesiology/intensive care, cardiothoracic surgery, and interventional radiology. The team convenes in real time (via a platform such as WhatsApp or text messages) to communicate clinical data, discuss the options and provide consensus for a course of management. By directly involving the expert clinicians, the team facilitates the immediate implementation of the care plan [4].

2 Description of the Pathway

In most cases, patients with PE present with dyspnea, chest pain, pre-syncope or syncope, or hemoptysis. However, in other cases, the signs and symptoms may be non-specific.

A. **Acute management of hemodynamically unstable patients** (Fig. 2)

The first action is to assess the hemodynamic status in any patient with suspected PE. Hemodynamic instability is defined as one of the following:

1. Presentation following cardiac arrest or current need for cardiopulmonary resuscitation.
2. Obstructive shock—defined as systolic BP <90 mmHg or vasopressors required to achieve a BP >90 mmHg despite adequate filling status AND end organ hypoperfusion (altered mental status, cold, clammy skin, oligo-anuria, increased serum lactate).
3. Persistent hypotension- defined as systolic BP <90 mmHg or systolic BP drop >40 mmHg from baseline, lasting longer than 15 min and not caused by a new onset arrhythmia, hypovolemia or sepsis.

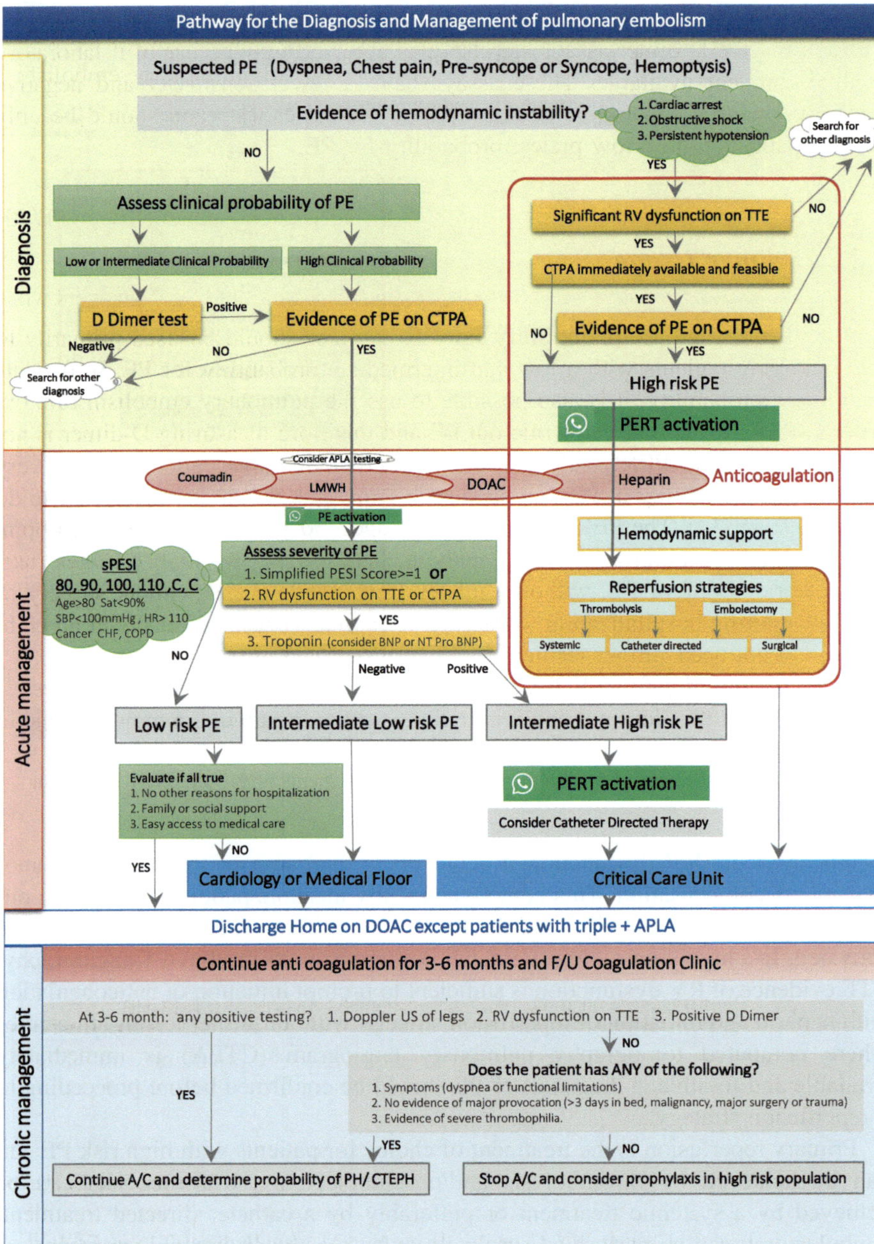

Fig. 1 Pathway for the diagnosis and management of pulmonary embolism

In patients with hemodynamic instability, the most useful initial test is bedside transthoracic echocardiography (TTE). The bedside TTE will show evidence of

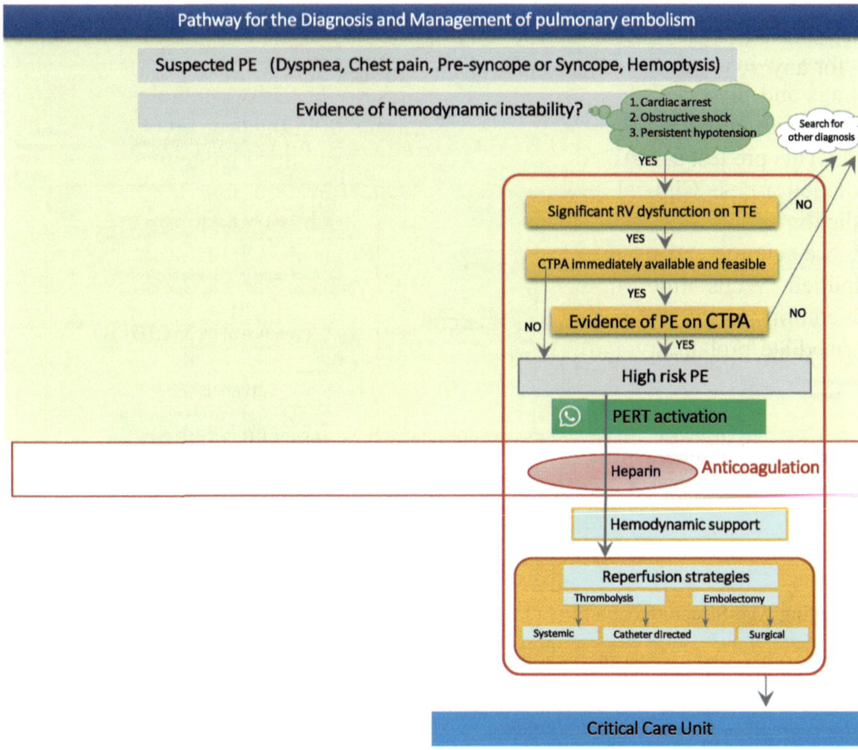

Fig. 2 Acute management of hemodynamically unstable patients with pulmonary embolism

significant acute RV dysfunction if acute PE is the cause of the patient's hemodynamic decompensation. This hemodynamically unstable patient is defined in our pathway as a "High Risk PE" and the PE Response Team (PERT team) should be activated. In a highly unstable patient, who cannot be mobilized to CT angiography, TTE evidence of RV dysfunction is sufficient to prompt initiation of anticoagulation with heparin and initiation of reperfusion strategy without further testing. In centres where computed tomography pulmonary angiogram (CTPA) is immediately available and feasible, a diagnosis of PE should be confirmed before proceeding to a reperfusion strategy.

Primary reperfusion is the treatment of choice for patients with high risk PE and can be achieved by thrombolysis and/or embolectomy. Thrombolysis can be achieved by a systemic treatment or preferably by a catheter directed treatment. Embolectomy can be performed surgically or by a catheter directed approach.

Following reperfusion treatment and hemodynamic stabilization, the patient should be hospitalized in a critical care unit. As patients continue to recover, they can be switched from parenteral to oral anticoagulation before discharge home.

B. **Acute management of hemodynamically stable patients** (Fig. 3)

In patients who are hemodynamically stable, the combination of symptoms, clinical findings and presence of predisposing factors for VTE allows the classification of patients with suspected PE into distinct categories of clinical or pretest probability of PE. This pre test assessment can be done either by clinical judgement or by using prediction rules. Clinical judgment lacks standardization and therefore several prediction scores have been developed. Of those the most frequently used and the ones we recommend using are the simplified "Revised Geneva" rule [5] and the simplified "Wells" rule [6]. Regardless of the score used, the proportion of patients with conformed PE is expected to be 10% in the low probability group, 30% in the Intermediate probability and 60% in the high probability groups [7].

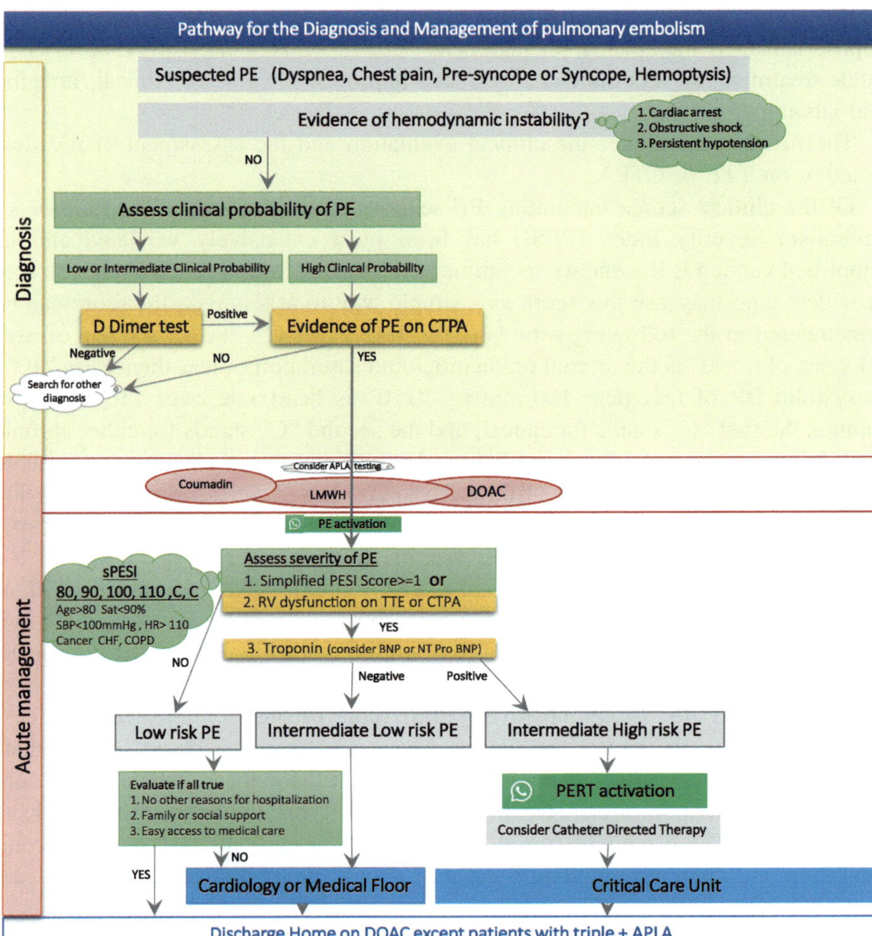

Fig. 3 Acute management of hemodynamically stable patients with pulmonary embolism

We recommend multidetector CTPA as a first line test in patients with a high clinical probability of PE. CTPA is considered to be diagnostic of PE when it shows a clot at least involving the segmental level of the pulmonary arterial tree. In patients with low or intermediate clinical probability of PE, we recommend measuring the plasma D-dimer as a first step and then proceeding to CTPA in patients with an elevated D-dimer level [2, 8].

For most cases of acute PE without hemodynamic compromise, parenteral or oral anticoagulation is adequate treatment. We suggest testing these stable patients for anti-phospholipid antibodies (APLA), for those with positive APLA tests, especially triple positive APLA, we recommend starting treatment with low molecular weight heparin (LMWH) and long term treatment with warfarin [9]. Otherwise treatment with direct oral anticoagulants (DOACS) is generally recommended.

Risk stratification of patients with acute PE is mandatory for determining the appropriate next therapeutic management step. In order to assess PE severity to guide treatment we recommend a two-step approach integrating clinical, imaging and laboratory findings.

The first step combines the clinical evaluation and the assessment of RV dysfunction on TTE or CTPA.

Of the clinical scores integrating PE severity and comorbidity, the Pulmonary Embolism Severity Index (PESI) has been most extensively validated and its simplified version is the one we recommend in our algorithm [9]. To aid health care providers who may use this score as a simple way to assess risk, the score can be remembered in the following way: "80, 90, 100, 110 CC". "80" is the age of over 80 years old, "90" is the arterial oxyhemoglobin saturation of less than 90%, "100" is systolic BP of less than 100 mmHg, "110" is heart rate over 110 beats per minute, the first "C" stands for cancer, and the second "C" stands for either chronic heart failure or chronic pulmonary disease. Each of these six parameters gets a score of one so the total score ranges from zero to six. Based on the simplified version score [10], 0 total points translates to 30 day mortality risk of 1% while a score of 1 or more translates to 30 day mortality risk of 10.9%.

In patients with either sPESI score of at least 1 and/or RV dysfunction on TTE or CTPA, further work up should include assessment of cardiac biomarkers for evidence of myocardial injury: elevated troponin or myocardial stretch-B type natriuretic peptide (BNP) and N-terminal (NT) proBNP.

Patients who are "triple" positive (sPESI score of one or more with RV dysfunction on imaging and positive cardiac biomarkers) are considered "intermediate high-risk PE". The PERT team should be activated for these patients with consideration of initiation of catheter directed therapy, typically catheter directed local thrombolysis. These patients are at a higher risk of early hemodynamic decompensation and circulatory collapse and they should be monitored in a critical care unit.

Patients who have either sPESI score of one or more and/or RV dysfunction on TTE or CTPA, but their cardiac biomarkers are negative are considered "intermediate low risk". These patients do not require additional reperfusion strategy beyond their anticoagulation therapy and they should be admitted to a general cardiology or medical floor.

There is a small group of patients with acute PE in whom the sPESI score is 0 and imaging modalities exclude RV dysfunction. These patients are considered as “low risk PE”. Early discharge and continuation of anticoagulant treatment at home should be considered if they meet the following three criteria: 1. There are no other reasons for hospitalization. 2. There is adequate family or social support. 3. There is easy access to medical care.

To summarize the diagnosis and management of patients with acute PE we have developed the HADASSAH mnemonic to help health care providers memorize the key points in our algorithm (Fig. 4). The key points are: Hemodynamic instability, Akinetic RV and Assessment probability of PE, D-dimer test and Defect on CTPA, Anti coagulation and Activation of PERT team, Simplified Severity Score of PE, Angiogram for catheter directed therapy and Hospital location to Home.

C. **Chronic management of patients with acute PE** (Fig. 5)

The goal of anticoagulation after acute PE is to complete the treatment of the acute episode and to prevent recurrence of VTE over the long term. Oral anticoagulants are highly effective in preventing recurrent VTE during treatment, but they do not eliminate the risk of subsequent recurrence after discontinuation of the treatment. Considering the bleeding risk of anticoagulation treatment, the key question is how to select patients for extended or indefinite anticoagulation.

Based on the 2019 ESC guidelines for the diagnosis and management of PE, all patients with PE should be treated with anticoagulation for at least 3 months [2, 11]. We recommend continued anticoagulation for a period of 3–6 months and following these patients in a specialty coagulation clinic if available. The direct oral anticoagulation (DOAC) agents are recommended by our team as a first choice based on their excellent safety profile and their excellent extended treatment data [12–14].

The key question at this point is to define who will benefit from an extended therapy beyond the first 3 to 6 months of anticoagulation. We recommend two steps work up:

Fig. 4 HADASSAH mnemonic for the diagnosis and management of pulmonary embolism

HADASSAH acronym for PE management

H Hemodynamic instability
A Akinetic RV, Assessment probability of PE
D D dimer test, Defect on CTPA
A Anti coagulation, Activation of PERT team
SS Simplified Severity Score of PE
A Angiogram for catheter directed therapy
H Hospital location to Home

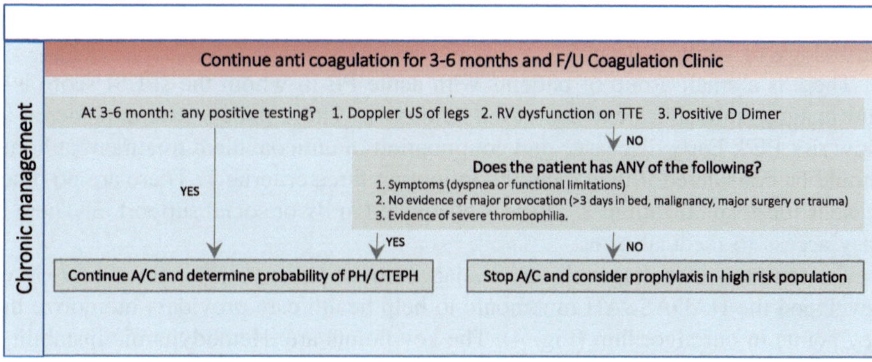

Fig. 5 Chronic management of patients with acute pulmonary embolism

The first step involves 3 tests: Duplex ultrasound to rule out lower extremities DVT, TTE to assess the RV function and pulmonary hypertension and a blood test for D-dimer. A positive finding in any of these tests will mandate continuation of anticoagulation for a longer period of time.

The second step is the clinical assessment of these patients in regards to persistence of symptoms (dyspnea and persistent functional limitations), evidence of severe thrombophilia and exclusion of a prior major provocation (>3 days in bed, malignancy or a major surgery or trauma).

If the entire work up is negative, we recommend discontinuing the anticoagulation therapy but to consider prophylaxis in high-risk situations.

The patency of the pulmonary arterial bed is restored in the majority of PE survivors within the first few months following the acute episode; therefore, no routine follow-up CTPA imaging is needed. However, in a very small group of patients, thrombi become persistent and organized, which in rare cases may result in chronic thromboembolic pulmonary hypertension (CTEPH), a potentially life-threatening condition. We recommend that these patients be followed in a CTEPH specialty clinic.

References

1. Raskob GE, Angchaisuksiri P, Blanco AN, Buller H, Gallus A, Hunt BJ, Hylek EM, Kakkar A, Konstantinides SV, McCumber M, Ozaki Y, Wendelboe A, Weitz JI. Thrombosis: a major contributor to global disease burden. Arterioscler Thromb Vasc Biol. 2014;34:2363–71.
2. Konstantinides SV, Meyer G. 2019 ESC Guidelines for the diagnosis and management of acute pulmonary embolism developed in collaboration with the European Respiratory Society (ERS): the Task Force for the diagnosis and management of acute pulmonary embolism of the European Society of Cardiology (ESC). Eur Respir J. 2019;54(3):1901647.
3. Herzog E, Elbaz-Greener G, Planer D, Koren T, Amir O, Shapiro J, Kalish Y. Pathway for the diagnosis and management of pulmonary embolism. Crit Pathw Cardiol. 2021;20:57–62.

4. Dudzinski DM, Piazza G. Multidisciplinary pulmonary embolism response teams. Circulation. 2016;133:98–103.
5. Klok FA, Mos IC, Nijkeuter M, Righini M, Perrier A, Le Gal G, Huisman MV. Simplification of the revised Geneva score for assessing clinical probability of pulmonary embolism. Arch Intern Med. 2008;168:2131–6.
6. Gibson NS, Sohne M, Kruip MJHA, Tick LW, Gerdes VE, Bossuyt PM, Wells PS, Buller HR, Christopher Study Investigators. Further validation and simplification of the Wells clinical decision rule in pulmonary embolism. Thromb Haemost. 2008;99:229–34.
7. Ceriani E, Combescure C, Le Gal G, Nendaz M, Perneger T, Bounameaux H, Perrier A, Righini M. Clinical prediction rules for pulmonary embolism: a systematic review and meta-analysis. J Thromb Haemost. 2010;8:957–70.
8. Kearon C, de Wit K, Parpia S, Schulman S, Afilalo M, Hirsch A, Spencer FA, Sharma S, D'Aragon F, Deshaies JF, Le Gal G, Lazo-Langner A, Wu C, Rudd-Scott L, Bates SM, Julian JA, PEGeD Study Investigators. Diagnosis of pulmonary embolism with d-Dimer adjusted to clinical probability. N Engl J Med. 2019;381(22):2125–34.
9. Pengo V, Hoxha A, Andreoli L, Tincani A, Silvestri E, Prisco D, Fierro T, Gresele P, Cafolla A, De Micheli V, Ghirarduzzi A, Tosetto A, Falanga A, Martinelli I, Testa S, Barcellona D, Gerosa M, Denas G. Trial of Rivaroxaban in AntiPhospholipid Syndrome (TRAPS): two-year outcomes after the study closure. J Thromb Haemost. 2020;00:1–5. https://doi.org/10.1111/jth.15158.
10. Jimenez D, Aujesky D, Moores L, Gomez V, Lobo JL, Uresandi F, Otero R, Monreal M, Muriel A, Yusen RD, RIETE Investigators. Simplification of the pulmonary embolism severity index for prognostication in patients with acute symptomatic pulmonary embolism. Arch Intern Med. 2010;170:1383–9.
11. Boutitie F, Pinede L, Schulman S, Agnelli G, Raskob G, Julian J, Hirsh J, Kearon C. Influence of preceding length of anticoagulant treatment and initial presentation of venous thromboembolism on risk of recurrence after stopping treatment: analysis of individual participants' data from seven trials. BMJ. 2011;342:d3036.
12. Schulman S, Kearon C, Kakkar AK, Schellong S, Eriksson H, Baanstra D, Kvamme AM, Friedman J, Mismetti P, Goldhaber SZ. Extended use of dabigatran, warfarin, or placebo in venous thromboembolism. N Engl J Med. 2013;368:709–18. 351.
13. Weitz JI, Lensing AWA, Prins MH, Bauersachs R, Beyer-Westendorf J, Bounameaux H, Brighton TA, Cohen AT, Davidson BL, Decousus H, Freitas MCS, Holberg G, Kakkar AK, Haskell L, van Bellen B, Pap AF, Berkowitz SD, Verhamme P, Wells PS, Prandoni P, EINSTEIN CHOICE Investigators. Rivaroxaban or aspirin for extended treatment of venous thromboembolism. N Engl J Med. 2017;376:1211–22.
14. Agnelli G, Buller HR, Cohen A, Curto M, Gallus AS, Johnson M, Porcari A, Raskob GE, Weitz JI, AMPLIFY-EXT Investigators. Apixaban for extended treatment of venous thromboembolism. N Engl J Med. 2013;368:699–708.

Epidemiology, Pathophysiology and Predisposing Factors of Pulmonary Embolism and Deep Vein Thrombosis

Dean Nachman, Arthur Pollack, and Eyal Herzog

1 Introduction

The prevalence of venous thromboembolism (VTE) had increased in recent years, leading to a substantial morbidity and mortality. Alongside ischemic heart disease and Ischemic stroke, VTE plays a prominent role in the cardiovascular disease burden. Pulmonary embolism (PE) and deep vein thrombosis (DVT) are the two interplaying entities that encompass VTE, sharing epidemiology, risk factors, and several basic pathophysiological processes.

Various trends are presently modifying our knowledge of VTE. The aging population, more invasive medical treatments, and the recent Coronavirus Disease 2019 (COVID-19) are among the recent developments in the epidemiology of VTE. Insights into inflammatory mechanisms, together with the classic Virchow's triad, adjust our understanding of the pathophysiology of VTE and may pave the route to novel treatment strategies. Importantly, as the risk factors for VTE become more abundant, it is of great importance that healthcare providers remain up to date with the present-day knowledge in the field.

This chapter will review the epidemiology pathophysiology, and risk factors of VTE, with particular emphasis on recent developments.

D. Nachman (✉) · A. Pollack · E. Herzog
Department of Cardiology, Heart Institute, Hadassah Hebrew University Medical Center, Jerusalem, Israel
e-mail: Dean@hadassah.org.il

E. Herzog (ed.), *Pulmonary Embolism*,
https://doi.org/10.1007/978-3-030-87090-4_2

2 Epidemiology

VTE is a common condition affecting the practice of healthcare providers from most disciplines of medicine on a daily basis. VTE incidence varies widely across different geographic populations, sex, age and ethnic origin, reflecting differences in exposure to risk factors and medical care availability. Moreover, comprehensive large population epidemiological studies are scarce, and the data differs according to methodological circumstances.

The annual rate of VTE in the high-income countries of western Europe, North America, and Australia is 0.75–2.69 per 1000 individuals [1]. In the United states an estimated 1.2 million VTE cases occurred in 2016, of them 370,000 PE cases and 875,000 cases of DVT [2]. The incidence was higher among African Americans and lower in Asian and Native Americans [3]. Studies from high-income south-eastern countries such as Taiwan and Hong-Kong found a lower incidence of VTE, similar to that of the Asian American population [1].

VTE, especially PE, is a substantial cause of mortality, ranking high among other cardiovascular diseases. 100,000–300,000 deaths yearly are associated with VTE in the US, and similar numbers have been reported from a similar size European population [4]. Furthermore, VTE leads to 7.6 Disability Adjusted Life Years per 100,000, an index that combines the sum of years lost and years lived with disability [4]. Considerable financial burden to the health care system is related to VTE, estimated to be as high as 70 billion US Dollars a year in the US alone [5]. As 60–75% of all VTE cases are hospital-acquired, applying prevention means, when appropriate, may drastically decrease the disease encumbrance [5].

VTE is rare before late adolescence and infrequent before middle age [3]. The incidence rises sharply in the seventh decade of life, up to six times the incidence at 50 years old [6]. The Differences in incidence between sexes are less pronounced, with a slight advantage for females over males, 110 versus 130 per 100,000 respectively. Higher incidence in females before 55 years of age was noticed, correlating to the deleterious thrombogenic effects of childbearing and pre-menopausal estrogen changes [4].

Recurrence of VTE is common and regarded as one of the most vital predisposing factors for VTE, with an estimated 30% of patients suffer from another episode during a long follow-up period. The risk of recurrence declines steeply as the time from the index episode passes. The vast majority of recurrent attacks take place during the first year [3].

Statistical data from recent decades had shown an increasing VTE rates, mainly PE, nearly doubling in the last four decades [7]. This incline may be related to the aging population, increasedcancer risk, and better availability and sensitivity of diagnosis modalities. Alongside this trend, the case fatality rate is declining, probably due to better treatment options, adherence to guidelines, and the spread of imaging devices leading to clinically insignificant disease diagnosis [8].

3 Pathophysiology

The pathophysiology of PE usually starts with the formation of a thrombus in the deep veins of the lower legs, developing to thrombus propagation and embolization into the pulmonary arteries. In half of the PE cases, a DVT is evident as well. At the pulmonary artery level, if significant, the emboli induce gas exchange abnormalities and potentially deleterious hemodynamic alterations. It is of importance that PE may also result from the embolization of non-blood clot material such as fat, amniotic fluid or cancerous cells in relevant much rarer clinical scenarios.

A. **Thrombus formation**

The Virchow's triad, including venous stasis, hypercoagulability, and endothelial damage is the cornerstone of thrombus generation and most patients with VTE fill at least some of the components. At the local level venous stasis at the venous sinuses or valves or damaged endothelium promotes the formation of a clot. The clot will extend in case of imbalance between coagulation and anti-coagulation factors and fibrinolysis and might eventually detach and travel to the pulmonary arteries.

Inflammation, although not included in the original Virchow triad, is another vital component in the generation of a thrombus. Inflammatory mediators alongside bacterial lipopolysaccharides induce endothelial damage accompanied by platelet activation. Furthermore, these activated platelets release procoagulant and proinflammatory substrates and attach to neutrophils, triggering them to release Neutrophil Extracellular Traps (NETs). The NETs constitute from expelled DNA fragments, Histones, and granules, forming a procoagulant network promoting platelet aggregation and thrombus formation [9]. Clinical evidence suggests that proinflammatory status, as indicated by high CRP levels, promotes VTE and anti-inflammatory interventions may prevent this association [10].

B. **Cardiopulmonary Hemodynamics**

PE might have detrimental hemodynamic effect, mainly through Right Ventricular (RV) pressure overload. Therefore, PE are categorized according to their effect on the RV function. Hypotension indicating massive (or unstable) PE, RV strain on imaging or serum biomarkers (Troponin, Brain Natriuretic Peptide) imply a submissive (or stable) PE, and no evidence of hypotension or RV strain or elevation in serum bio-markers, suggesting a non-massive PE. These categories have direct treatment and outcomes implications.

The pulmonary artery thrombus increases Pulmonary Vascular Resistance (PVR) by both the mechanical occlusion and vasoactive substances such as Serotonin and thromboxane-A2 from platelets, Histamine and Endothelin from lung tissue. Using compensation mechanisms such as, tachycardia, increased contractility and pulmonary vascular recruitment, a healthy RV can withstand an obstruction of up to 50% of the vascular tree, generating up to a mean pulmonary artery pressure of 40 mmHg. Obstruction above this level, might initiate the cascade of pathophysiological mechanisms eventually evolving to hemodynamic collapse. It is important to stress that in previously diseased cardiopulmonary system, the threshold for failure might be lower. Pressure overload generates RV dilatation and wall tension elevation that translates to RV ischemia by several pathways- reduced coronary perfusion pressure, increased RV work, cardiac output drop and hypotension via decreased Left Ventricular (LV) filling due to bulging of the interventricular septum to the left. This mechanistic vicious cycle, if not abruptly terminated, leads to secondary neurohormonal activation and inflammatory stress resulting in a delayed cardiovascular failure, that might progress to death [8, 11].

C. **Gas exchange**

Several modifications in gas exchange ensue following the advent of a PE. Redistribution of blood flow along the pulmonary vascular bed from obstructed to non-involved vessels generating a ventilation-perfusion (V/Q) mismatch. In the event of totally obstructed pulmonary arteries a ventilatory dead space arises. Existing right to left shunts, such as a patent foramen ovale, might emerge as right sided pressure elevates. Atelectasis or pulmonary hemorrhage may also influence via a shunt mechanism. These processes eventually contribute to the commonly noticed hypoxemia that accompanies a significant PE. Hypoxemia might aggravate in cases of low cardiac output due to the low mixed venous oxygen saturation. Respiratory alkalosis is frequently seen secondary to an accompanying hyperventilation, even though dead space is elevated in PE owing to the obstructed arteries [12].

4 Predisposing Factors

Multiple predisposing factors contribute to the occurrence of VTE, starting from reversible medical conditions to genetic influences, medications, and lifestyle preferences. These predisposing factors reflect different aspects in the mechanisms of thrombus formation. Some have a sizeable impact on the likelihood of VTE. Other, which are very prevalent conditions, have no more than a modest impact on the individual level but a considerable epidemiological effect attributable to their abundance at the community level (Table 1).

Provoked VTE constitutes one half to two thirds of cases as they correlate to strong trigger such as immobility, trauma,cancer, surgery or indwelling catheter. The rest are considered unprovoked. This dichotomy might have a significant effect when deciding on the length of anticoagulation treatment.

A. **Venous Stasis**

Prolonged immobility is a key predisposing factor for VTE by facilitating venous stasis. Immobility can evolve in diverse medical conditions and every-day situations. Numerous studies found an association between prolonged or even short-term inactivity, sedentary lifestyle, and the risk for VTE.

Table 1 Predisposing factors for venous thromboembolism. (Partially [36] adapted from Anderson FA, et al.

Predisposing factor	Odds ratio
Venous stasis	
Physical inactivity	2.6
Spending free time sedentary	1.4
Orthopedic disorders (fractures, amputations)	2.1–2.8
Long distance air travel	<2
Hospitalization (specifically heart failure or arrythmia)	>10
Hypercoagulable state	
Prothrombin gene mutation G20210A	3–7
Factor V Leiden	3–11
Antiphospholipid antibody syndrome	5.3
Nephrotic syndrome	
Polycythemia Vera	
Pregnancy and puerperium	4–20
Oral contraceptive and hormone replacement	3–4
Overweight and obesity	3–6
Inflammatory bowel disease	3
Rheumatoid arthritis	4.9
Lupus	9.8
Cancer	2–9
Endothelial damage	
Infection	2–9
Respiratory and urinary	2.5
Gram positive bacteria	7.5
Staphylococcus aureus	1.2
Gram negative bacteria	
Influenza	
Coronavirus Disease 2019	
Major trauma	>10
Central venous lines and indwelling medical devices	2–9

Inconsistency regarding the effect of physical activity on VTE risk arises from population-based studies. Physical activity improves venous flow but tends to raise the risk for orthopedic injuries [13]. In contrast, the association of physical inactivity is widely acceptable. It was found that women spending more than 40 hours inactive at home per week have a 2.6-fold risk for VTE compared to those spending less than 10 hours a week [14]. Interestingly, it was found that for every 2 hours a day watching television, the hazard ratio for PE related mortality increases by 1.4 [15]. The prevalence of PE in flights is neglectable, yet the incidence of PE in Long-distance air travel of more than 10,000 km is

4.8 per million passengers compared to 0.01 cases with flight length of less than 5000 km [16].

Orthopedic disorders induce considerable immobility. The incidence of VTE in the 90 days following surgery for fractured bone or amputation is 2.8 and 2.1 higher, respectively [17]. Other orthopedic injuries such as sprains and dislocations have a less prominent relationship to VTE [17]. Without thromboprophylaxis, the incidence of VTE after hip and knee arthroplasty is high. Prophylactic anticoagulation adjacent to the surgery lowers the incidence to 0.5–1%, of them 0.14–0.27% PE [18].

VTE is highly associated with hospitalization; it was estimated that 59–75% of all VTE are acquired during hospitalization, particularly during the month following the index hospitalization. A large proportion (80%) of VTE attacks during a hospital stay are considered preventable. The cost of hospital-acquired VTE in the USA is estimated at 5–27 billion US Dollars annually, hence the great interest in early preemptive detection of the at-risk patient and applying prophylactic measures [5].

B. **Hypercoagulable states and inflammation**

Various acquired and heritable factors have a vital impact on the potential for developing VTE through the induction of a hypercoagulable state. As a general statement, acquired states belong to diverse medical fields and have a proven immediate effect on first and recurring VTE attack, in some, alongside arterial thrombosis. In contrast, genetic predispositions generally result from a mutation in a clotting factor gene leading to an elevated VTE rate, with equivocal recurrence rates.

Inherited thrombophilia contributes to an elevated VTE risk by a variety of mechanisms. The prevalence of the two most common inherited thrombophilia is 2–4% for the prothrombin gene mutation G20210A and 4–5% for Factor V Leiden (FVL). The prothrombin gene mutation G20210A elevates the factor concentration, contributing to a 3–7-fold increase in the risk of VTE. Clotting factor 5 is resistant to the inhibitory effect of protein C in FVL and an 3–11 Relative Risk (RR) for VTE. Other less common genetic disorders include-deficiency in the coagulation inhibitors protein C (1 in 200–500) and protein S (1:250) and antithrombin (1:600–5000) [19].

Eventhough many hopes were raised, the clinical value of genetic testing for thrombophilia is questionable. It has been shown that the risk for recurrence depends less on inherited factors and more on the presence of transient provoking risk factors, so the decision on treatment length cannot be made on the sole principle of carried genetic risk. In the future, specific genetic predispositions may have a role in choosing the specific anticoagulation drug [20].

Antiphospholipid Antibody (APLA) syndrome is the most common acquired thrombophilia. The syndrome is characterized by frequent miscarriages, intrauterine growth retardation, venous and arterial thrombosis alongside autoimmune phenomena, such as hemolytic anemia, thrombocytopenia, and valvular heart disease. Diagnosis of APLA necessitates obstetric or thrombotic

episodes combined with two positive antibody tests (anticardiolipin, lupus anticoagulant, and anti-β2-glycoprotein) separated by 12 weeks or more [21] The prevalence of APLA was 10% in VTE patients under the age of 50, and the risk for VTE is 5–8% higher in patients positive to APLA antibodies. It is important to stress that using Direct Oral Anti Coagulants (DOAC) demonstrated worse thrombotic outcomes compared to Vitamin K antagonists [22].
In Nephrotic syndrome, the loss of anticoagulant protein factors in the diseased glomeruli alongside the inflammatory activation contributes to thrombotic attacks that classically occur in the renal vein. Certain hematological conditions, such as Polycythemia vera and Paroxysmal Nocturnal Hemoglobinuria, also provoke venous and arterial thrombosis [20].
Active malignancy, especially during the first year of diagnosis and treatment, is a significant contributor to VTE risk, and a high level of suspicion should be taken when relevant symptoms present. Adenocarcinoma, and metastatic disease, exerts an exceptionally high VTE risk. It is of interest that no increased risk was noted in patients withcancer on remission following treatment [23]. The hypercoagulable effect arises from several routes; it has been shown thatcancer cells produce specific procoagulant substances such as tissue factor. Cancer mass can also protrude to a vessel inducing local stasis and endothelial damage, or emboli and clog a distant blood vessel.
VTE is four to twenty times more frequent during pregnancy and puerperium, with PE more dominant during the puerperal period. The rate of VTE was found to be 1.72 for 1000 deliveries with a higher risk with aging, obesity, and background thrombophilia. Furthermore, a death rate of 1.1 deaths per 100,000 was noted [24]. Pregnant women undergo a shift towards a procoagulant state by induction of clotting factors (VII, VIII, X, von Willebrand, and fibrinogen) in conjunction with reduced anticoagulation by a drop in protein S and acquired activated protein C resistance. It is presumed that these adjustments aim to prevent the increased bleeding during delivery and puerperium [11]. Direct pressure of the growing womb leading to lower body venous stasis is another relevant mechanism of heightened VTE chance.
Oral contraceptive (OC) agents are the most widespread predisposing factor for VTE in young females, yet the absolute chance remains exceptionally low. OC differs in the likelihood of VTE based on their specific components. The hazard for VTE using a combined estrogen and progesterone pill increases by a magnitude of 3–4, mostly during the first three months and with a pill containing the newer generation of progestins. The risk particularly increases when OC are administered to a woman with other risk factors, such as obesity, smoking, or genetic thrombophilia. Progesterone-only pills were not linked with increased risk [25]. Postmenopausal hormone replacement therapy may also increase the risk, particularly during the first year of treatment [26].
Over-weight and obesity are prevalent on a scale of a pandemic in some parts of the world and have an essential relevance to VTE. Numerous studies displayed a practically linear correlation of Body Mass Index (BMI) to the Relative Risk

(RR), with a RR of 1.08 for every 1 kg/m^2 increment. The risk was apparent even in the considered normal range of BMI (22.5–25 kg/m^2) but dramatically pronounced with morbid obesity (BMI >35 kg/m^2, RR = 6) [27]. In a mechanistic point of view, obesity is linked to a general inflammatory state, higher tissue factor activity, and tend to be less physically active and suffer from numerous VTE-related comorbidities [27].

Rheumatologic disorders have a strong link to VTE. The relationship has been notably described in Inflammatory Bowel Disease (IBD) (RR = 3), Rheumatoid arthritis (RR = 4.9), and Systemic Lupus Erythematosus (SLE) even without APLA (RR = 9.8) [28]. There is a tendency towards more VTE attacks early after diagnosis and during a flare of the inflammatory disease. Moreover, the survival of rheumatologic patients who suffer from VTE worsens [29].

C. **Endothelial damage**

Acute infection, rather in the hospital or community settings provoke VTE risk mainly within the first month following the index infection, and a twofold increment was observed during the subsequent year. Respiratory and urinary infections, viral or bacterial, result in the greatest thrombogenic impact. Gram positive yields higher risk than Gram negative (OR = 2.5 vs. 1.2), particularly *Staphylococcus aureus* (OR = 7.5) [30]. Influenza and the recent COVID-19 viral infections stimulate a remarkably elevated threat for VTE, at least partially modulated by vaccination in the case of Influenza [31]. Combination of host defense mechanisms such as interleukins tumor necrosis factor and complement components tissue factor and bacterial lipopolysaccharides induces a procoagulant state by direct damage to the endothelial integrity and activation of clotting factors [17, 32, 33].

Major Trauma and surgery are known to have a prothrombotic effect, generated by the direct venous injury but also by the systemic inflammation and secondary immobility. The risk for DVT/PE varies widely according to the literature from 0.35 to 24% [34]. Significant burns, alongside oncologic, neurosurgical, orthopedic, cardiac surgeries or renal transplantation disproportionally contribute to VTE probability.

Central venous lines induce vessel wall damage, promote fibrin, biofilm, and coagulation factors to propagate, eventually inducing thromboembolism. Similarly, pacemaker or defibrillator leads may contribute in the same manner. The extended use of these long-term indwelling vascular devices in recent years is accompanied by a growth in upper arm DVT [35].

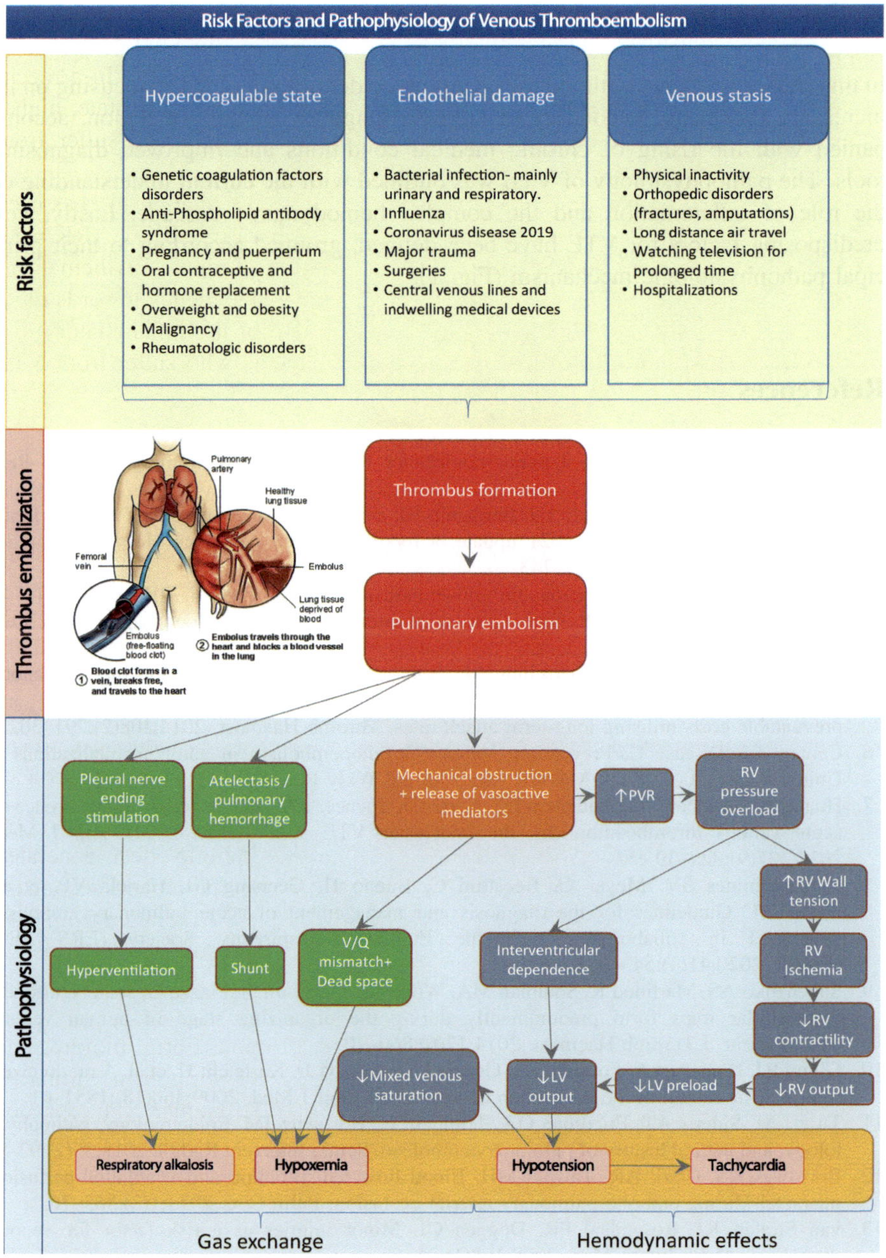

Fig. 1 Risk factors and pathophysiology of venous thromboembolism. RV—Right ventricle, LV—left ventricle, PVR—pulmonary vascular resistance, V/Q—ventilation perfusion

5 Summary

In this chapter we have outlined the changing epidemiology of VTE, focusing on its increasing prevalence secondary to increase longevity of the population, accompanied with the rising of chronic medical conditions and improved diagnosing tools. The pathophysiology of VTE was outlined with the current understanding of the role of inflammation and the complex hemodynamic cascade. Lastly, key predisposing factors for VTE have been defined, grouped according to their principal pathophysiologic mechanism (Fig. 1).

References

1. Day ISCfWT. Thrombosis: a major contributor to global disease burden. Thromb Res. 2014;134(5):931–8.
2. Virani SS, Alonso A, Aparicio HJ, Benjamin EJ, Bittencourt MS, Callaway CW, et al. Heart disease and stroke statistics-2021 update: a report from the American Heart Association. Circulation. 2021;143(8):e254–743.
3. Heit JA. Epidemiology of venous thromboembolism. Nat Rev Cardiol. 2015;12(8):464–74.
4. Wendelboe AM, Raskob GE. Global burden of thrombosis: epidemiologic aspects. Circ Res. 2016;118(9):1340–7.
5. Mahan CE, Borrego ME, Woersching AL, Federici R, Downey R, Tiongson J, et al. Venous thromboembolism: annualised United States models for total, hospital-acquired and preventable costs utilising long-term attack rates. Thromb Haemost. 2012;108(2):291–302.
6. Centers for Disease C, Prevention. Venous thromboembolism in adult hospitalizations—United States, 2007–2009. MMWR Morb Mortal Wkly Rep. 2012;61(22):401–4.
7. Huang W, Goldberg RJ, Anderson FA, Kiefe CI, Spencer FA. Secular trends in occurrence of acute venous thromboembolism: the Worcester VTE study (1985–2009). Am J Med. 2014;127(9):829–39 e5.
8. Konstantinides SV, Meyer G, Becattini C, Bueno H, Geersing GJ, Harjola VP, et al. 2019 ESC Guidelines for the diagnosis and management of acute pulmonary embolism developed in collaboration with the European Respiratory Society (ERS). Eur Heart J. 2020;41(4):543–603.
9. Savchenko AS, Martinod K, Seidman MA, Wong SL, Borissoff JI, Piazza G, et al. Neutrophil extracellular traps form predominantly during the organizing stage of human venous development. J Thromb Haemost. 2014;12(6):860–70.
10. Glynn RJ, Danielson E, Fonseca FA, Genest J, Gotto AM Jr, Kastelein JJ, et al. A randomized trial of rosuvastatin in the prevention of venous. N Engl J Med. 2009;360(18):1851–61.
11. Turetz M, Sideris AT, Friedman OA, Triphathi N, Horowitz JM. Epidemiology, pathophysiology, and natural history of pulmonary embolism. Semin Intervent Radiol. 2018;35(2):92–8.
12. Burrowes KS, Clark AR, Tawhai MH. Blood flow redistribution and ventilation-perfusion mismatch during embolic pulmonary arterial occlusion. Pulm Circ. 2011;1(3):365–76.
13. van Stralen KJ, Rosendaal FR, Doggen CJ. Minor injuries as a risk factor for venous thrombosis. Arch Intern Med. 2008;168(1):21–6.
14. Kabrhel C, Varraso R, Goldhaber SZ, Rimm E, Camargo CA, Jr. Physical inactivity and idiopathic pulmonary embolism in women: prospective study. BMJ. 2011;343:d3867.
15. Shirakawa T, Iso H, Yamagishi K, Yatsuya H, Tanabe N, Ikehara S, et al. Watching television and risk of mortality from pulmonary among Japanese men and women: The JACC study (Japan Collaborative Cohort). Circulation. 2016;134(4):355–7.

16. Lapostolle F, Surget V, Borron SW, Desmaizieres M, Sordelet D, Lapandry C, et al. Severe pulmonary embolism associated with air travel. N Engl J Med. 2001;345(11):779–83.
17. Rogers MA, Levine DA, Blumberg N, Flanders SA, Chopra V, Langa KM. Triggers of hospitalization for venous thromboembolism. Circulation. 2012;125(17):2092–9.
18. Januel JM, Chen G, Ruffieux C, Quan H, Douketis JD, Crowther MA, et al. Symptomatic in-hospital deep vein and pulmonary following hip and knee arthroplasty among patients receiving recommended prophylaxis: a systematic review. JAMA. 2012;307(3):294–303.
19. Stern RM, Al-Samkari H, Connors JM. Thrombophilia evaluation in pulmonary embolism. Curr Opin Cardiol. 2019;34(6):603–9.
20. Moran J, Bauer KA. Managing thromboembolic risk in patients with hereditary and acquired thrombophilias. Blood. 2020;135(5):344–50.
21. Garcia D, Erkan D. Diagnosis and management of the antiphospholipid syndrome. N Engl J Med. 2018;378(21):2010–21.
22. Cerda P, Becattini C, Iriarte A, Hernandez JC, Corbella X, Riera-Mestre A. Direct oral anticoagulants versus vitamin K antagonists in antiphospholipid syndrome: a meta-analysis. Eur J Intern Med. 2020;79:43–50.
23. Stein PD, Beemath A, Meyers FA, Skaf E, Sanchez J, Olson RE. Incidence of venous thromboembolism in patients hospitalized with cancer. Am J Med. 2006;119(1):60–8.
24. James AH, Jamison MG, Brancazio LR, Myers ER. Venous thromboembolism during pregnancy and the postpartum period: incidence, risk factors, and mortality. Am J Obstet Gynecol. 2006;194(5):1311–5.
25. Barsoum MK, Heit JA, Ashrani AA, Leibson CL, Petterson TM, Bailey KR. Is progestin an independent risk factor for incident venous thromboembolism? A population-based case-control study. Thromb Res. 2010;126(5):373–8.
26. Giordano NJ, Jansson PS, Young MN, Hagan KA, Kabrhel C. Epidemiology, pathophysiology, stratification, and natural history of pulmonary embolism. Tech Vasc Interv Radiol. 2017;20(3):135–40.
27. Kabrhel C, Varraso R, Goldhaber SZ, Rimm EB, Camargo CA. Prospective study of BMI and the risk of pulmonary in women. Obesity (Silver Spring). 2009;17(11):2040–6.
28. Murthy SK, Robertson McCurdy AB, Carrier M, McCurdy JD. Venous thromboembolic events in inflammatory bowel diseases: a review of current evidence and guidance on risk in the post-hospitalization setting. Thromb Res. 2020;194:26–32.
29. Yusuf HR, Hooper WC, Grosse SD, Parker CS, Boulet SL, Ortel TL. Risk of venous thromboembolism occurrence among adults with selected autoimmune diseases: a study among a U.S. cohort of commercial insurance enrollees. Thromb Res. 2015;135(1):50–7.
30. Dalager-Pedersen M, Sogaard M, Schonheyder HC, Thomsen RW, Baron JA, Nielsen H. Venous thromboembolism after community-acquired bacteraemia: a 20-year danish cohort study. PLoS One. 2014;9(1):e86094.
31. Zhu T, Carcaillon L, Martinez I, Cambou JP, Kyndt X, Guillot K, et al. Association of influenza vaccination with reduced risk of venous thromboembolism. Thromb Haemost. 2009;102(6):1259–64.
32. Musil D. Acute infections, venous thrombosis, and recommended thromboprophylaxis. Vnitr Lek. 2020;66(8):17–23.
33. Smeeth L, Cook C, Thomas S, Hall AJ, Hubbard R, Vallance P. Risk of deep vein thrombosis and pulmonary embolism after acute infection in a community setting. Lancet. 2006;367 (9516):1075–9.
34. Bahloul M, Dlela M, Bouchaala K, Kallel H, Ben Hamida C, Chelly H, et al. Post-traumatic pulmonary embolism: incidence, physiopathology, risk factors of early occurrence, and impact outcome. A narrative review. Am J Cardiovasc Dis. 2020;10(4):432–43.
35. Greene MT, Flanders SA, Woller SC, Bernstein SJ, Chopra V. The association between PICC use and venous thromboembolism in upper and lower extremities. Am J Med. 2015;128 (9):986–93 e1.
36. Anderson FA Jr, Spencer FA. Risk factors for venous thromboembolism. Circulation. 2003;107(23 Suppl 1):I9-16.

Non-imaging Diagnosis of Pulmonary Embolism

Israel Gotsman and Eyal Herzog

1 Introduction

In this chapter, the clinical manifestations of acute pulmonary embolism (PE) and the non-imaging tests that help in the assessment of the clinical probability of PE are described. Based on this clinical probability, further biomarker evaluation or imaging is indicated. Cardiac biomarkers and their importance in management of PE are also discussed.

2 Clinical Presentation

Pulmonary Embolism (PE) is a common phenomenon that can lead to significant clinical manifestations and sequelae. Prompt diagnosis is imperative to enable early treatment and improve outcome. The clinical presentation varies considerably, dependent on the severity of the obstruction as well as the background clinical status of the patient. It can vary from being completely asymptomatic or lead to cardiogenic shock and sudden death. The most common clinical symptoms are shortness of breath and pleuritic chest pain with or without symptoms of deep vein thrombosis (DVT). However, the clinical spectrum is very diverse including absence of symptoms and symptoms that are not specific; therefore, ***the key to the diagnosis is a high index of suspicion***, particularity if risk factors for thromboembolic disease are present.

I. Gotsman (✉) · E. Herzog
Heart Institute, Hadassah Hebrew University Medical Center, Jerusalem, Israel
e-mail: igotsman@bezeqint.net

E. Herzog (ed.), *Pulmonary Embolism*,
https://doi.org/10.1007/978-3-030-87090-4_3

3 Symptoms and Signs

Table 1 describes the common presenting symptoms and signs that are manifestations of PE. Data is based on a diverse cohort of patients with PE in the Prospective Investigation of Pulmonary Embolism Diagnosis I and II (PIOPED I and II) [1, 2]. The most common symptoms include shortness of breath at rest or effort, pleuritic chest pain, cough, orthopnea, symptoms of DVT i.e., calf or thigh pain or swelling, wheezing and hemoptysis. Common presenting signs on examination include tachypnea, tachycardia and signs of DVT including calf or thigh swelling, erythema, edema, tenderness or palpable cords. Other signs include rales, decreased breath sounds, accentuated pulmonic component of the second heart sound and jugular venous distension.

The presence of these clinical symptoms and signs can help raise the clinical suspicion for PE, however, the sensitivity and specificity of making a diagnosis based on clinical symptoms and signs alone is fairly low [3], therefore if there is a

Table 1 Common symptoms and signs of pulmonary embolism

Symptoms	PIOPED I (%)	PIOPED II (%)	Signs	PIOPED I (%)	PIOPED II (%)
Dyspnea	73	73	Temperature >38.5 °C	7	1
Pleuritic pain	66	44	Abnormal Cardiac examination	–	21
Cough	37	34	Increased P2	23	15
Leg swelling	28	41	Right ventricular lift	4	4
Leg pain	26	44	Jugular venous distension	–	14
Hemoptysis	13	–	Abnormal Lung examination	–	29
Palpitations	10	–	Rales (crackles)	51	18
Wheezing	9	21	Wheezes	5	2
Angina-like pain	4	–	Rhonchi	–	2
Signs			Decreased breath sounds	–	17
Tachypnea ($\geq$20/min)	70	54	Pleural friction rub	3	0
Tachycardia (>100/min)	30	24	Calf or thigh DVT signs	11	47
Diaphoresis	11	2	Calf and thigh DVT signs		14
Cyanosis	1	0			

Data from published Prospective Investigation of Pulmonary Embolism Diagnosis I and II (PIOPED I and II) studies [1, 2]

clinical suspicion, risk assessment for the probability of diagnosis should be performed and further testing conducted based on this, primarily a blood test for the biomarker D-dimer.

4 Thromboembolic Risk

Predisposing factors for venous thromboembolism (VTE) are important to evaluate, as their presence increases significantly the clinical probability of PE. The probability increases with the number of VTE predisposing factors present. Predisposing factors include major surgery, multiple trauma, hip fracture, or lower extremity paralysis because of spinal cord injury. Additional risk factors include previous VTE, increasing age, cardiac or respiratory failure, prolonged immobility, presence of central venous lines, estrogens, and a wide variety of inherited and acquired hematological conditions [4]. However, it is important to keep in mind that a non-significant minority of patients with PE ($\sim$40%), do not have any apparent predisposing factors.

5 Pretest probability Scores for the Diagnosis of PE

When PE is suspected, it is important to classify patients according to the probability of a diagnosis of PE. This is based on symptoms, clinical signs and predisposing factors for VTE. This probability assessment is imperative as it will dictate further steps to make the most efficient pathway to diagnosis or exclusion of PE. It is possible to use clinical acuity or 'gestalt', based on clinical experience to asses probability. Clinical judgement has shown to have value. A more accurate and standardized way to calculate the risk of PE is based on several validated scores estimating the probability for PE. The scores include the Wells, modified Wells, simplified Wells, the revised Geneva or simplified Geneva Score [5–8] as shown in Table 2. The sensitivity of these scores ranged from 88 to 96% with lower specificity from 48 to 53% [9]. Pretest probability of PE using one of these scores is recommended to classify the clinical probability risk as low, intermediate or high. Based on this classification, further evaluation is indicated, including D-dimer or imaging studies. We recommend using the simplified Geneva or simplified Wells scores.

Table 2 Clinical scores to estimate the probability of pulmonary embolism

Variable	Wells	Simplified Wells	Variable	Revised Geneva	Simplified Geneva
Clinical signs and symptoms of DVT	3	1	Pain on lower limb deep venous palpation and unilateral edema	4	1
			Unilateral lower-limb pain	3	1
Alternative diagnosis less likely	3	1			
Heart rate >100 beats per minute	1.5	1	Heart rate ≥ 95 beats per minute	5	2
			Heart rate 75–94 beats per minute	3	1
Previous DVT/PE	1.5	1	Previous DVT/PE	3	1
Immobilization (≥ 3 days) or surgery in the previous four weeks	1.5	1	Surgery under general anesthesia or fracture of the lower limbs within one month	2	1
Malignancy	1	1	Active malignancy (last year)	2	1
Hemoptysis	1	1	Hemoptysis	2	1
			Age >65 years	1	1
Clinical probability			*Clinical probability*		
High	≥ 7	–	High	≥ 11	≥ 5
Intermediate	2–6	–	Intermediate	4–10	2–4
Low	<2	–	Low	0–3	0–1
Two-level score (modified wells)			Two-level score		
PE likely	≥ 5	≥ 2	PE likely	≥ 6	≥ 3
PE unlikely	0–4	0–1	PE unlikely	0–5	0–2

Adapted from the published scores [5–8]

6 Biomarkers

6.1 D-dimer

D-dimer is a fibrin degradation product that is produced with acute thrombosis and is a very sensitive biomarker of acute PE. Acute thrombosis is initiated by

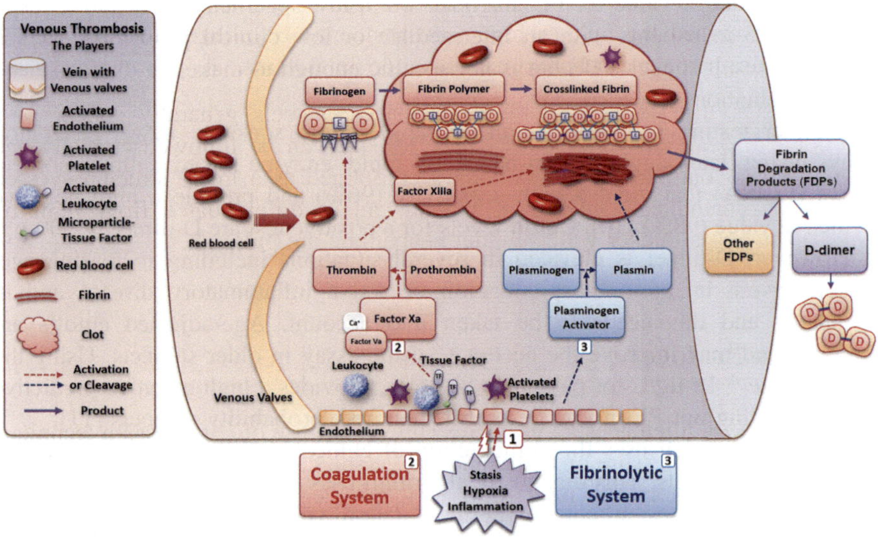

Fig. 1 Thrombus formation involving coagulation and fibrinolysis systems that produce D-dimer

activation of the coagulation system with subsequent activation of the fibrinolysis system, causing breakdown of fibrin clot into fibrin degradation products including D-dimer. Figure 1 depicts the production of D-dimer in venous thrombosis due to activation of the coagulation and fibrinolysis systems. Thrombus formation starts by activation of the endothelium (step 1 in Fig. 1) caused by inflammation or hypoxia that occurs downstream to venous valves due to stasis. This leads to adhesion of leukocytes and thrombocytes and expression of tissue factor on adhered activated leukocytes, microparticles and possibly on the endothelium, that activates the coagulation system. The coagulation system (step 2 in Fig. 1) is initiated by factor Xa on these activated thrombocytes as part of the prothrombinase complex including calcium and factor Va. This complex converts prothrombin (factor II) to active thrombin (factor IIa), an active serine protease that cleaves fibrinogen, producing fibrin molecules. The fibrin molecules form complexes producing a fibrin polymer. This is stabilized by crosslinking of the D parts of the fibrin molecule mediated by factor XIII which is also activated by thrombin, resulting in an insoluble mesh that strengthens the blood clot. The fibrinolytic system (step 3 in Fig. 1) is activated by plasminogen activator, a serine protease on endothelial cells that converts plasminogen into plasmin. This enzyme plasmin cleaves the fibrin polymer into fibrin degradation products (FDPs). One of the FDPs is D-dimer containing two D fragments of the fibrin protein joined by a cross-link.

Increased D-dimer concentration in the blood is therefore highly suggestive of thrombosis. The assay is very sensitive to any increase in fibrinolysis and is ***primarily used in ruling out acute PE***. D-dimer has a high sensitivity and a high negative predictive value for PE diagnosis but a low specificity. A negative result rules out PE in patients with an intermediate or low clinical probability of PE. A positive result suggests PE but is not specific enough to make the diagnosis and further evaluation is needed.

D-dimer testing is best done using rapid highly sensitive newer-generation assays using latex-agglutination-based or rapid enzyme-linked immunosorbent assays (ELISA) that yield a high sensitivity (96%) and provide a high negative predictive value (98%) [10]. Cutoff levels for a positive test are D-dimer ≥ 500 μg/L. However, D-dimer is elevated in several situations including increasing age, cancer, severe infection, hospitalization or active inflammatory disease and in pregnancy and this needs to be taken into account. Age-adjusted cutoffs are available and may improve the accuracy of the assay in older subjects. Using the cutoff of age * 10 μg/L for patients >50 years, provides a high negative predictive value for ruling out PE in low to intermediate risk probability subjects [11].

Another approach uses the combination of clinical probability and D-dimer at different cutoff levels. This diagnostic algorithm uses the YEARS clinical decision rule that incorporates differential D-dimer cutoff values at presentation in conjunction with 3 clinical items including clinical signs of DVT, hemoptysis, and whether pulmonary embolism is the most likely diagnosis. PE can be excluded in patients without YEARS items and D-dimer <1000 ng/mL, or in patients with one or more YEARS items and D-dimer <500 ng/mL. This strategy was efficient and safe in excluding PE and reduced the need for further imaging by 14% [12].

Point-of-care D-dimer assays are also available and may be useful if laboratory facilities are not available. These assays have a lower sensitivity and negative predictive value compared to laboratory-based D-dimer tests and should be only used in patients with a low pretest probability for PE.

6.2 D-dimer Usage

Low and intermediate probability for PE D-dimer should be used primarily to rule-out PE in patients with a low and intermediate probability for PE. In patients with a low probability, it is also possible to use the pulmonary embolism rule out criteria (PERC) rule that helps rule out PE and therefore measuring D-dimer is not required [13]. The PERC rule was constructed to identify patients with a very low clinical probability of PE that have such a low risk that it is unnecessary to do further testing [14]. The PERC score includes age <50 years, heart rate <100 bpm, oxyhemoglobin saturation $\geq 95\%$, without hemoptysis, without estrogen use, without prior DVT or PE, without unilateral leg swelling and without surgery or trauma requiring hospitalization within the prior four weeks. Patients with all eight criteria do not need further testing and PE can be ruled out.

High probability for PE Patients with a high probability risk *do not need a D-dimer test*, as this does not have enough sensitivity to rule-out completely, and in

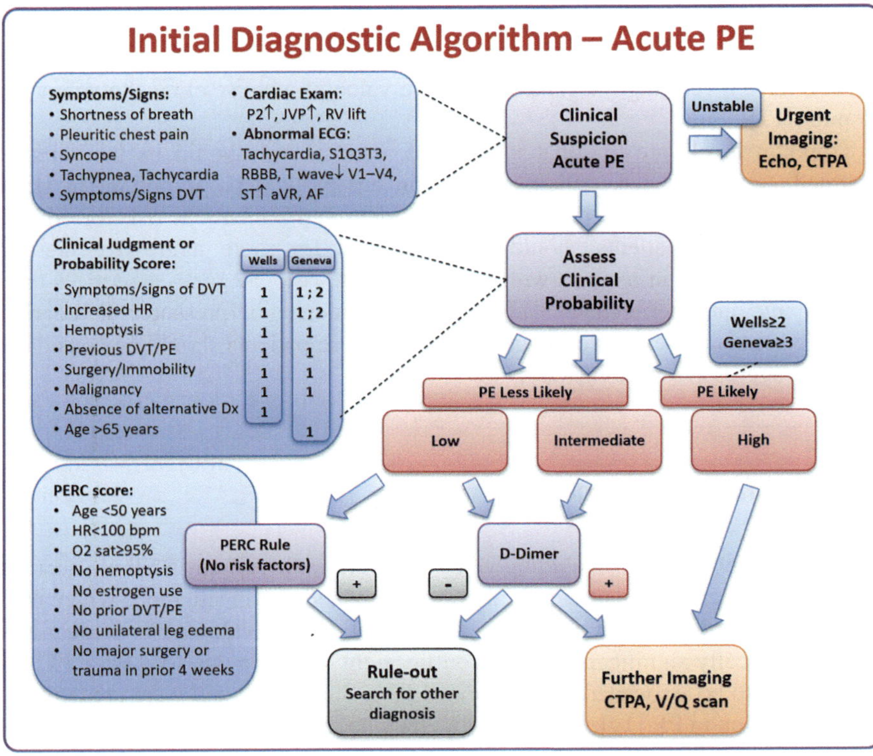

Fig. 2 Initial diagnostic flow chart (prior to imaging) to assess patients with suspected PE

high probability patients particularly unstable patients, further evaluation with imaging is mandatory in any case. Figure 2 provides a diagnostic algorithm flow chart to assess patients with suspected PE.

6.3 *Troponin*

Troponin I and T levels are the most sensitive and specific biomarkers of myocardial injury. In the context of PE, they signify RV strain and dysfunction, suggesting a larger and possibly a hemodynamically significant PE. While Troponin levels do not have diagnostic utility in PE, they provide important prognostic information. Between 30 and 60% of patients with a PE have elevated troponin levels, depending on the sensitivity of the assay used. Elevated troponin levels identify patients at high risk of short-term death and adverse outcome events. A metanalysis demonstrated a five-fold increase in mortality in patients with a positive troponin test and this was also seen in a subgroup of hemodynamically stable patients [15]. In addition, troponin was shown to add prognostic information to the simplified pulmonary embolism severity index and echocardiography, identifying patients at higher risk [16]. Moreover, normal high-sensitivity troponin T levels have a very high negative predictive value of adverse clinical outcomes in hospital [17].

Troponin levels are optional in low-risk patients but should be measured in intermediate or high-risk patients. Troponin are particularly important in stable patients with intermediate risk, as troponin identified patients at risk for adverse events and these patients should be considered for more aggressive therapy. A positive troponin in patients with an intermediate risk category categorizes these patients into an intermediate - high level if evidence of pressure on the right ventricle is also present on echocardiography. These patients should be considered for more aggressive lytic therapy.

6.4 *Natriuretic Peptides*

Natriuretic peptides (NP) including BNP or N-terminal (NT)-proBNP are secreted from cardiac chambers, particularly the ventricles, and rise in situations where there are elevated cardiac filling pressures. These peptides are valuable in evaluating a hemodynamically significant pressure on the right ventricle due to a large PE. NP were shown to be associated with increased RV volume [18] and were predictive of RV dysfunction in PE [19]. Like troponin, they have low diagnostic yield. They are not recommended as part of the standard initial evaluation of acute PE.

NP testing may be useful in estimating prognosis of patients with a large PE. A metanalysis demonstrated that a positive NP test (BNP >100 pg/mL; NT-proBNP >600 ng/L) was associated with an increased risk of between 6 to 16 for all-cause in-hospital or short-term mortality in patients with acute PE [19]. Moreover, NP have a high negative predictive value [20]. This may help identify patients with a lower risk and better prognosis. In stable patients with acute PE, NP levels were shown to have a sensitivity and specificity of 60% and 62% respectively, for predicting early recurrent VTE or fatal outcome [21]. This relatively low prediction rate suggests that NP levels are not accurate enough to guide clinical management for lytic therapy. While these biomarkers have been shown to have prognostic value and can be used as such, they have yet to be clinically predictive enough to guide treatment decisions. Therefore, current guidelines do not recommend NP testing as part of the standard evaluation of patients with PE.

7 Electrocardiogram

The Electrocardiogram (ECG), although non-specific, may increase the index of suspicion for PE as well as provide prognostic information. Its main purpose is to suggest alternative diagnoses that need to be recognized and treated. Classical

Table 3 Electrocardiogram manifestations of PE

Electrocardiogram signs of PE
Tachycardia[a]
T-wave inversion in lead V1[a]
ST elevation in lead aVR[a]
S1Q3T3 pattern: Prominent S wave in lead I, Q wave and inverted T wave in lead III[a]
Complete RBBB
Inverted T waves in V1–V4[a]
Atrial arrhythmias; Atrial fibrillation[a]
Incomplete RBBB
Rightward shift of the QRS axis
P-pulmonale

[a]Signs of RV strain and findings associated with a massive PE and increased risk of circulatory shock and death [19]

electrocardiographic abnormalities of pulmonary embolism are helpful in suggesting PE; however, the absence of such abnormalities has a low predictive value. Table 3 provides a list of the ECG manifestations of acute PE and Fig. 3 depicts the classical findings of the ECG in acute PE. The most common abnormalities found on the ECG in acute PE are tachycardia (38%) Fig. 3a, T-wave inversion in lead V1 (38%), Fig. 3b, and ST elevation in lead aVR (36%), Fig. 3c. The classical McGinn-White *S1Q3T3* pattern consisting of a prominent S wave in lead I, Q wave and inverted T wave in lead III (Fig. 3d) is specific and suggestive of PE, however it is insensitive, occurring in only 15–25% of patients with PE. More importantly, this sign is predictive of RV strain and increases the risk of adverse events. Additional findings suggesting PE are new-onset complete or incomplete RBBB (Fig. 3e), inverted T waves in V1–V4 (Fig. 3f), P-pulmonale, rightward shift of the QRS axis and atrial arrhythmias, particularly atrial fibrillation.

Beyond raising the suspicion of PE, the ECG can provide important information regarding the severity of the PE by estimating the hemodynamic significance on the right ventricle (RV) and provide prognostic value. A 21-point ECG scoring system based on ECG findings was constructed by Daniel and was shown to highly correlate with the severity of pulmonary hypertension in acute PE [22] as well as predict the risk of developing hemodynamic collapse. A modification of this score demonstrated six findings that are most indicative of RV strain. These include tachycardia, S1Q3T3, complete right bundle-branch block, inverted T waves in V1–V4, ST elevation in aVR, and atrial fibrillation. The findings are associated with a massive PE and increase the risk of circulatory shock and death [23].

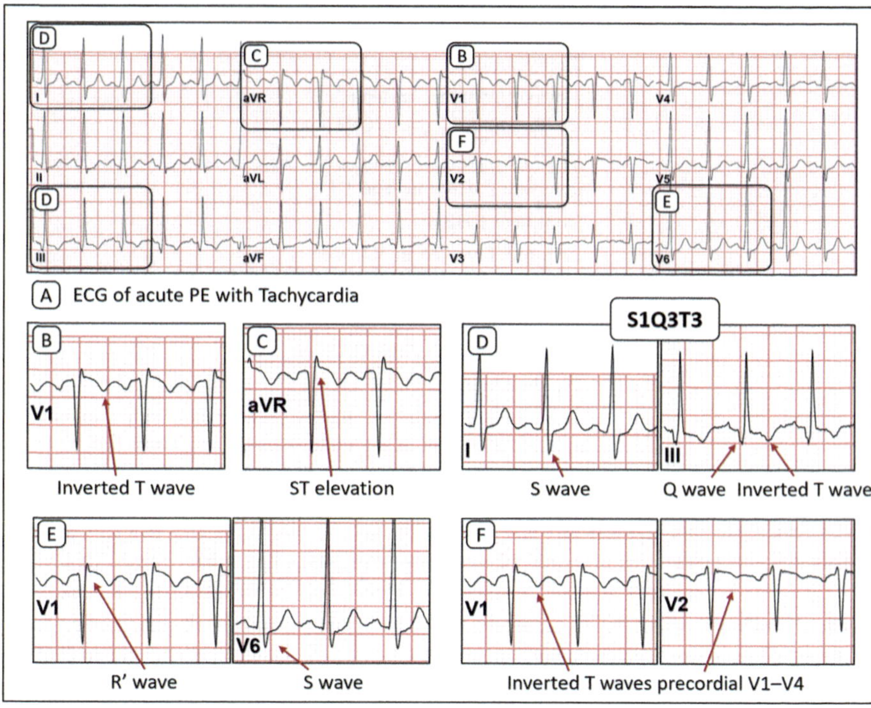

Fig. 3 ECG manifestations of Acute PE. **a** ECG of acute PE with Tachycardia. **b** T wave inversion in V1. **c** ST elevation in aVR. **d** The classical McGinn-White *S1Q3T3* pattern consisting of a prominent S wave in lead I, Q wave and inverted T wave in lead III. **e** Incomplete right bundle branch block (IRBBB) with QRS duration between 100 and 120 ms, SR' pattern in V1 and noticeable S wave in V6. **f** Inverted T waves in precordial leads V1–V4

8 Chest X-ray

The chest X-ray is not specific and may be normal in a quarter of patients with PE. The most common abnormal findings on the X-ray are cardiac enlargement (27%), pleural effusion (23%), elevated hemidiaphragm (20%), pulmonary artery enlargement (19%), atelectasis (18%) and parenchymal pulmonary infiltrates (17%) [24]. However, cardiac enlargement or pulmonary artery enlarged were neither sensitive or specific for RV dysfunction. The chest X-ray is more helpful in excluding other causes of shortness of breath or chest pain.

9 Arterial Blood Gases

Arterial blood gas, while not specific for PE, is usually abnormal and can provide prognostic information regarding the severity of the PE. Hypoxemia without obvious lung findings on physical examination and chest X-ray, should raise the index of suspicion for PE. The most common findings seen with PE are hypoxemia, widened alveolar-arterial gradient for oxygen and low CO_2. However, the blood gas may be also be normal. Hypoxemia usually suggests a more extensive PE and oxygen saturation below 95% increases the risk of complications as well as death [25].

References

1. Stein PD, Beemath A, Matta F, Weg JG, Yusen RD, Hales CA, et al. Clinical characteristics of patients with acute pulmonary embolism: data from PIOPED II. Am J Med. 2007;120 (10):871–9.
2. Stein PD, Terrin ML, Hales CA, Palevsky HI, Saltzman HA, Thompson BT, et al. Clinical, laboratory, roentgenographic, and electrocardiographic findings in patients with acute pulmonary embolism and no pre-existing cardiac or pulmonary disease. Chest. 1991;100 (3):598–603.
3. Lucassen W, Geersing GJ, Erkens PM, Reitsma JB, Moons KG, Buller H, et al. Clinical decision rules for excluding pulmonary embolism: a meta-analysis. Ann Intern Med. 2011;155(7):448–60.
4. White RH. The epidemiology of venous thromboembolism. Circulation. 2003;107(23 Suppl 1):I4-8.
5. Wells PS, Anderson DR, Rodger M, Ginsberg JS, Kearon C, Gent M, et al. Derivation of a simple clinical model to categorize patients probability of pulmonary embolism: increasing the models utility with the SimpliRED D-dimer. Thromb Haemost. 2000;83(3):416–20.
6. Le Gal G, Righini M, Roy PM, Sanchez O, Aujesky D, Bounameaux H, et al. Prediction of pulmonary embolism in the emergency department: the revised Geneva score. Ann Intern Med. 2006;144(3):165–71.
7. Gibson NS, Sohne M, Kruip MJ, Tick LW, Gerdes VE, Bossuyt PM, et al. Further validation and simplification of the Wells clinical decision rule in pulmonary embolism. Thromb Haemost. 2008;99(1):229–34.
8. Klok FA, Mos IC, Nijkeuter M, Righini M, Perrier A, Le Gal G, et al. Simplification of the revised Geneva score for assessing clinical probability of pulmonary embolism. Arch Intern Med. 2008;168(19):2131–6.
9. Hendriksen JM, Geersing GJ, Lucassen WA, Erkens PM, Stoffers HE, van Weert HC, et al. Diagnostic prediction models for suspected pulmonary embolism: systematic review and independent external validation in primary care. BMJ. 2015;351:h4438.
10. Stein PD, Hull RD, Patel KC, Olson RE, Ghali WA, Brant R, et al. D-dimer for the exclusion of acute venous thrombosis and pulmonary embolism: a systematic review. Ann Intern Med. 2004;140(8):589–602.
11. Righini M, Van Es J, Den Exter PL, Roy PM, Verschuren F, Ghuysen A, et al. Age-adjusted D-dimer cutoff levels to rule out pulmonary embolism: the ADJUST-PE study. JAMA. 2014;311(11):1117–24.

12. van der Hulle T, Cheung WY, Kooij S, Beenen LFM, van Bemmel T, van Es J, et al. Simplified diagnostic management of suspected pulmonary embolism (the YEARS study): a prospective, multicentre, cohort study. Lancet. 2017;390(10091):289–97.
13. Raja AS, Greenberg JO, Qaseem A, Denberg TD, Fitterman N, Schuur JD. Evaluation of patients with suspected acute pulmonary embolism: best practice advice from the clinical guidelines committee of the American college of physicians. Ann Intern Med. 2015;163 (9):701–11.
14. Kline JA, Webb WB, Jones AE, Hernandez-Nino J. Impact of a rapid rule-out protocol for pulmonary on the rate of screening, missed cases, and pulmonary vascular imaging in an urban US emergency department. Ann Emerg Med. 2004;44(5):490–502.
15. Becattini C, Vedovati MC, Agnelli G. Prognostic value of troponins in acute pulmonary embolism: a meta-analysis. Circulation. 2007;116(4):427–33.
16. Kaeberich A, Seeber V, Jimenez D, Kostrubiec M, Dellas C, Hasenfuss G, et al. Age-adjusted high-sensitivity troponin T cut-off value for risk stratification of pulmonary embolism. Eur Respir J. 2015;45(5):1323–31.
17. Lankeit M, Jimenez D, Kostrubiec M, Dellas C, Hasenfuss G, Pruszczyk P, et al. Predictive value of the high-sensitivity T assay and the simplified Pulmonary Embolism Severity in hemodynamically stable patients with acute pulmonary embolism: a prospective validation study. Circulation. 2011;124(24):2716–24.
18. Pasha SM, Klok FA, van der Bijl N, de Roos A, Kroft LJ, Huisman MV. NT-pro-BNP levels in patients with acute pulmonary embolism are correlated to right but not left ventricular volume and function. Thromb Haemost. 2012;108(2):367–72.
19. Cavallazzi R, Nair A, Vasu T, Marik PE. Natriuretic peptides in acute pulmonary embolism: a systematic review. Intensive Care Med. 2008;34(12):2147–56.
20. Coutance G, Cauderlier E, Ehtisham J, Hamon M. The prognostic value of markers of right ventricular dysfunction in pulmonary embolism: a meta-analysis. Crit Care. 2011;15(2):R103.
21. Sohne M, Ten Wolde M, Boomsma F, Reitsma JB, Douketis JD, Buller HR. Brain natriuretic peptide in hemodynamically stable acute pulmonary embolism. J Thromb Haemost. 2006;4 (3):552–6.
22. Daniel KR, Courtney DM, Kline JA. Assessment of cardiac stress from massive pulmonary embolism with 12-lead ECG Chest. 2001;120(2):474–81.
23. Shopp JD, Stewart LK, Emmett TW, Kline JA. Findings from 12-lead electrocardiography that predict circulatory shock from pulmonary embolism: systematic review and meta-analysis. Acad Emerg Med. 2015;22(10):1127–37.
24. Elliott CG, Goldhaber SZ, Visani L, DeRosa M. Chest radiographs in acute pulmonary embolism. Results from the International Cooperative Pulmonary Embolism Registry. Chest. 2000;118(1):33–8.
25. Kline JA, Hernandez-Nino J, Newgard CD, Cowles DN, Jackson RE, Courtney DM. Use of pulse oximetry to predict in-hospital complications in normotensive patients with pulmonary. Am J Med. 2003;115(3):203–8.

Imaging Modalities in Pulmonary Embolism: Echocardiography

Ronen Beeri, David Leibowitz, Eyal Herzog, and Edgar Argulian

1 Introduction

Pulmonary embolism (PE) is a common, but underdiagnosed condition which acutely affects both respiration and circulation alike. In particular it may affect right ventricular function acutely. Unfortunately, many of the clinical signs of PE are underdiagnosed.

The right ventricle (RV) has thin walls and is very compliant. The RV is much more sensitive than the left ventricle (LV), to increased afterload and responds with a drop in systolic contraction and stroke volume [1]. In pulmonary embolism, an acute increase in RV afterload due to partial obstruction of the pulmonary circulation leads to an upsurge in pulmonary pressure, accompanied in many cases by a decrease in RV systolic function due to the inability to overcome abrupt increases in afterload. This may also induce reduced perfusion of the RV muscle, further hindering RV function. An acute increase in mean pulmonary artery pressure above 40 mmHg is generally not tolerated [2]. There is significant interdependence between the RV and LV, both in systole and diastole. Systolic interdependence may actually partially preserve RV function due to preserved septal contraction, while diastolic interdependence in the setting of acute RV dilatation may impair LV diastolic filling with an acutely deviated septum bulging to the left, reducing LV diastolic volume (the "Reverse Bernheim" phenomenon) [3], LV stroke volume and peripheral perfusion [4].

The degree of increase in pulmonary pressure is highly dependent on the relative surface-area of the occluded pulmonary arteries, and hence on clot mass.

R. Beeri (✉) · D. Leibowitz · E. Herzog
Diagnostic Cardiology Unit and Department of Cardiology, Heart Institute, Hadassah Hebrew University Medical Center, Jerusalem, Israel
e-mail: rbeeri@Hadassah.org.il

E. Argulian
Department of Cardiology, Mount Sinai Morningside Hospital, New York, NY, USA

E. Herzog (ed.), *Pulmonary Embolism*,
https://doi.org/10.1007/978-3-030-87090-4_4

Pulmonary pressures did not exceed 20 mmHg in 58% of the patients enrolled in the PIOPED I trial. In 85% of these patients, PA systolic pressure was less than 30 mmHg [5].

1. **Echocardiography in acute pulmonary embolism**

The utility of echocardiography in pulmonary embolism varies widely based on specific clinical settings. Although studies have focused on both diagnostic and prognostic yield of echocardiography, several considerations are important when applying the evidence base to clinical practice. First, pulmonary embolism presents with a complex spectrum of disease severity ranging from frank obstructive shock, to a low risk condition with no measurable hemodynamic effect. The diagnostic yield of echocardiography follows this spectrum: in patients with hemodynamic instability, when other imaging studies are not feasible, bedside echocardiography can effectively rule out pulmonary embolism by demonstrating a normal sized and contractile right ventricle as well as potentially identify other etiologies of shock. Similarly, a dilated and hypokinetic right ventricle in these settings strongly suggests the diagnosis. On the other hand, in low-risk patients with low clot burden, echocardiography is unlikely to be of significant diagnostic and prognostic value. Since echocardiography mostly identifies the downstream hemodynamic effects of pulmonary vascular obstruction, the study findings investigating the role of echocardiography in pulmonary embolism are very dependent on the severity spectrum of the recruited population. Studies also vary in their qualitative and quantitative approaches to echocardiographic findings and by the experience of the provider obtaining and interpreting the images. Non-specific definitions of 'right ventricular strain' or 'right ventricular hypokinesis' in some studies, although practical, introduce reproducibility issues. Finally, echocardiography can be ordered in patients with pulmonary embolism to investigate other comorbid cardiac conditions since many admitted patients are elderly with a high co-morbidity burden.

Echocardiographic findings in pulmonary embolism can be broadly divided into the following categories: anatomic findings (thrombi in transit), measures of chamber size, measures of function and global/regional contractility, and Doppler derived estimates of regurgitation, pressure and resistance [6].

Figure 1 outlines an apical 4-chamber view of the ventricles in a patient with acute pulmonary embolus.

A. **Thrombi in transit**

Thrombi in transit seen in the right heart chamber are an uncommon echocardiographic finding in patients with pulmonary embolism. The prevalence of this finding is 2–4% in different registries of consecutive patients, but it is likely higher in high risk patients [6]. Right heart thrombi are most typically seen in hypotensive patients with enlarged and hypokinetic right ventricle. They likely indicate a high clot burden in the pulmonary arteries, but the thrombi also have potential to cross the interatrial septum through a foramen ovale opened by high right atrial pressures and cause systemic embolic events.

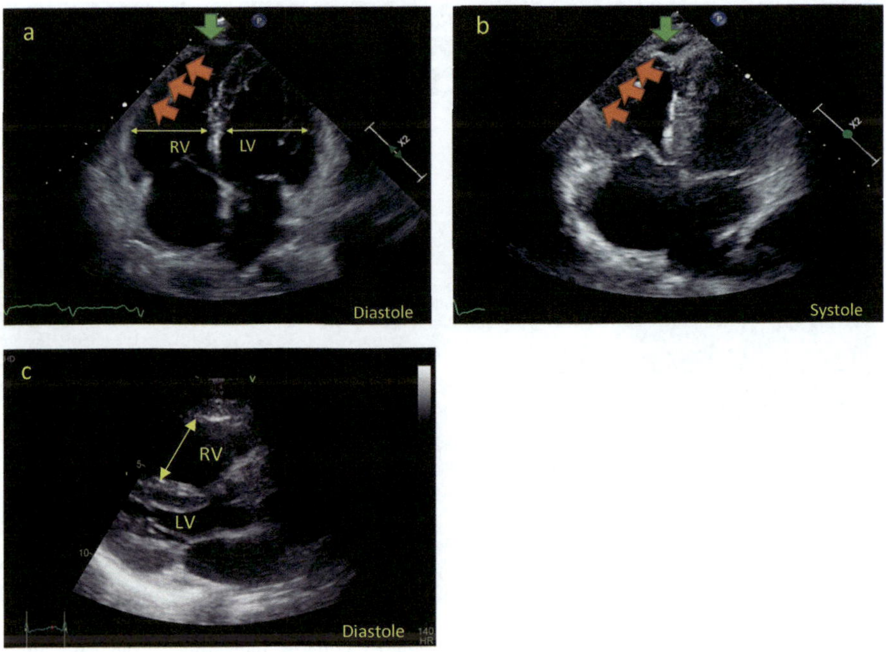

Fig. 1 Apical 4-chambers view of the ventricles in a patient with acute pulmonary embolus. Note the enlargement of the right ventricle in diastole (panel A—yellow arrow), akinesis of the right ventricular free wall (panel B—orange arrows) with normal contraction of the right ventricular apex (panel green arrow)—the **Mc Connell sign**. In panel C (parasternal long axis view), there is diastolic compression of the LV by the dilated RV

Right heart thrombi have been consistently associated with poor prognosis, increasing short-term mortality with an odds ratio of 3.0 [7].

B. **Right heart side enlargement with volume and pressure overload**
Right ventricular enlargement was measured in different studies as either right ventricular end-diastolic diameter or right ventricle to left ventricle ratio (>0.9–1.0). Right ventricular end-diastolic diameter is likely the most sensitive echocardiographic finding of pulmonary embolism with pooled sensitivity exceeding 80% [8]. Right ventricle to left ventricle ratio is less sensitive (close to 50%) but has a high specificity exceeding 90%, both in laboratory-performed and point-of-care ultrasound studies [8]. Not surprisingly, the presence and degree of these abnormalities are dependent on the severity of the disease [9]. Right ventricle to left ventricle ratio was an independent marker of mortality among patients with pulmonary embolism admitted to the intensive care unit [10]. Right atrial enlargement is as well an independent prognostic variable associated with pulmonary-embolism related mortality [11]. Figure 2 demonstrates a dilated inferior vena cava with no inspiratory collapse indicating elevated RV filling pressures in a patient with acute pulmonary embolus. Figure 3 shows a parasternal short-axis view at the mid-left ventricular level in

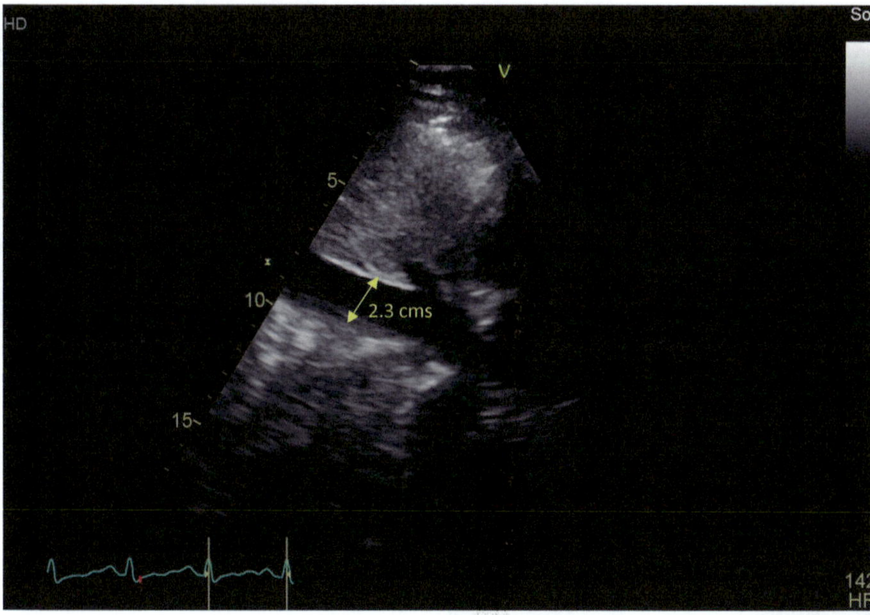

Fig. 2 A dilated inferior vena cava with no inspiratory collapse indicating elevated RV filling pressures in a patient with acute pulmonary embolus (subcostal short-axis view)

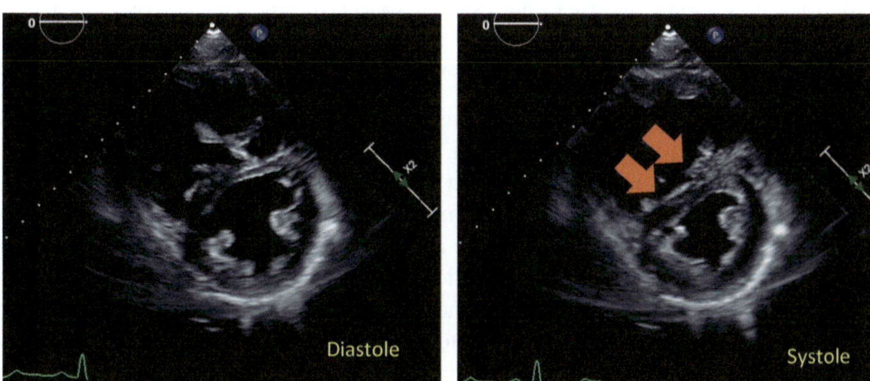

Fig. 3 Parasternal short-axis view at mid left ventricular level in a patient with acute pulmonary emboli, showing systolic flattening of the of inter-ventricular septum, signifying right ventricular pressure overload

a patient with acute pulmonary embolism, showing systolic flattening of the of inter-ventricular septum, signifying right ventricular pressure overload.

C. **Measures of global and regional contractility**
Measures of global and regional contractility include right ventricular free wall hypokinesis/'strain', McConnell sign (lateral wall hypokinesis with preservation of contractile 'echocardiographic' apex), abnormal septal motion, decreased fractional area change, decreased s' velocity and decreased tricuspid annular plane systolic excursion (TAPSE). More advanced techniques have also been used such as right ventricular ejection fraction derived from 3D echocardiographic datasets, and 2D right ventricular longitudinal strain measured by speckle tracking. Overall qualitative impression of 'right heart strain' had moderate sensitivity but high specificity, including in emergency department and point-of-care ultrasound studies. Sensitivity of these findings depends on the severity of the disease. In one large echocardiographic study, McConnell sign and septal flattening were present in 20 and 18% of all pulmonary embolism patients but 75 and 69% of high risk patients, respectively [9]. Interestingly, many contractility measures appear to carry high specificity, including lateral wall hypokinesis, McConnell sign, and abnormal septal motion, but only in the right clinical settings [12].

Tricuspid annular plane systolic excursion (TAPSE) (seen in Fig. 4) has been studied as a marker of adverse prognosis in patients with acute pulmonary embolism. In hemodynamically stable patients on admission, TAPSE $\leq$ 15 mm identified patients with an increased 30-day pulmonary embolism-related mortality and was superior to right ventricle to left ventricle ratio [13]. It may also be a better prognostic marker compared to TV annulus tissue Doppler s' wave velocity [14, 15].

Advanced echocardiographic measures of right ventricular deformation have not been well studied in patients with acute pulmonary embolism, but the existing evidence shows some promise. In one study of hemodynamically stable patients, right ventricular free wall strain was an independent predictor of in-hospital adverse events (death, inotropic support, thrombolysis or surgery), with the cutoff global strain value of -15.9% showing optimal prognostic performance [16]. Another study of non-hypotensive patients showed that changes in 3D right ventricular ejection fraction and mid-free wall longitudinal strain were the most sensitive predictors of adverse events and were independently associated with adverse outcomes [17].

In the modern management of pulmonary embolism, echocardiography is typically used in the context of clinical risk stratification tools and other test findings, namely CT angiography and cardiac biomarkers. CT angiography was sensitive but non-specific in detecting right ventricular dysfunction identified by echocardiography, and echocardiography offered incremental prognostic value compared to CT in predicting clinical deterioration [18]. Echocardiography also improves risk stratification for intermediate-high risk patients with pulmonary embolism compared to clinical assessment and CT angiography [19]. A low stroke volume index

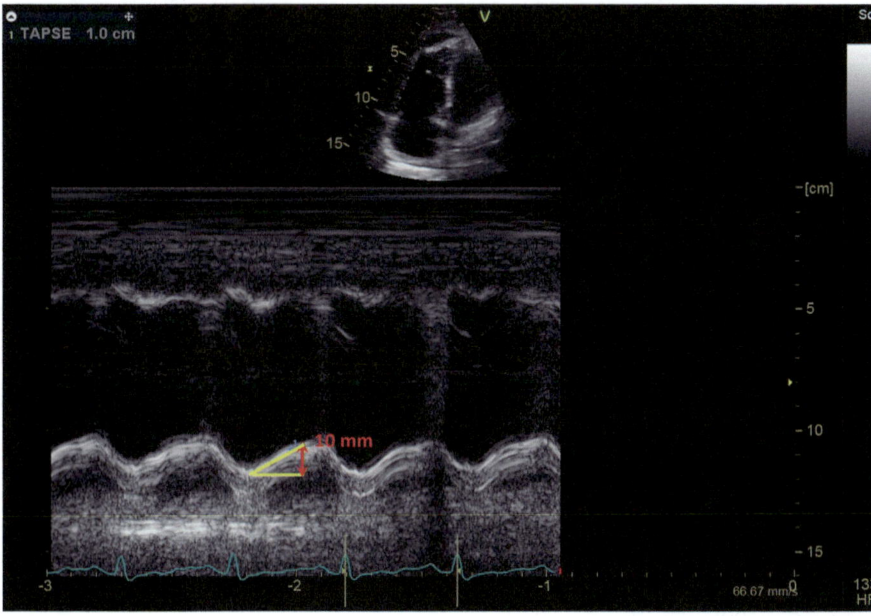

Fig. 4 M-mode of the lateral annulus of the tricuspid valve (apical 4-chamber RV-focused view) in a patient with acute pulmonary embolus. Tricuspid annular peak-systolic excursion (TAPSE) is measured at 10 mm (reduced)

(below 20 mL/m^2), determined using Doppler velocity–time integral at either the LVOT or RVOT, is associated with in-hospital mortality and cardiopulmonary decompensation in normotensive PE patients [20]. On the other hand, the role of echocardiography in combination with cardiac biomarkers (troponin and brain natriuretic peptide levels) is less clear. Cardiac biomarkers may provide better risk stratification than echocardiographic markers of right ventricular overload. In one study of normotensive patients with acute pulmonary embolism, echocardiography added no independent prognostic value to a multivariate prediction score, including the simplified Pulmonary Embolism Severity Index (sPESI), cardiac troponin I, brain natriuretic peptide (BNP), and lower limb ultrasound [21].

2. **Specific echocardiographic signs of acute pulmonary embolism**

A. **"McConnell sign"**

McConnell et al. described a regional pattern of RV dysfunction in patients with PE of akinesia of the RV free wall but normal or even hyperdynamic function of the apex (Fig. 1) [22]. This finding was in contrast to other causes of RV dysfunction which generally led to diffusely abnormal wall motion. In this study, the "McConnell sign" had a positive predictive value of 71% and a negative predictive value of 96% for the diagnosis of PE. The authors postulated three potential mechanisms for this finding. First, tethering of the RV apex to a hyperdynamic left ventricular apex, second localized ischemia of the RV free wall due to increased wall stress and third, geometric changes due to the acute increase in RV afterload. The same group demonstrated that regional RV dysfunction seen in acute PE could be reversed with thrombolytic therapy strengthening the association between this echocardiographic finding and acute hemodynamic changes due to PE [23]. Interestingly, despite the 2D appearance of apical hyperkinesis, apical strain has been demonstrated to be reduced in patients with the McConnell sign with and without PE [24].

More recent studies have called into question the diagnostic accuracy of the "McConnell sign". In a study based on an emergency room database comparing patients with a diagnosis of "massive or submassive" PE and those with right ventricular infarction, the McConnell sign carried a sensitivity of 70% but a specificity of only 33% for the diagnosis of PE [25]. In patients with moderate PE presenting to the ER, there was a sensitivity of 20% and a specificity of 100% [26]. While only a minority of patients in another study had a McConnell sign, 75% of patients with hemodynamic instability demonstrated a McConnell sign [9]. In summary, the diagnostic value of this sign appears valuable mainly as a specific sign of PE in patients with suspected acute massive PE and hemodynamic compromise. Conversely, the utility of this sign alone to predict prognosis in patients with PE is limited. In 211 patients with PE, the presence of a McConnell sign on admission did not predict short or long term mortality [10]. In a prospective study of patients with PE who were hemodynamically stable on admission, a McConnell sign was predictive of mortality and rescue thrombolysis on univariable but not multivariable analysis [13].

B. **"60/60" sign**

Torbicki et al. described a modified RV ejection pattern in patients with proximal pulmonary emboli [27]. They described a significantly shorter time interval, generally less than 60 ms, from the onset of forward flow into the pulmonary artery to the peak velocity of this flow in patients with acute PE. This finding tended to occur without significantly elevated pulmonary artery pressures. A short ejection time of less than 60 ms together with a tricuspid valve pressure gradient less than 60 mmHg (the "60/60" sign—Fig. 5) had a sensitivity of 48% and specificity of 98% for acute PE. The authors also described a characteristic mid systolic deceleration, or "early systolic notching" (ESN) pattern found in 96% of acute PE patients as compared to 56% of patients with chronic lung disease and 83% with idiopathic pulmonary hypertension. In 67 patients with confirmed PE, the "60/60" sign had a sensitivity of only 25% but an excellent specificity of 94% leading to a positive predictive value of 90% and a negative predictive value of 38%. When the 60/60 criterion was combined with the presence of a McConnell sign, sensitivity was slightly improved to 36% without a significant change in specificity. The results were not significantly different in patients with or without previous known cardiorespiratory diseases. Patients with a 60/60 sign were more hypoxemic, suggesting a possible association with more severe PE. Similarly to the McConnell sign, the 60/60 sign appears to be a reliable but not sensitive sign of PE [28]. Alfonso et al.

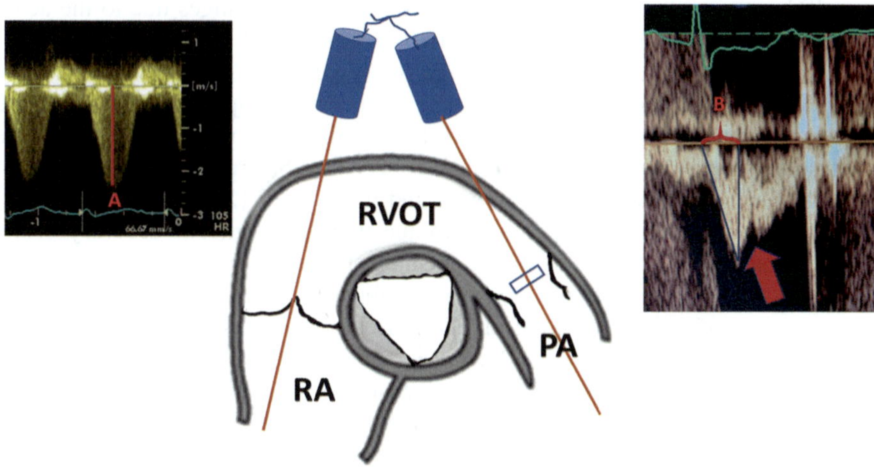

Fig. 5 The 60/60 and early systolic notching of RVOT flow (from the high parasternal short-axis view). 1. **60/60 sign:** A TR pressure gradient (by CW Doppler) smaller or equal 60 mmHg, with **B.** RVOT acceleration time (from start of ejection to peak RVOT flow) by pulsed-wave Doppler shorter or equal 60 ms. The sample volume is placed just below the pulmonic valve. 2. **Early systolic notching** (red arrow): a dip is seen in early systole in RVOT flow, with a more gradual flow subsequently ("Spike and dome")

retrospectively analyzed the diagnostic utility of ESN in PE patients diagnosed by CT scanning [29]. In this study, ESN was considered present if the Doppler envelope exhibited a narrow peaked initial wave (spike) with early deceleration producing a sharp notch within the first half of systole (initial 50% of ejection (Fig. 4)). This was then followed by a second, more curvilinear Doppler wave. In patients with massive or sub-massive PE, this finding had 92% sensitivity and 99% specificity with a positive and negative value of 98% and 96% respectively. In the same population the McConnell sign and the 60/60 sign had lower diagnostic accuracy. The authors postulated, based on animal studies, that the site of obstruction in the pulmonary vascular tree affects the systolic flow velocity curve. Proximal thromboemboli cause early return of reflected pressure waves potentially causing notching and a cutoff of the peak velocity. This sign was absent in patients with left sided, post capillary pulmonary hypertension. It is important to note that ESN had little diagnostic value in patients with low risk, subsegmental PE.

2. **Transesophageal echocardiography**
   TEE can directly image the right-sided cardiac structures, the main pulmonary artery, a significant portion of the right pulmonary artery and the proximal portion of the left pulmonary artery. The ability of TEE to directly visualize central pulmonary emboli has been well documented [30]. Several trials have examined the utility of TEE particularly in patients with hemodynamic instability or documentation of RV overload on TTE or CT in which the presence of

central PE is more likely. A pooled analysis of these early studies showed a sensitivity of 70% and a specificity of 81% for TEE [31]. A higher diagnostic accuracy with 80% sensitivity and specificity of 97% was demonstrated in a single center study [32]. Given the need for esophageal intubation, use of TEE may be more relevant in certain subgroups of patients with suspected PE. The utility of TEE has been examined in patients with unexplained hemodynamic instability in non-cardiac surgical patients and been shown to be effective in managing these complex patients [33]. TEE can be safely performed during resuscitation and a prospective study using TEE in patients with unexplained sudden cardiac arrest demonstrated that in 25 patients with pulseless electrical activity (PEA), TEE revealed evidence of PE in 8 (22%) of whom 2 survived to hospital discharge [34]. The authors suggest early use of TEE in patients with unexplained PEA may help improve outcomes in this population. The ability of TEE to directly image pulmonary artery thrombi enables assessment of thrombus mobility. In a prospective registry study of 47 patients, Podbregar et al. showed that immobile thrombi noted on TEE were associated with lower cardiac index and higher pulmonary resistance [35]. Patients with immobile thrombi had a worse short term prognosis. The authors postulated that immobile thrombi were more organized and therefore more resistant to therapy than non-mobile thrombi.

3. **Patent foramen ovale**
   The prevalence of a patent foramen ovale (PFO) detected by color Doppler or agitated saline injection appears to be increased in patients with PE and correlates with a worse prognosis. Konstantinides et al. performed agitated saline studies in 139 consecutive patients with PE and evidence of right-sided pressure overload. PFO (with right to left shunt diagnosed with agitated saline injection) was noted in 35% of patients and in hospital mortality in this group was 33% compared to 14% in patients without PFO. Patients with PFO had a significantly higher incidence of ischemic stroke (13% vs. 2.2%) and peripheral embolism 15% vs. 0%), presumably due to paradoxical embolism [36]. Clergeau et al. also demonstrated a significant increase in silent brain infarctions detected by MRI (33.3% vs. 2.2%) in patients with PE and PFO demonstrated on agitated saline study [37]. A recent study from the RIETE registry showed that 67% of all-comers with acute PE had no TTE performed on admission, and among the remaining patients 26% had a PFO. Patients with PFO were more likely to have chronic heart failure, prior myocardial infarction or ischemic stroke, and had a higher rate of subsequent ischemic stroke than those without PFO. The authors suggest that TTE is under-performed in this population despite the excess risk derived from the presence of PFO [38].
4. **Other ultrasound technologies**
   Limited reports have examined the use of invasive intravascular echocardiographic techniques such as intravascular ultrasound (IVUS) and intracardiac echocardiography (ICE) in the diagnosis and management of PE. In a study of 11 patients comparing IVUS to invasive angiography, IVUS detected thrombus

formation in 38% of angiographically normal segments. In addition, IVUS was able to differentiate mobile from non-mobile thrombi [39]. ICE has demonstrated the ability in several case reports to detect incidental PE during electrophysiologic procedures [40]. Given their invasive nature, these techniques have a limited role in the routine management of PE.

5. **Point of care echocardiography (POCUS) and cardiopulmonary ultrasound (CPUS)**
   The availability of mobile echocardiography devices, with 2D and color Doppler imaging, has made echocardiographic signs, sometime in combination with lung ultrasound, a valuable bedside tool, where pulmonary CTA and/or full echocardiographic studies are not available [41]. Many standard echocardiographic signs of pulmonary emboli are readily seen on 2D imaging, and do not require sophisticated Doppler analyses. A negative POCUS (including TAPSE, septal flattening (Fig. 5), MConnell's sign and tricuspid regurgitation severity) significantly lowered the likelihood of PE diagnosis in a majority of hemodynamically unstable patients with suspected PE in a large multicenter study [42]. In particular, in the subgroup of patients with heart rates above 110 beats/min, POCUS was 100% sensitive and 63% specific for the diagnosis, making it a good screening test for hemodynamically significant PE.

Lung ultrasound (LUS) is a promising technique to image lung parenchyma and the pleural space. Pulmonary localized sub-pleural consolidations are localized to areas of pulmonary infarctions. In a prospective study, LUS demonstrated a sensitivity of 80%, specificity of 92%, and a positive and negative predictive value of 95% and 72% respectively [43]. Other studies showed lower sensitivity and specificity values [44]. In particular, lung ultrasound may be valuable to rule-out other causes of dyspnea. Point of care vascular ultrasound of the femoral and popliteal veins can be easily performed at the bedside, and by using only 2D compression technique yields a sensitivity and specificity of 93% for the diagnosis for significant deep-vein thrombosis when performed by a non-sonographer [45].

Nazerian et al. performed multi-organ point of care CPUS, diagnosing PE if DVT, multiple subpleural consolidations and RV dilatation were found. Sensitivity and specificity for PE were 90% and 86.2% respectively. Thus, multiorgan CPUS is more sensitive than single-organ point of care US in diagnosing PE, and may obviate the need for CTA in suspected PE [46].

References

1. Haddad FO, Hunt SA, Rosenthal DN, Murphy DJ. Right ventricular Function in cardiovascular disease Part I. Circulation. 2008;117(11):1436–48.
2. Haddad FO, Doyle R, Murphy DJ, Hunt SA. Right ventricular function in cardiovascular disease Part II. Circulation. 2008;117(13):1717–31.
3. Santamore WP, Dell'Italia LJ. Ventricular interdependence: significant left ventricular contributions to right ventricular systolic function. Prog Cardiovasc Dis. 1998;40(4):289–308.

4. Alpert JS. Effect of Right Ventricular Dysfunction on Left Ventricular Function. In: Left ventricular dysfunction. International symposium. Jerusalem; 1985. pp. 25–34. Adv Cardiol.
5. Stein DP. Relation of right-sided pressures to clinical characteristics of patients with no prior cardiopulmonary disease. In: Stein DP, editor. Pulmonary embolism. Malden, Mass: Wiley-Blackwell; 2007.
6. Dabbouseh NM, Patel JJ, Bergl PA. Role of echocardiography in managing acute pulmonary embolism. Heart. 2019;105(23):1785–92.
7. Barrios D, Rosa-Salazar V, Morillo R, Nieto R, Fernandez S, Zamorano JL, Monreal M, Torbicki A, Yusen RD, Jimenez D. Prognostic significance of right heart thrombi in patients with acute symptomatic pulmonary embolism: systematic review and meta-analysis. Chest. 2017;151(2):409–16.
8. Fields JM, Davis J, Girson L, Au A, Potts J, Morgan CJ, Vetter I, Riesenberg LA. Transthoracic echocardiography for diagnosing pulmonary embolism: a systematic review and meta-analysis. J Am Soc Echocardiogr 2017;30(7):714–23e4.
9. Kurnicka K, Lichodziejewska B, Goliszek S, Dzikowska-Diduch O, Zdończyk O, Kozłowska M, Kostrubiec M, Ciurzyński M, Palczewski P, Grudzka K, Krupa M, Koć M, Pruszczyk P. Echocardiographic pattern of acute pulmonary embolism: analysis of 511 consecutive patients. J Am Soc Echocardiogr. 2016;29(9):907–13.
10. Khemasuwan D, Yingchoncharoen T, Tunsupon P, Kusunose K, Moghekar A, Klein A, Tonelli AR. Right ventricular echocardiographic parameters are associated with mortality after acute pulmonary embolism. J Am Soc Echocardiogr. 2015;28(3):355–62.
11. Bikdeli B, Lobo JL, Jimenez D, Green P, Fernandez-Capitan C, Bura-Riviere A, Otero R, DiTullio MR, Galindo S, Ellis M, Parikh SA, Monreal M, Investigators R. Early Use of Echocardiography in Patients With Acute Pulmonary Embolism: Findings From the RIETE Registry. J Am Heart Assoc 2018;7(17):e009042.
12. Wright L, Dwyer N, Power J, Kritharides L, Celermajer D, Marwick TH. Right ventricular systolic function responses to acute and chronic pulmonary hypertension: assessment with myocardial deformation. J Am Soc Echocardiogr. 2016;29(3):259–66.
13. Pruszczyk P, Goliszek S, Lichodziejewska B, Kostrubiec M, Ciurzyński M, Kurnicka K, Dzikowska-Diduch O, Palczewski P, Wyzgal A. Prognostic value of echocardiography in normotensive patients with acute pulmonary embolism. JACC Cardiovasc Imaging. 2014;7(6):553–60.
14. Kurnicka K, Lichodziejewska B, Ciurzynski M, Kostrubiec M, Goliszek S, Zdonczyk O, Dzikowska-Diduch O, Palczewski P, Skowronska M, Koc M, Grudzka K, Pruszczyk P. Peak systolic velocity of tricuspid annulus is inferior to tricuspid annular plane systolic excursion for 30 days prediction of adverse outcome in acute pulmonary embolism. Cardiol J. 2020;27(5):558–65.
15. Lobo JL, Holley A, Tapson V, Moores L, Oribe M, Barron M, Otero R, Nauffal D, Valle R, Monreal M, Yusen RD, Jimenez D, Protect, investigators R. Prognostic significance of tricuspid annular displacement in normotensive patients with acute symptomatic pulmonary embolism. J Thromb Haemost 2014;12(7):1020–7.
16. Lee K, Kwon O, Lee E-J, Sin M-J, Lee JS, Lee S, Kang D-H, Song J-K, Song J-M. Prognostic value of echocardiographic parameters for right ventricular function in patients with acute non-massive pulmonary embolism. Heart Vessels. 2019;34(7):1187–95.
17. Vitarelli A, Barilla F, Capotosto L, D'Angeli I, Truscelli G, De Maio M, Ashurov R. Right ventricular function in acute pulmonary embolism: a combined assessment by three-dimensional and speckle-tracking echocardiography. J Am Soc Echocardiogr. 2014;27(3):329–38.
18. Dudzinski DM, Hariharan P, Parry BA, Chang Y, Kabrhel C. Assessment of right ventricular strain by computed tomography versus echocardiography in acute pulmonary embolism. Acad Emerg Med. 2017;24(3):337–43.
19. Barrios D, Morillo R, Lobo JL, Nieto R, Jaureguizar A, Portillo AK, Barbero E, Fernandez-Golfin C, Yusen RD, Jimenez D, investigators P. Assessment of right ventricular function in acute pulmonary embolism. Am Heart J 2017;185:123–9.

20. Prosperi-Porta G, Solverson K, Fine N, Humphreys CJ, Ferland A, Weatherald J. Echocardiography-derived stroke volume index is associated with adverse in-hospital outcomes in intermediate-risk acute pulmonary embolism. Chest. 2020;158(3):1132–42.
21. Jimenez D, Kopecna D, Tapson V, Briese B, Schreiber D, Lobo JL, Monreal M, Aujesky D, Sanchez O, Meyer G, Konstantinides S, Yusen RD, On Behalf Of The Protect I. Derivation and validation of multimarker prognostication for normotensive patients with acute symptomatic pulmonary embolism. Am J Respir Crit Care Med 2014;189(6):718–26.
22. McConnell MV, Solomon SD, Rayan ME, Come PC, Goldhaber SZ, Lee RT. Regional right ventricular dysfunction detected by echocardiography in acute pulmonary embolism. Am J Cardiol. 1996;78(4):469–73.
23. Nass N, McConnell MV, Goldhaber SZ, Chyu S, Solomon SD. Recovery of regional right ventricular function after thrombolysis for pulmonary embolism. Am J Cardiol 1999;83(5):804–6, a10.
24. Mediratta A, Addetia K, Medvedofsky D, Gomberg-Maitland M, Mor-Avi V, Lang RM. Echocardiographic diagnosis of acute pulmonary embolism in patients with McConnell's sign. Echocardiography. 2016;33(5):696–702.
25. Casazza F, Bongarzoni A, Capozi A, Agostoni O. Regional right ventricular dysfunction in acute pulmonary embolism and right ventricular infarction. Eur J Echocardiogr. 2005;6(1):11–4.
26. Dresden S, Mitchell P, Rahimi L, Leo M, Rubin-Smith J, Bibi S, White L, Langlois B, Sullivan A, Carmody K. Right ventricular dilatation on bedside echocardiography performed by emergency physicians aids in the diagnosis of pulmonary embolism. Ann Emerg Med. 2014;63(1):16–24.
27. Torbicki A, Kurzyna M, Ciurzynski M, Pruszczyk P, Pacho R, Kuch-Wocial A, Szulc M. Proximal pulmonary emboli modify right ventricular ejection pattern. Eur Respir J. 1999;13(3):616–21.
28. Kurzyna M, Torbicki A, Pruszczyk P, Burakowska B, Fijałkowska A, Kober J, Oniszh K, Kuca P, Tomkowski W, Burakowski J, Wawrzyńska L. Disturbed right ventricular ejection pattern as a new Doppler echocardiographic sign of acute pulmonary embolism. Am J Cardiol. 2002;90(5):507–11.
29. Afonso L, Sood A, Akintoye E, Gorcsan J 3rd, Rehman MU, Kumar K, Javed A, Kottam A, Cardozo S, Singh M, Palla M, Ando T, Adegbala O, Shokr M, Briasoulis A. A Doppler echocardiographic pulmonary flow marker of massive or submassive acute pulmonary embolus. J Am Soc Echocardiogr. 2019;32(7):799–806.
30. Rittoo D, Sutherland GR, Samuel L, Flapan AD, Shaw TR. Role of transesophageal echocardiography in diagnosis and management of central pulmonary artery thromboembolism. Am J Cardiol. 1993;71(12):1115–8.
31. Kline JA, Johns KL, Colucciello SA, Israel EG. New diagnostic tests for pulmonary embolism. Ann Emergency Med. 2000;35(2):168–80.
32. Wittlich N, Erbel R, Eichler A, Schuster S, Jakob H, Iversen S, Oelert H, Meyer J. Detection of central pulmonary artery thromboemboli by transesophageal echocardiography in patients with severe pulmonary embolism. J Am Soc Echocardiogr. 1992;5(5):515–24.
33. Vieillard-Baron A, Qanadli SD, Antakly Y, Fourme T, Loubières Y, Jardin F, Dubourg O. Transesophageal echocardiography for the diagnosis of pulmonary embolism with acute cor pulmonale: a comparison with radiological procedures. Intensive Care Med. 1998;24(5):429–33.
34. Krivec B, Voga G, Zuran I, Skale R, Pareznik R, Podbregar M, Noc M. Diagnosis and treatment of shock due to massive pulmonary embolism: approach with transesophageal echocardiography and intrapulmonary thrombolysis. Chest. 1997;112(5):1310–6.
35. Podbregar M, Voga G, Krivec B. Morphologic characteristics of central pulmonary thromboemboli predict haemodynamic response in massive pulmonary embolism. Intensive Care Med. 2004;30(8):1552–6.

36. Konstantinides S, Geibel A, Kasper W, Olschewski M, BlüMel L, Just HR. Patent foramen ovale is an important predictor of adverse outcome in patients with major pulmonary embolism. Circulation. 1998;97(19):1946–51.
37. Clergeau M-R, Hamon ML, Morello RM, Saloux E, Viader F, Hamon M. Silent cerebral infarcts in patients with pulmonary embolism and a patent foramen ovale. Stroke. 2009;40(12):3758–62.
38. Lacut K, Le Moigne E, Couturaud F, Font C, Vázquez FJ, Cañas I, Díaz-Peromingo JA, Gil-Díaz A, Bucherini E, Monreal M. Outcomes in patients with acute pulmonary embolism and patent foramen ovale: Findings from the RIETE registry. Thromb Res. 2021;202:59–66.
39. Gorge G, Schuster S, Ge J, Meyer J, Erbel R. Intravascular ultrasound in patients with acute pulmonary embolism after treatment with intravenous urokinase and high-dose heparin. Heart. 1997;77(1):73–7.
40. Asbach S, Biermann J, Blanke P, Pache G, Bode C, Faber TS. Incidental finding of a pulmonary embolus by intracardiac echocardiography during an atrial fibrillation ablation procedure. EP Europace. 2010;12(8):1199–200.
41. Kagima J, Stolbrink M, Masheti S, Mbaiyani C, Munubi A, Joekes E, Mortimer K, Rylance J, Morton B. Diagnostic accuracy of combined thoracic and cardiac sonography for the diagnosis of pulmonary embolism: A systematic review and meta-analysis. PLoS One 2020;15(9):e0235940.
42. Daley JI, Dwyer KH, Grunwald Z, Shaw DL, Stone MB, Schick A, Vrablik M, Kennedy Hall M, Hall J, Liteplo AS, Haney RM, Hun N, Liu R, Moore CL. Increased sensitivity of focused cardiac ultrasound for pulmonary embolism in emergency department patients with abnormal vital signs. Acad Emerg Med. 2019;26(11):1211–20.
43. Reissig A, Heyne J-P, Kroegel C. Sonography of lung and pleura in pulmonary embolism. Chest. 2001;120(6):1977–83.
44. Pfeil A, Reissig A, Heyne J-P, Wolf G, Kaiser WA, Kroegel C, Hansch A. Transthoracic sonography in comparison to multislice computed tomography in detection of peripheral pulmonary embolism. Lung. 2010;188(1):43–50.
45. Canakci ME, Acar N, Bilgin M, Kuas C. Diagnostic value of point-of-care ultrasound in deep vein thrombosis in the emergency department. J Clin Ultrasound. 2020;48(9):527–31.
46. Nazerian P, Vanni S, Volpicelli G, Gigli C, Zanobetti M, Bartolucci M, Ciavattone A, Lamorte A, Veltri A, Fabbri A, Grifoni S. Accuracy of point-of-care multiorgan ultrasonography for the diagnosis of pulmonary embolism. Chest. 2014;145(5):950–7.

Imaging Modalities in Venous-Thromboembolism: Ultrasound for Lower Extremity Deep Venous Thrombosis

Gal Ben-Arie and Liat Appelbaum

1 Introduction

Venous thromboembolic disease (VTE) is a spectrum of conditions ranging from small deep-vein thrombosis (DVT) up to pulmonary emboli (PE) which is a life-threatening disease and is a common cause of morbidity and mortality in hospitalized patients. It is presumed that most PE's arise in the deep veins of the lower limbs and pelvis emphasizing the importance of DVT diagnosis [1–4].

Ultrasound (US) is the standard imaging test for patients suspected of having lower limb DVT. However, there is a wide disagreement regarding the required components of this test in the literature. This chapter will cover the basic constitutes of venous US including anatomical knowledge, transducer choosing, technique, and expected results and pitfalls. It is based on the Recommendations of the Society of Radiologist in Ultrasound Consensus Multidisciplinary Conference [5].

As always with imaging and with US in particular, theoretical knowledge cannot substitute for practice. In any case of doubt do not hesitate and consult an expert radiologist.

G. Ben-Arie
Department of Radiology, Soroka University Medical Center, Beer Sheva, Israel

L. Appelbaum (✉)
Department of Radiology, Hadassah Hebrew University Medical Center, Jerusalem, Israel
e-mail: liata@hadassah.org.il

E. Herzog (ed.), *Pulmonary Embolism*,
https://doi.org/10.1007/978-3-030-87090-4_5

2 Exam Protocol

2.1 *Anatomy*

As outlined in Fig. 1, the following veins should be included in the study (Fig. 1):

- Bilateral common femoral veins (CFV)
- Sapheno-femoral junction
- Great Saphenous Vein
- Proximal Deep Femoral Vein
- Proximal femoral vein (FV)
- Mid FV
- Distal FV
- Popliteal vein
- Posterior tibial veins
- Peroneal veins.

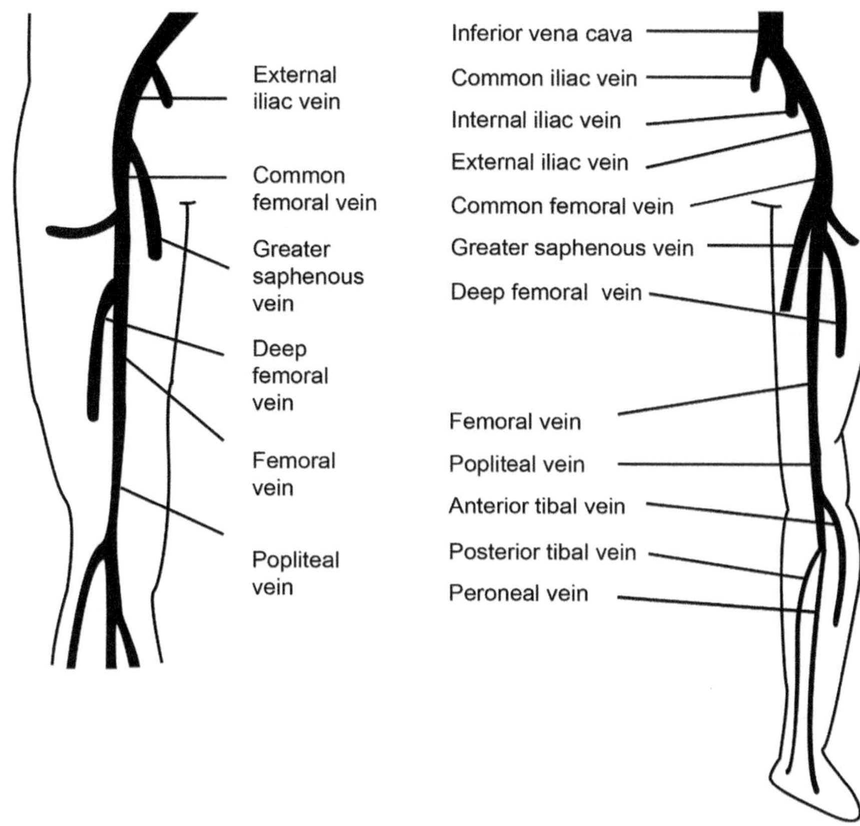

Fig. 1 Venous anatomy of the lower limb

The CFV should be the first vessel documented, and as a rule of thumb, it is the most medial vessel depicted in the groin. Documentation of more proximal veins is recommended if there is a CFV thrombus, and then it is advisable to follow the external iliac and common iliac veins up to the Inferior vena cava (IVC). The deep pelvic veins are frequently obscured by bowel gas, but at least parts of them are usually visible.

The calf veins, below the Popliteal vein (PV) show a wide anatomical variance. The exam protocol should include at least the posterior tibial and peroneal veins, and could be extended according to symptomatology, such as focal pain, area of redness or string-like sensitive structure [5–7].

2.2 *Image Acquisition and Techniques*

Transducer selection—A linear, typically 5–10 MHz transducer should be used. When the vessels are deeper than expected, such as in cases of severe edema or swelling of the legs, or significant obesity, a lower frequency transducer may be required, sometimes even a 2–5 MHz curvilinear—"abdominal" transducer. The later would be the appropriate transducer for examining the pelvic veins, if necessary [8].

The operator should position the transducer perpendicularly to the skin in a transverse/short axis orientation (Fig. 2) and maintain the probe marker facing the right side of the patient along the test to avoid direction mistakes when examining the images later.

Patient positioning—the optimal way to view the veins would be with the patient in a supine position, with the examined leg externally rotated and the knee flexed (Fig. 3). If possible, position the bed in a reverse Trendelenburg direction to increase venous filling and allowing an easier examination. The lateral decubitus

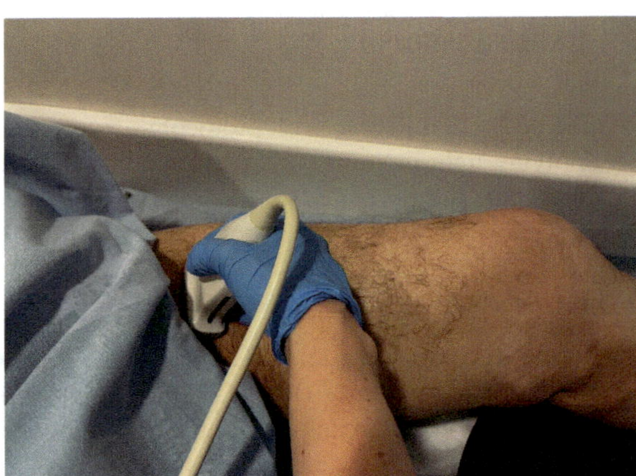

Fig. 2 Photograph demonstrating appropriate patient positioning during ultrasound evaluation of the femoral vein. Notice a 5–10 MHz transducer is used, perpendicularly to the skin in a transverse/short axis orientation, with the probe marker facing the right side of the patient

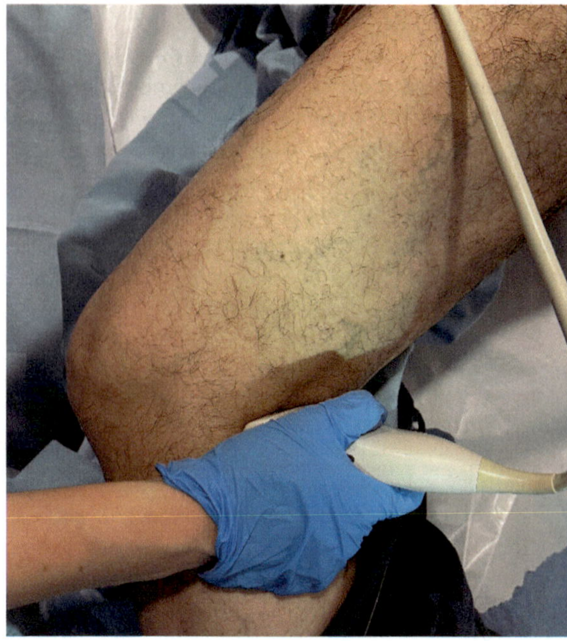

Fig. 3 Photograph demonstrating appropriate patient positioning for the popliteal area evaluation, with the examined leg externally rotated and the knee flexed. Alternatively, lateral decubitus or prone position may be utilized

(with the examined leg up), or prone position, may be utilized to visualize the popliteal vein, peroneal and proximal posterior tibial veins.

Imaging—On the US screen, in axial images, vessels generally appear as a well-defined, oval, anechoic (black) structure and can be followed cranially and caudally. In a longitudinal image it may be defined as a linear structure–vessel. Apart from anatomical knowledge, arteries can be differentiated from veins by typically having a thicker wall, rounder shape, and are pulsatile.

3 Exam Protocol

Despite protocol differences all protocols support the use of compression technique i.e. applying light pressure on the examined vessel, confirming its compressibility. Healthy veins are normally fully compressible under light pressure while arteries and acute thrombotic veins are not. Failure to fully compress the venous lumen is the hallmark for the diagnosis of acute DVT even if the thrombi is not visualized or flow is detected while using color Doppler [5].

Complete duplex ultrasound (CDUS) is the preferred venous ultrasound test for the diagnosis of acute DVT. CDUS is compression of the deep veins from the inguinal ligament to the ankle (including posterior tibial and peroneal veins in the calf), performed at 2 cm intervals. Usually only the symptomatic leg is examined,

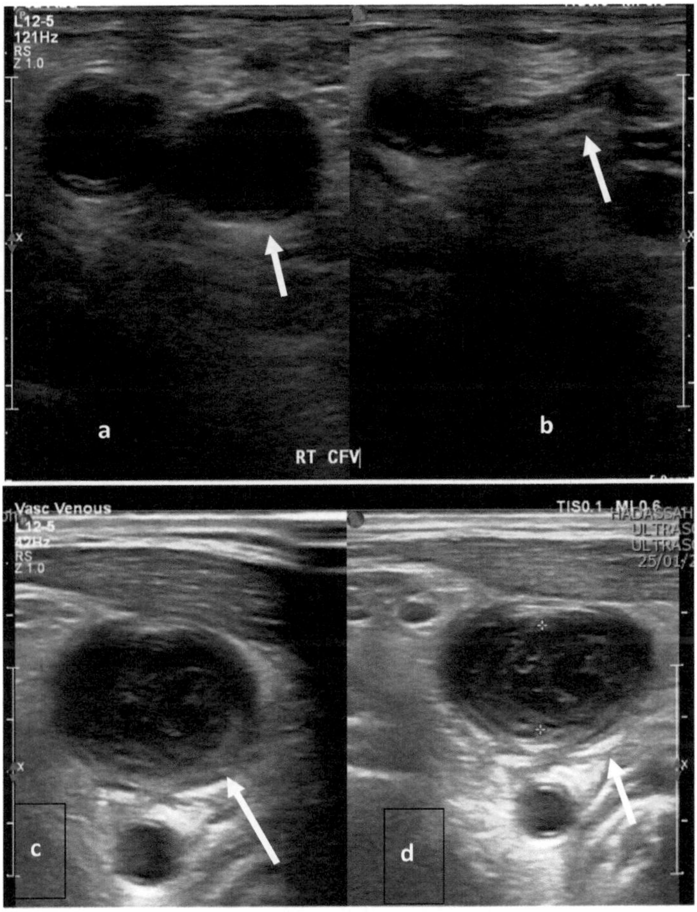

Fig. 4 Normal femoral vein, without (**a**) and with (**b**) normal compression, and acute DVT of the popliteal vein, without (**c**) and with (**d**) compression. The artery is seen next to the vein, with a thicker wall. After compression, the normal vein is completely collapsed, indicating normal compressibility. **c** and **d**, Ultrasound images of acute popliteal vein thrombus without (**c**) and with (**d**) compression. The acute DVT is heterogeneous. It expands the vein. After compression (**d**), the vein does not collapse but has an oval shape indicating an acute DVT based on the noncompressible but deformable vein

but the CFV is an exception and should be examined bilaterally [5]. Figure 4, outlines the normal femoral vein, with and without compression (Fig. 4 a and b respectively), and figures Fig. 4c and d demonstrate acute popliteal vein thrombosis.

Sliding along the CFV the operator should recognize the GSV branch and examine at least its proximal part, as demonstrated in Fig. 5.

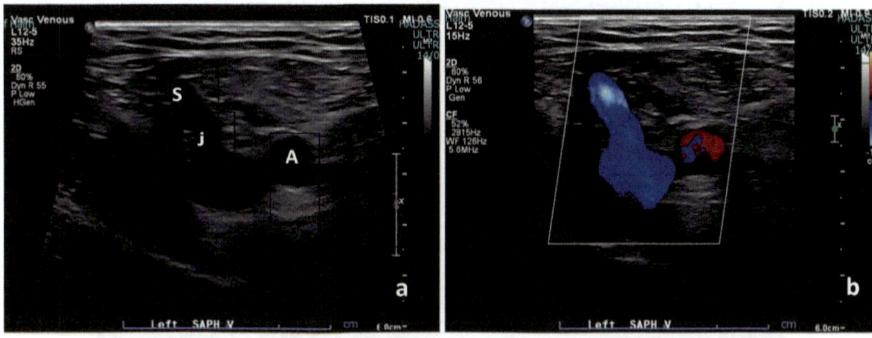

Fig. 5 Ultrasound image visualizing the femoral artery and the saphenous and common femoral vein junction

In the next step, the operator should move caudally along the CFV identifying lateral perforator veins and follow the CFV till it divides to the FV and DFV (note that typically the CFA divides before the CFV). The operator should than follow and examine the FV to the distal thigh where it enters the adductor canal and cannot be further followed. The operator should then, place the transducer within the popliteal fossa and examine the PV (note that typically the PV is superficial or lateral to the PA). The PV should be followed caudally to the trifurcation of the PV into the Anterior and Posterior Tibial Veins and the Peroneal vein. Finally, the operator should examine the Posterior Tibial and the Peroneal vein as well as the main branches—the calf muscles veins to their tiniest part.

Color and Spectral Doppler—Color Doppler ultrasound can detect complete versus incomplete obstruction. It may also help identify smaller and pelvic veins, in particular if augmentation is used [8].

Spectral waveform assessment is performed in the long axis at least in two points—for the CFV bilaterally, and for the popliteal vein. It is not required to angle correct unless measuring velocities. If angle correction is utilized, 45–60° angles must be maintained and aligned with the vessel wall. The normal waveform varies with respiration and during the cardiac cycle. Spectral Doppler abnormalities can be used to identify obstruction in the vein segments central to the sample site. Spectral Doppler assessment of both common femoral or external iliac veins for phasicity and symmetry may yield important information [9]. Figure 6, outlines normal popliteal vein waveform.

An abnormal spectrum, particularly a flat (continuous) waveform, has good specificity for iliocaval venous obstruction that may be the result of central thrombosis, scarring, or extrinsic compression from pelvic pathology. Routine spectral Doppler distal augmentation is not necessary to diagnose DVT [10].

Symptomatic areas in the examined leg, such as points of local pain, redness, or palpable string-like structures, should be evaluated to determine if there is superficial venous thrombosis or other pathology, in particular if the assessment of the

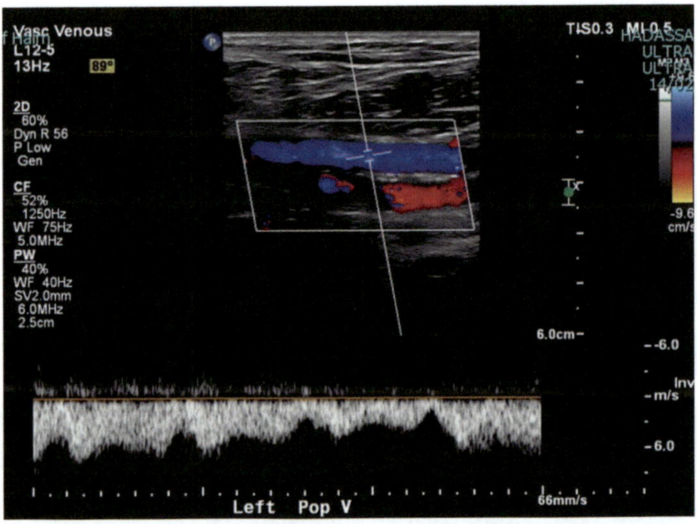

Fig. 6 Normal popliteal vein waveforms. Long-axis spectral Doppler images of the popliteal vein, showing a normal waveform which varies with respiration and during the cardiac cycle flowing toward the heart (away from the transducer, below the baseline)

deep veins is normal. Figure 7, demonstrates a focal swollen sensitive red area in the inner anterior mid-calf (7a), with the ultrasound images showing a tubular tortious structure with echogenic content, no compressibility and no flow in color doppler.

Point-Of-Care-Ultrasound (POCUS)—Point-Of-Care-Ultrasound (POCUS), is routinely practiced today all over the world. DVT diagnosis has become part of the POCUS arsenal, and under some circumstances, (for example—in centers where the ultrasound lab does not give 24/7 service to the emergency department, in rural areas, etc.) it is the best solution and should be performed by a competent practitioner. It has certain drawbacks, which include the use of a limited protocol, a different ultrasound scanner than the high-end premium scanner used usually in the ultrasound unit, and often is used by less experienced operators.

Most of the devices used for POCUS lack the ability to perform duplex (both spectral and color Doppler images). They are often equipped with a limited number of transducers, and in some circumstances such as thick-edematous leg, the study becomes very limited. The limited protocol used usually in POCUS—a limited compression test (encompassing only upper part of the leg) is often not enough, and has a relatively high false-negative rate [11, 12]. Thus, a second study 5–7 days following the initial one should be performed to safely exclude DVT.

In regard to operator experience, several studies have demonstrated that training emergency physicians, to perform Extended compression ultrasound (ECUS) is possible [11]. The extent of required training, has not been defined yet. Even though many studies show good competency after a short, focused course, others

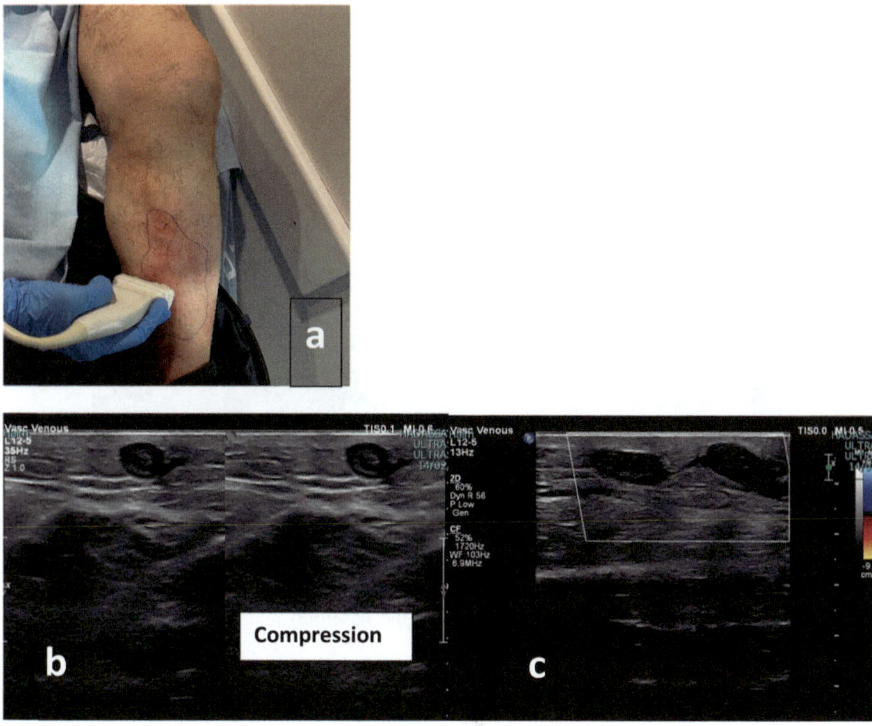

Fig. 7 Symptomatic area—(**a**) a red, warm and sensitive area, with a string-like palpable finding. Incompressible, varicose, peripheral vein with internal echoes (**b**) and no flow (**c**)

show a large discrepancy between the ED physicians and the "gold-standard" Radiology Ultrasound [12]. In a study by Zitek [12], among 260 cases who were deemed to be negative for DVT by ultrasound performed in the Radiology Department, 10 were falsely thought to be positive by ED residents using two-point compression. Overall, the Emergency Department (ED) residents had a sensitivity of 57.1% (95% [CI 38.8–75.5]) and a specificity of 96.1% (95% CI [93.8–98.5]) for identification of proximal lower extremity DVT.

4 Pitfalls and Mimickers

The main pitfall when performing a DVT study is failing to identify the correct vessels. It is important to identify that both the artery and the vein are running together to ensure the correct location. In overweight patients, or patients with edematous legs, the relatively shallow depth of the high-frequency probe may be inadequate limiting the ability to obtain adequate images.

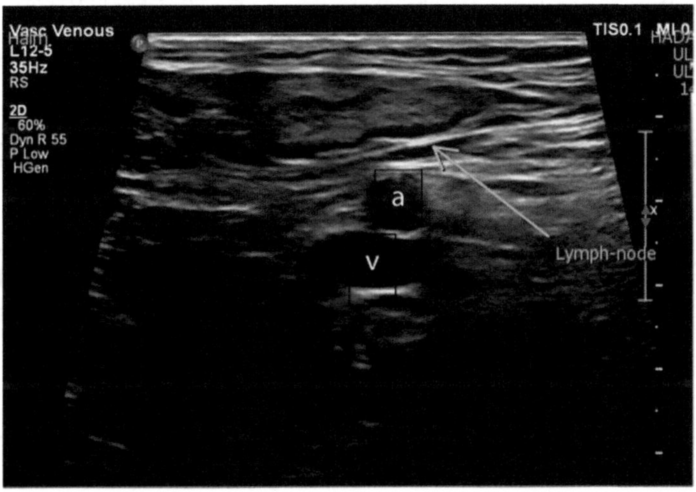

Fig. 8 Ultrasound imaging of the groin, demonstrating the appearance of a lymph node, which can sometimes be mistaken as a thrombus, by less experienced operators

Another problem which may be encountered is misdiagnosing another anatomical structure, such as lymph-nodes in the femoral region (a common mimicker, demonstrated at Fig. 8) or a Baker's cyst in the popliteal fossa, confusing them with a thrombosed vein. An attempt to follow the structure will reveal the boundaries of either one rather than an elongated vessel.

Operator should keep in mind that a non-compressible vein can result from technical matters rather than DVT. A lack of firm compression, an obese patient or edematous limb may all lead to such misdiagnosis.

References

1. Kearon C, Akl EA, Ornelas J, Blaivas A, Jimenez D, Bounameaux H, et al. Antithrombotic therapy for VTE disease: CHEST guideline and expert panel report. Chest. 2016;149(2):315–52.
2. Katz DS, Hon M. Current DVT imaging. Tech Vasc Interv Radiol. 2004;7(2):55–62.
3. Williams MT, Aravindan N, Wallace MJ, Riedel BJCJ, Shaw ADS. Venous thromboembolism in the intensive care unit. Crit Care Clin. 2003;19(2):185–207.
4. Büller HR, Agnelli G, Hull RD, Hyers TM, Prins MH, Raskob GE. Antithrombotic therapy for venous thromboembolic disease: the Seventh ACCP Conference on Antithrombotic and Thrombolytic Therapy. Chest. 2004;126(3 Suppl):401S–28S.
5. Needleman L, Cronan JJ, Lilly MP, Merli GJ, Adhikari S, Hertzberg BS, et al. Ultrasound for lower extremity deep venous thrombosis: Multidisciplinary recommendations from the society of radiologists in ultrasound consensus conference. Circulation. 2018;137(14):1505–15.
6. Schellong SM. Distal DVT: worth diagnosing? Yes. J Thromb Haemost. 2007;5(Suppl 1):51–4.
7. Henry JC, Satiani B. Calf muscle venous thrombosis: a review of the clinical implications and therapy. Vasc Endovascular Surg. 2014;48(5–6):396–401.

8. AIUM Practice Parameter for the Performance of a Peripheral Venous Ultrasound Examination. J ultrasound Med Off J Am Inst Ultrasound Med. 2020;39(5):E49–56.
9. Lin EP, Bhatt S, Rubens D, Dogra VS. The importance of monophasic Doppler waveforms in the common femoral vein: a retrospective study. J ultrasound Med Off J Am Inst Ultrasound Med. 2007;26(7):885–91.
10. Lockhart ME, Sheldon HI, Robbin ML. Augmentation in lower extremity sonography for the detection of deep venous thrombosis. AJR Am J Roentgenol. 2005;184(2):419–22.
11. Situ-LaCasse E, Guirguis H, Friedman L, Patanwala AE, Cohen SE, Adhikari S. Can emergency physicians perform extended compression ultrasound for the diagnosis of lower extremity deep vein thrombosis? World J Emerg Med. 2019;10(4):205–9.
12. Zitek T, Baydoun J, Yepez S, Forred W, Slattery DE. Mistakes and pitfalls associated with two-point compression ultrasound for deep vein thrombosis. West J Emerg Med. 2016;17(2):201–8.

Imaging Modalities in Acute Pulmonary Embolism: Computerized Tomography

Dotan Cohen and Dorith Shaham

1 Introduction

Computerized tomography pulmonary angiography (CTPA) is currently the imaging modality of choice for the workup of suspected acute pulmonary embolism (PE). The PIOPEDII trial has reported CTPA sensitivity and specificity for the diagnosis of PE of 83% and 96% respectively, positive predictive values of 96% for high or low clinical probabilities and 92% for intermediate clinical probability, based mainly on 4-detector CT machines [1]. At approximately the same time the clinical validity of using CTPA to rule-out PE was shown to be similar to that reported for conventional pulmonary angiography, with a negative predictive value of 99% [2]. In the following years CT technology has greatly advanced with faster acquisitions, higher spatial resolution, better image reconstruction algorithms and the advent of dual energy CT and artificial intelligence algorithms for automatic PE detection and timely diagnosis. Hence, a recent meta-analysis of CT accuracy for the diagnosis of PE reported pooled estimates for CTPA sensitivity and specificity of 94 and 98% respectively [3].

After intra-venous injection of iodinated contrast medium, CTPA enables direct visualization of pulmonary arteries lumen and of possible emboli. CTPA can readily assess emboli load and signs of right pressure overload. CT is an excellent imaging modality of pulmonary parenchyma, and can clearly demonstrate parenchymal effects of PE (i.e. pulmonary infarcts, hemorrhage and perfusion defects).

Furthermore, CT can detect many of the alternative diagnoses of PE, namely pneumonia, thoracic neoplasm, pneumothorax, aortic dissection/intra-mural hematoma and acute coronary syndrome. When clinically indicated, lower limb

D. Cohen (✉) · D. Shaham
Department of Radiology, Hadassah Medical Center and Faculty of Medicine, Hebrew University of Jerusalem, Jerusalem, Israel

E. Herzog (ed.), *Pulmonary Embolism*,
https://doi.org/10.1007/978-3-030-87090-4_6

CT venography may be performed with no additional contrast injection to assess deep vein thrombosis. Thus, CT may be used as an “all-in-one” test in the setting of suspected acute PE.

2 CTPA Protocol and Technical Considerations

Although the exact CTPA protocol may vary depending on scanner capabilities and patient parameters, several basic concepts can be recognized for performing a good quality CTPA.

Dense opacification of the pulmonary arteries is paramount for high diagnostic accuracy while avoiding artifacts and other factors leading to image degradation.

The minimal pulmonary arteries density required to distinguish thrombus from intra-luminal contrast material has been estimated at 93 Hounsfield units (HU) for acute PE and 211 HU for chronic PE [4]; However, common clinical experience shows 250 HU measured in the main pulmonary artery to be adequate for the detection of pulmonary emboli [5, 6, 9].

Dense opacification of the pulmonary arteries, or in other words peak contrast enhancement (PCE), mainly depends on contrast material delivery rate and volume, scan timing, peak tube potential and patient parameters [7, 8].

A. **Contrast material delivery rate**
   Contrast material is delivered via automatic injector, enabling rapid, yet safe and accurate, contrast material administration. A minimum of 20-gauge venous access is required, preferably antecubital [8].
   Contrast material delivery rate is the product of contrast concentration and infusion rate, both are directly proportional to PCE [7–9]. Hence, high concentrations of contrast material (e.g. 350–400 mg iodine/mL) seem to be beneficial, and high injection rates, at least 3–4 mL/s, are required [9]. An adequate iodine delivery rate is typically greater than 1.2–1.3 g/s [17].
B. **Contrast material volume**
   Contrast material volume is directly proportional to PCE [7]. Ideally contrast material should be adjusted to patient parameters such as weight and renal function and to scan duration [5, 15]. Practically many centers use a constant contrast material volume for most patients, that can range between 40 mL in new generation ultra-fast MDCT to 150 mL in older 4–16 slice scanners [9, 17, 18].
C. **Saline bolus chaser**
   The use of saline bolus chaser is recommended immediately following contrast material injection. The benefit of bolus chaser is threefold—it reduces the amount of dense contrast material within the superior vena cava and brachiocephalic veins which can cause artifacts and degrade arterial enhancement, it reduces the total volume of contrast material required to achieve the same

enhancement of the pulmonary arteries and it prolongs contrast enhancement plateau [7, 8].

D. **Peak tube potential**

Peak tube potential (kVp) is inversely proportional to PCE—lower kVp is closer to the k-absorption edge of iodine (33.2 keV), resulting in higher enhancement. Therefore, a 100 kVp scan, or even an 80kVp scan in certain scenarios, are usually preferred over a 120 kVp scan [9]. Dual energy CT scanners use this same principle to obtain images with ultra-low kVp ($\sim$50–80 kVp) and thus achieve excellent contrast enhancement as further discussed below.

E. **Scan timing**

Accurate scan timing is critical, as PCE is achieved during the first-pass of contrast material and is only a few seconds long. Although a second PCE appears in the recirculation phase of contrast material, it is not as high as the first PCE and usually not high enough for a diagnostic CTPA on standard CT machines. The use of dual energy CT, however, may achieve high enough PCE in the recirculation phase as has been recently reported [10].

Ideal scan acquisition timing is achieved by one of two methods—bolus tracking or test bolus. Both of these methods use the same principle of monitoring contrast enhancement in the main pulmonary artery during the administration of contrast material and prior to CTPA acquisition. A region of interest (ROI) is drawn on the main pulmonary artery, and a single slice, low-dose scan is initiated a few seconds after the start of contrast material injection and repeated in certain time intervals (e.g. every second). In the bolus tracking method, as contrast enhancement in the ROI crosses a predetermined threshold, CTPA acquisition begins (after an additional few seconds delay called the "post-threshold delay"). In the test bolus method, a small amount of contrast material (around 10–15 mL) is injected prior to the actual scan and time to peak enhancement is measured over the ROI. This time is subsequently used to initiate the CTPA scan at exactly the correct timing post injection of the full amount of contrast material.

F. **Patient parameters**

Patient habitus and cardiovascular dynamics affect contrast material bolus geometry and therefore may influence PCE as well [8].

Cardiac output is inversely proportional to PCE. High cardiac output, as during pregnancy, reduces contrast enhancement by increasing contrast material dilution [11]. Inversely, heart failure may result in increased PCE [7, 8].

The effect of body habitus on image quality is twofold—body weight has been shown to have negative correlation with PCE [5], likely due to contrast material dilution by increased blood volume and cardiac output in larger patients. In addition, increased body weight leads to higher image noise if radiation dose is not appropriately adjusted. In order to avoid these effects, several protocol modifications can be applied when scanning larger patients—higher contrast material volume and/or concentration, higher injection rates and increased

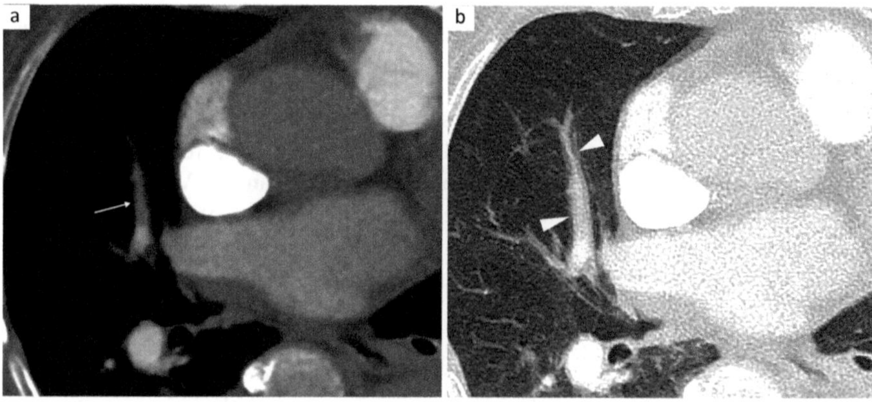

Fig. 1 Respiratory motion artifacts. **a** CTPA axial image shows a hypodense region in the medial segmental artery of the right middle lobe (arrow) mimicking PE. **b** Same image in lung window shows blurring of the vessel and duplication of its walls (arrowheads) indicating the hypodensity is likely related to respiratory motion rather than a pulmonary embolus

radiation dose. Several commonly used technological advents allow improving image quality while minimizing radiation dose increase, including certain image reconstruction algorithms and auto-modulation of radiation dose according to patient body habitus.

G. **Protocol considerations for reduction of scan artifacts**

Several types of artifacts may degrade image quality. Respiratory motion artifacts are perhaps the most frequent type to cause indeterminate CTPA [6] (Fig. 1) and can be reduced by fast gantry rotation time, oxygen supplement for dyspneic patients and scanning in caudal-cranial direction [9]—scanning lower lung regions earlier can potentially reduce respiratory artifacts in these regions where emboli are more frequent.

Another common artifact is transient contrast interruption. This physiological phenomenon occurs as a result of a patient's deep inspiration prior to breath-holding. The drop in thoracic pressure causes non-enhanced blood from the inferior vena cava (IVC) to flux into the right atrium and pulmonary arteries and dilute contrast material. The following Valsalva during breath holding increases intra-thoracic pressure, and reduces the flow of contrast material into the right atrium and pulmonary arteries. The combined effect may create areas with interrupted contrast material that may either mimic or obscure PE. Guiding patients for shallow, instead of deep, inspiratory breath-hold ("small breath in and hold"), or for expiratory breath-hold, has been shown to reduce this phenomenon [9, 12]. High pitch CT—a very fast scan, during shallow free breathing may also be used in dyspneic patients, reducing both breathing artifacts and contrast interruption [13].

Streak or beam-hardening artifacts are potentially caused by dense contrast material in the superior vena cava and brachiocephalic veins (Fig. 2). This

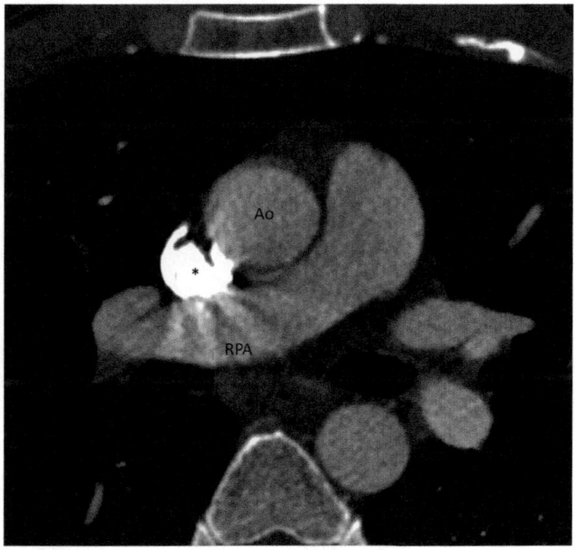

Fig. 2 Streak artifacts. CTPA axial image with dense contrast material within the superior vena cava (asterisk) causing typical appearance of streak artifacts, characterized by radiating non-anatomical bright and dark streaks, overlying the right pulmonary artery (RPA) and to lesser extent the ascending aorta (Ao)

artifact may be reduced by using saline bolus chaser as mentioned above. Streak artifacts may also be caused by metallic objects outside or within the patient's body (e.g. metallic implants, central catheters or a pacemaker).

Transmitted motion artifacts from cardiac pulsation occasionally limit assessment of peripheral pulmonary arteries in the lingula and right middle lobe. ECG gated CTPA has been shown to reduce these artifacts and improve image quality [14, 16]; However, no significant effect on diagnostic accuracy has been shown to justify the increased radiation dose [16, 17]. Therefore, this technique is usually reserved for cases in which coronary arteries and/or aortic pathologies are being considered as well ("triple-rule-out" protocol).

3 Normal Appearance and Anatomy of Pulmonary arteries on CTPA

CTPA enables exquisite demonstration of pulmonary arterial vasculature as well as surrounding structures. Imaging data is first acquired as thin axial images that can be subsequently reconstructed in various planes, and can be used to generate detailed 3 dimensional reconstructions. The following Figs. 3, 4, 5, 6, 7, 8, 9, 10, 11, 12, 13, and 14 depict normal pulmonary arteries appearance on CTPA, and demonstrate a few possible reconstructions. It should be noted that although the anatomy of the central pulmonary arterial vasculature is fairly constant, the course and branching patterns of the more peripheral lobar and certainly segmental branches are more variable.

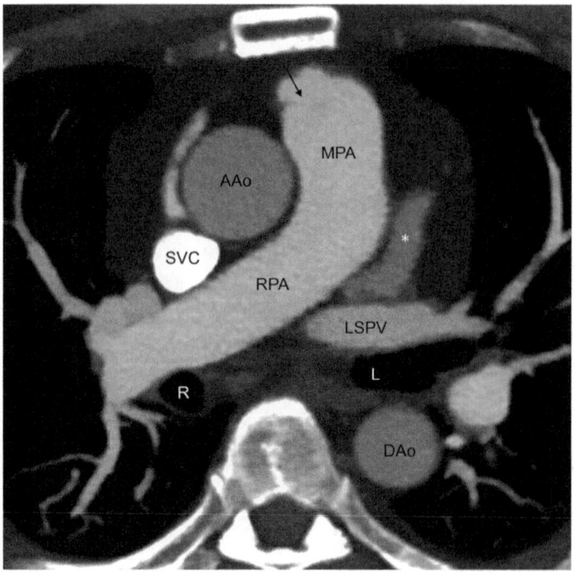

Fig. 3 Main pulmonary artery (MPA) origin. CTPA axial maximal intensity projection (MIP) image at the level of the MPA origin from the right ventricle. The pulmonary valve is partially seen (arrow). The MPA curves to the right giving rise to the right pulmonary artery (RPA), which courses anterior to the right main bronchus (R). The left pulmonary artery which takes a more cranial course (arching above the left main bronchus) is not included in this slice. Also seen are the left main bronchus (L), the ascending and descending aorta (AAo and DAo respectively), dense contrast material within the superior vena cava (SVC), the left superior pulmonary vein (LSPV) and the left atrial appendage (asterisk)

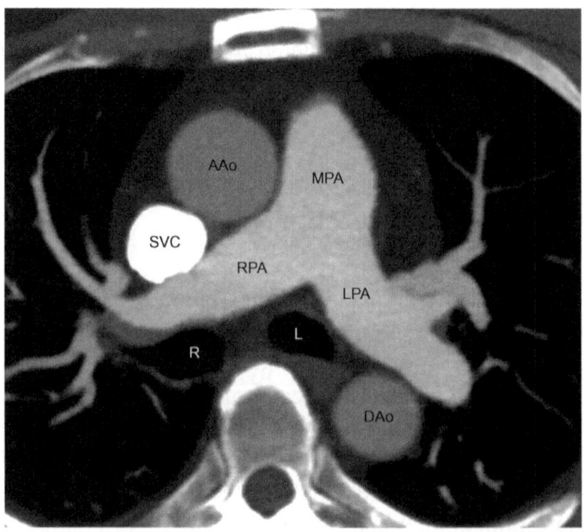

Fig. 4 Main pulmonary arteries. Axial CTPA MIP image at a slightly more cranial level than Fig. 3, showing the main pulmonary artery (MPA) and its bifurcation into the right pulmonary artery (RPA) and the left pulmonary artery (LPA). Also shown are the right and left main bronchi (R, L respectively), the ascending and descending aorta (AAo and DAo respectively) and dense contrast material within the superior vena cava (SVC)

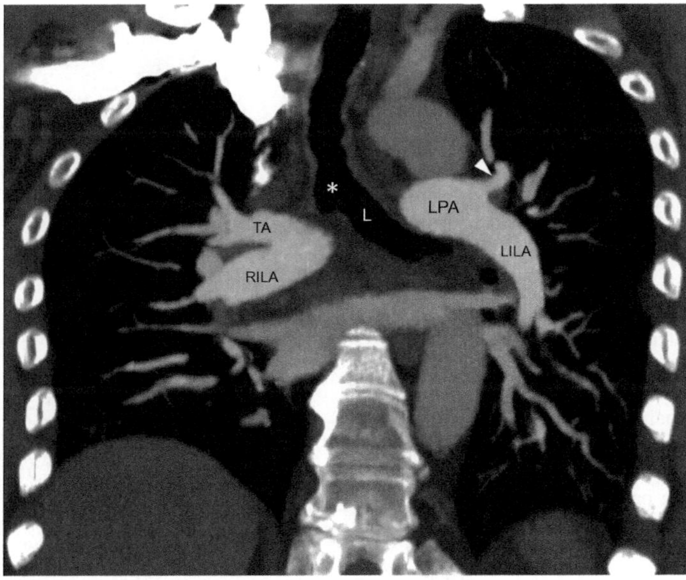

Fig. 5 Right and left pulmonary arteries and inter-lobar branches. CTPA oblique coronal MIP image demonstrates the higher position of the left pulmonary artery (LPA) compared to the right, arching above the left main bronchus (L) which is seen extending from the carina (asterisk). In this case, the LPA gives a short ascending branch (arrowhead) that subsequently branches into segmental arteries to the left upper lobe (not seen here), after which the left pulmonary artery is named the left inter-lobar artery (LILA) taking a vertical course to supply part of the upper lobe and the whole left lower lobe. On the right, the bifurcation of the right pulmonary artery is seen, giving an ascending branch—the truncus anterior (TA) which supplies the right upper lobe, and a descending branch—the right inter-lobar artery (RILA), which subsequently branches into the right middle and right lower lobar arteries (not seen here)

4 CTPA Findings in Acute PE

A. **Vascular findings**

CTPA enables direct visualization of pulmonary emboli. The low density emboli, on the background of high density, contrast enhanced, vessels cause partial or complete endoluminal filling defects, having a sharp interface with the intra-venous contrast. Emboli that fill the vessel lumen cause complete endoluminal filling defects and may enlarge the vessel compared to adjacent patent vessels (Fig. 15). Partial endoluminal filling defects caused by acute PE are typically central, with surrounding peripheral contrast enhancement of the vessel lumen creating the "polo mint" sign when viewed perpendicular to the long axis of the vessel (Fig. 16) and the "railway track" sign when viewed in

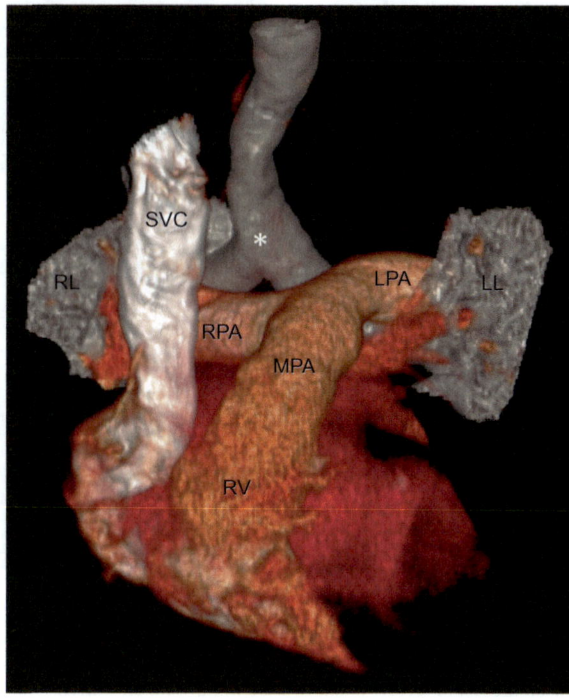

Fig. 6 CTPA 3D reconstruction (volume rendering) of the main pulmonary arteries and surrounding structures. The main pulmonary artery (MPA) originates from the right ventricle (RV), and bifurcates into the left pulmonary artery (LPA) which arches above the left main bronchus (carina marked in asterisk), and into the right pulmonary artery (RPA) which courses anterior to the right main bronchus and bifurcates behind the superior vena cava (SVC). Peri-hilar lung parenchyma is also seen bilaterally (RL, LL)

the long axis (Fig. 17). Less frequently, acute PE may be seen as an eccentric endoluminal filling defect, causing an acute angle with the vessel wall (in contrast to chronic thromboembolism having an obtuse angle with the vessel wall). An embolus caught at the branching of a pulmonary artery creates the saddle appearance (Fig. 18).

B. **Parenchymal findings**
Although most PE positive CTPA studies have been shown to contain at least one pleural or parenchymal abnormal finding, the only two parenchymal findings significantly associated with PE are wedge shaped opacities and parenchymal bands [19, 20]. A wedge shaped opacity, representing a pulmonary infarct (with or without parenchymal haemorrhage) is a roughly triangular area of increased attenuation (consolidation and/or ground-glass opacity) with a broad base abutting a pleural surface, and an apex pointing toward the para-hilar region (Fig. 19), correlating to the characteristic Hampton's hump sign on chest X-Rays. These opacities have a lower lobe predominance, occasionally creating a "reverse halo sign" or "atoll sign" on CT, in which a ground-glass opacity is surrounded by a rim of denser consolidation. The reported prevalence of a wedge shaped opacity in positive CTPA studies varies between 25 and 62% [19, 20]. Although associated with PE, wedge shaped opacities are not specific and may appear in other pathologies such as pneumonia, neoplasm, fibrosis, hemorrhage and pulmonary edema [20].

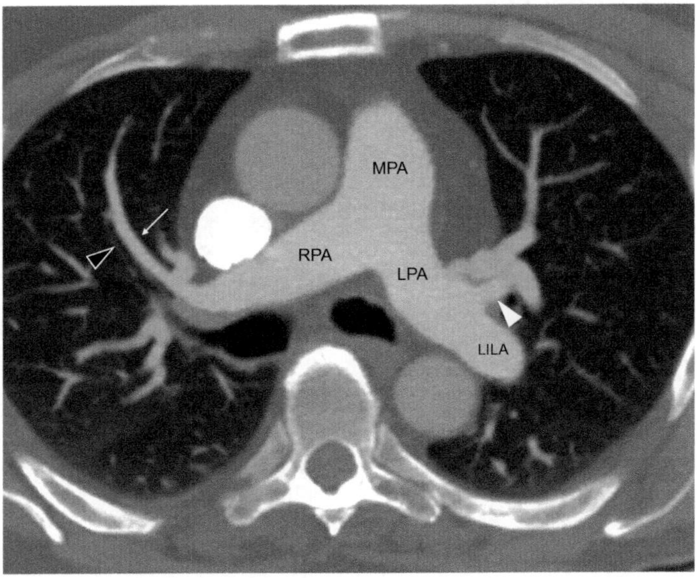

Fig. 7 Anterior segmental artery of the right upper lobe. CTPA axial MIP image shows the segmental artery supplying the anterior segment of the right upper lobe (white arrow). The accompanying segmental bronchus can be noted (black arrowhead). Also seen here are the main pulmonary artery (MPA), right and left pulmonary arteries (RPA and LPA respectively), the branching off of an ascending branch from the LPA (white arrowhead) as seen on Fig. 5 as well and the proximal part of the left inter-lobar artery (LILA)

Parenchymal bands are linear high attenuation opacities usually 1–3 mm thick that usually extend to the visceral pleura (Fig. 20). Parenchymal bands are non-specific for PE as well, and may appear in many pathologies associated with fibrosis or atelectasis.

5 Predictors of PE Severity and Clinical Outcome

CTPA is usually obtained very early in the management of patients with suspected acute PE. CTPA allows not only direct visualization of pulmonary emboli, but also excellent demonstration of cardiac structures, great vessels and contrast material dynamics. These in turn can be useful for early assessment of PE severity, hemodynamic significance and prognosis. Various CT parameters have been suggested as such predictors. Most clinically relevant are those assessing right ventricular dysfunction (RVD) and strain, enabling early risk stratification.

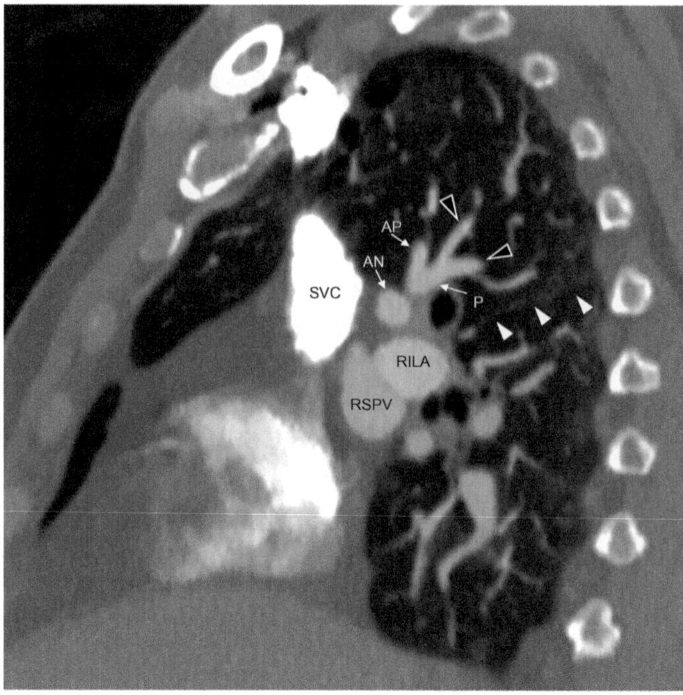

Fig. 8 Segmental arteries of the right upper lobe. CTPA sagittal reconstruction demonstrates the three segmental arteries of the right upper lobe close to their origin: AN—anterior segmental artery, AP—apical segmental artery, P—posterior segmental artery and two of its sub-segmental branches (black arrowheads). Also seen are the right inter-lobar artery (RILA) viewed perpendicular to its long axis, the right superior pulmonary vein (RSPV) and dense contrast material within the superior vena cava (SVC). The right major fissure is clearly seen as well (white arrowheads)

A. **RV to LV diameter and volume ratios**

RV:LV diameter ratio has the strongest predictive value and the most robust evidence base, for adverse clinical outcomes in patients with acute PE [21, 22]. RV:LV diameter ratio can be measured either on the original transverse images or on 4-chamber reconstructions, measuring the widest distance between endocardial borders, perpendicular to the long axis of the heart (Figs. 21 and 22). The cutoff point above which the RV is considered enlarged can be set to different values, ranging from 0.9 to 1.2 in various publications. Values of 0.9 on 4-chamber measurements and 1 on transverse plane measurements are most commonly used [22]. Naturally these parameters influence the statistical significance of the association between increased RV:LV diameter ratio and outcome [21]. CTPA derived RV:LV diameter ratio is a highly reproducible parameter [23] with good correlation with ECHO derived RV:LV diameter ratio, both have been shown to identify a similar proportion of subjects with

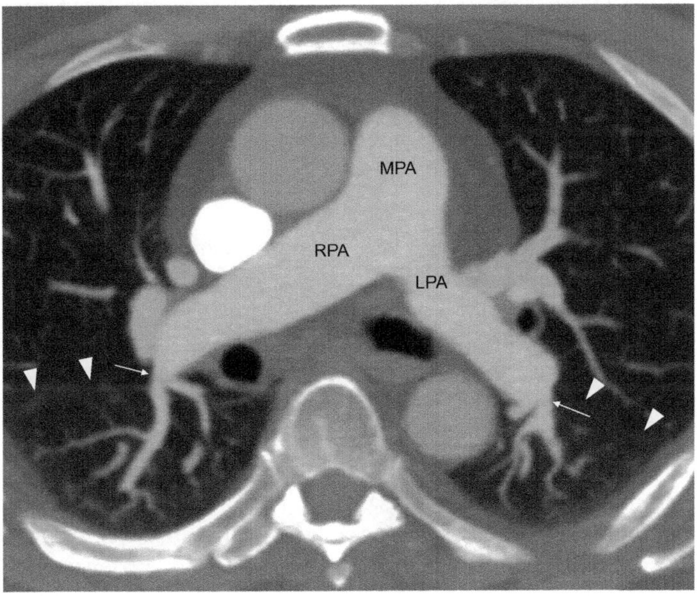

Fig. 9 Superior segmental arteries of the lower lobes. CTPA axial MIP image demonstrates the segmental arteries to the superior segments of both lower lobes (arrows). The bifurcation of the main pulmonary artery (MPA) into right and left pulmonary arteries (RPA, LPA respectively) and the right and left major fissures (arrowheads) can be seen as well

Fig. 10 Right common basal trunk. CTPA sagittal oblique MIP image showing the origin of the superior segmental artery of the right lower lobe (arrow) from the inter-lobar artery (black arrowhead), after which the artery is named the common basal trunk (CBT), which supplies the basal segments of the right lower lobe as its name indicates. The major fissure of the right lung can be seen as well (white arrowheads)

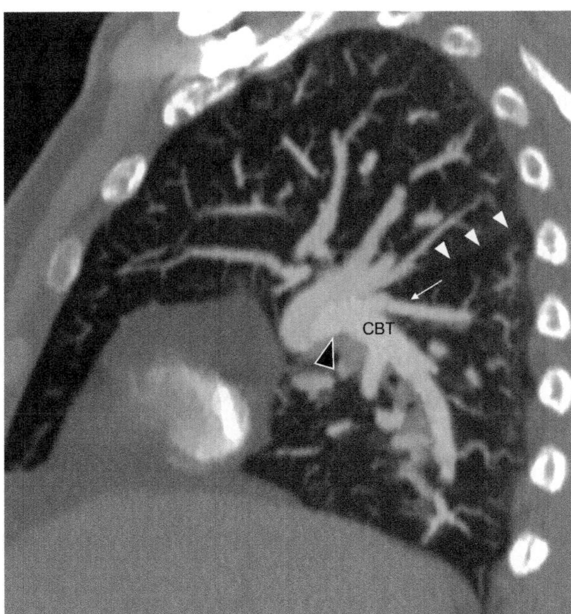

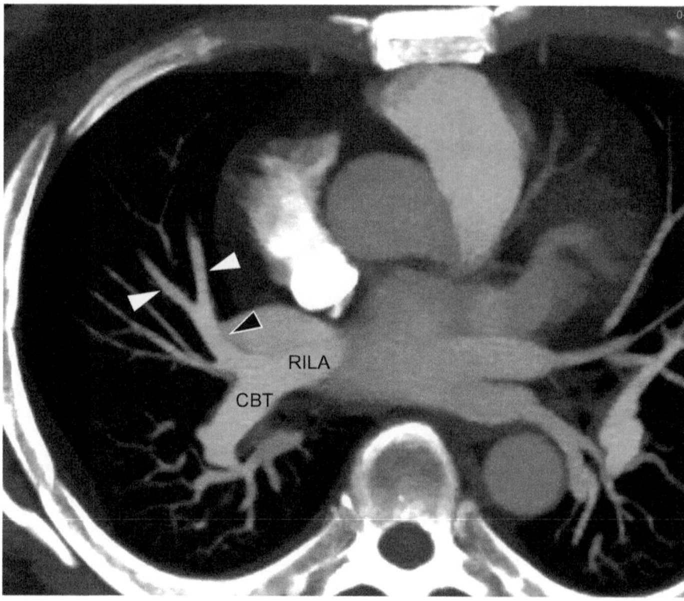

Fig. 11 Right middle lobar and segmental arteries and common basal trunk. CTPA axial MIP image shows the lobar artery to the right middle lobe (black arrowhead) branching off from the right inter-lobar artery (RILA), and more distally its bifurcation into two segmental arteries (white arrowheads) to the medial and lateral segments of the right middle lobe. The common basal trunk (CBT) continues to supply the basal segments of the right lower lobe as seen in Fig. 10 as well

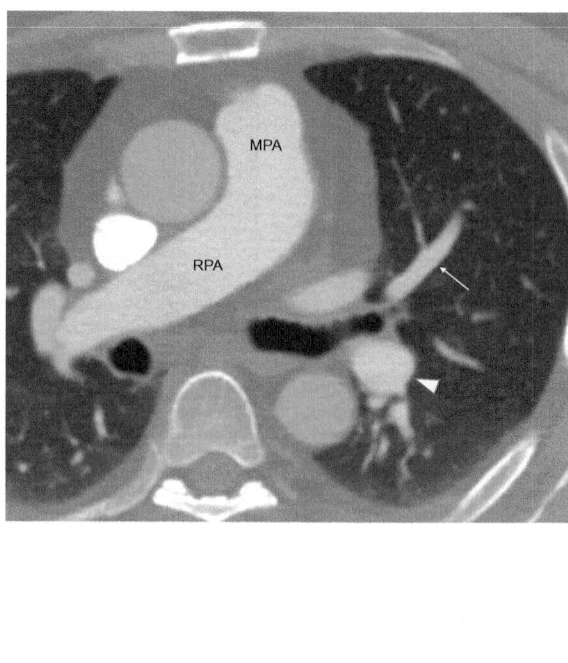

Fig. 12 Lingula artery. CTPA axial MIP image shows the artery to the lingula (arrow) and the lobar artery to the left lower lobe (arrowhead). The main pulmonary artery (MPA) and the right pulmonary artery (RPA) can be seen as well

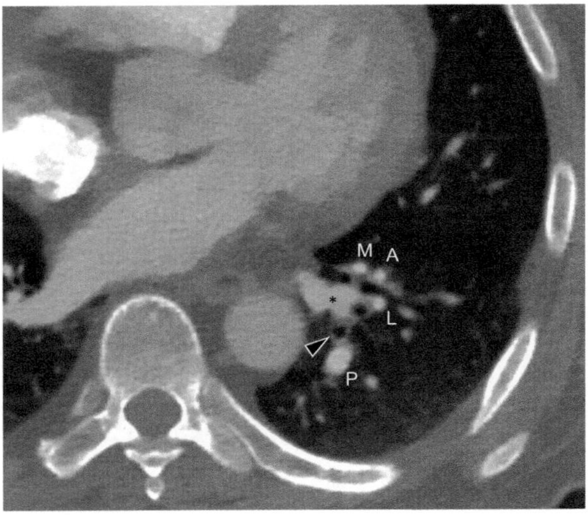

Fig. 13 Basal segmental arteries of the left lower lobe (LLL). CTPA axial image shows four segmental arteries in the basal LLL: P—posterior segmental artery, L—lateral segmental artery, and the medial (M) and anterior (A) segmental arteries that supply the anterior-medial segment. Accompanying segmental bronchi are nicely demonstrated (the arrowhead marks one, the posterior segmental bronchus). The inferior left pulmonary vein (asterisk) is seen as well

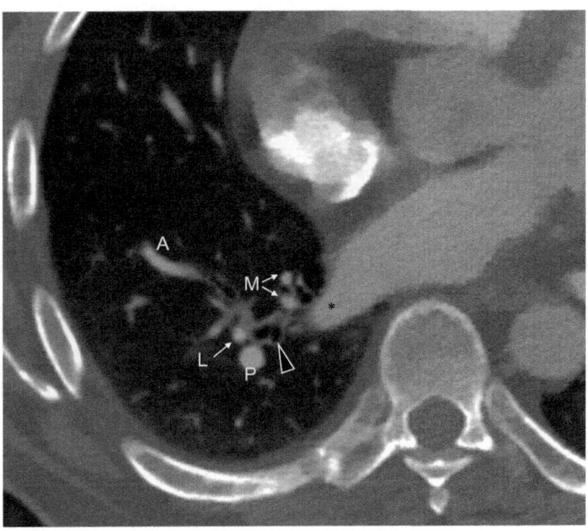

Fig. 14 Basal segmental arteries of the right lower lobe (RLL). CTPA axial image shows three segmental arteries and two sub-segmental arteries in the basal RLL: P—posterior segmental artery, L—lateral segmental artery, A—anterior segmental artery and two sub-segmental branches (M) of the medial segmental artery which has already bifurcated at a more cranial slice. Accompanying segmental bronchi are again clearly seen (the arrowhead marks one, the posterior segmental bronchus). The inferior right pulmonary vein (asterisk) is seen as well

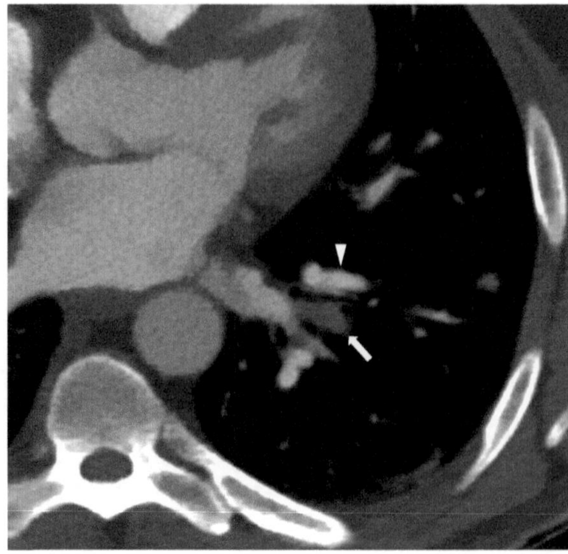

Fig. 15 Complete endoluminal filling defect in segmental PE. Axial CTPA image shows a complete endoluminal filling defect in the lateral segmental artery of the left lower lobe (arrow). The artery is enlarged compared to the adjacent anterior-medial segmental artery which is patent (arrowhead)

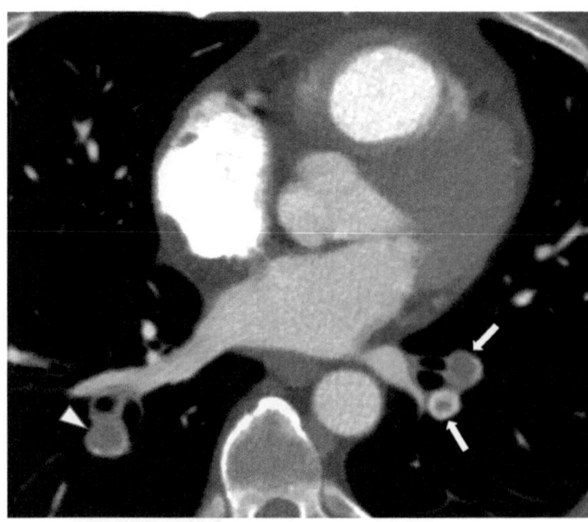

Fig. 16 Partial endoluminal filling defects in bilateral segmental PE. Axial CTPA image shows bilateral partial endoluminal filling defects causing the "polo mint" appearance—in the left lower lobe within a large common artery supplying the anterior-medial and lateral segments and posterior to it in the posterior segmental artery (arrows). In the right lower lobe within a large common artery supplying the posterior and lateral segments (arrowhead)

right ventricular dysfunction [24]. RV:LV volume ratio measurement may be more indicative than diameter ratio for right ventricular dysfunction; However, it is more time consuming and requires a dedicated software [25] (Fig. 23).

B. **Displacement of the interventricular septum**

Displacement of the interventricular septum is another parameter suggestive of RVD and strain. Normally the interventricular septum is convex toward the right ventricle. Straightening of the septum or convexity toward the left ventricle may indicate increased RV pressure (Fig. 22). Several studies have shown

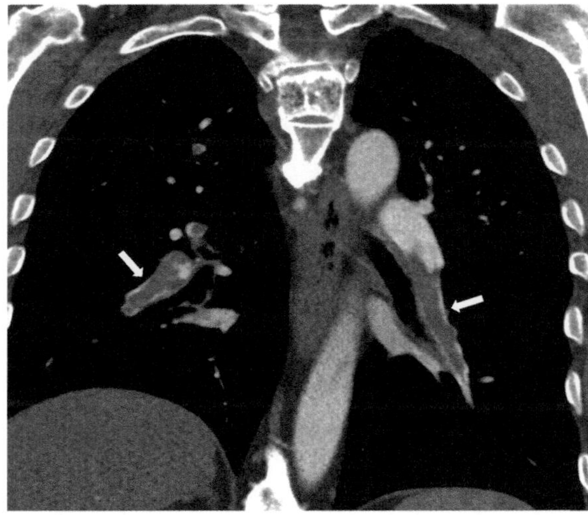

Fig. 17 Railway track sign. Coronal CTPA image demonstrates extensive partial filling defects in pulmonary arteries bilaterally. Partial filling defects seen in the long axis of the vessel give the appearance of "railway tracks" (arrows)

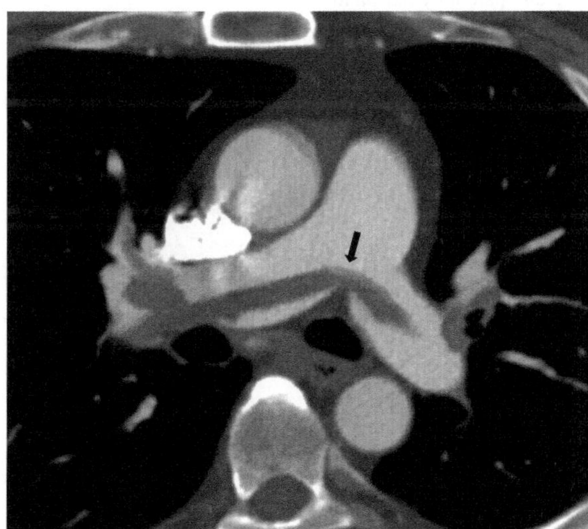

Fig. 18 Saddle pulmonary embolus. Axial CTPA image shows a large filling defect caught at the bifurcation of the main pulmonary artery (arrow) extending into the right and left pulmonary arteries. Additional emboli are seen in this image in the main and lobar pulmonary arteries bilaterally

an association between septal displacement and all-cause mortality, PE related mortality and adverse outcomes [21]. This parameter however was shown to have high inter observer variability [23].

C. **Contrast material reflux**

CTPA is acquired during the first pass of contrast material when recirculation has not yet occurred. Since contrast material is injected through an upper limb vein passing into the superior vena cava, right atrium and right ventricle, the IVC should not contain a significant amount of contrast material at this stage. However, occasionally contrast material is seen to reflux from the right atrium

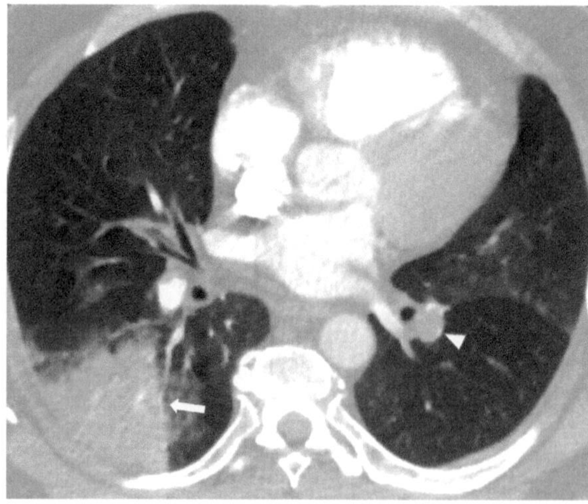

Fig. 19 Pulmonary infarct. Axial CTPA image in lung window shows a wedge shaped consolidation in the superior segment of the right lower lobe (arrow) consistent with a pulmonary infarct. The filling defect in the artery supplying this region is not included in this slice. However, another filling defect can be noted in the lobar artery of the left lower lobe (arrowhead), sub-optimally seen in lung window

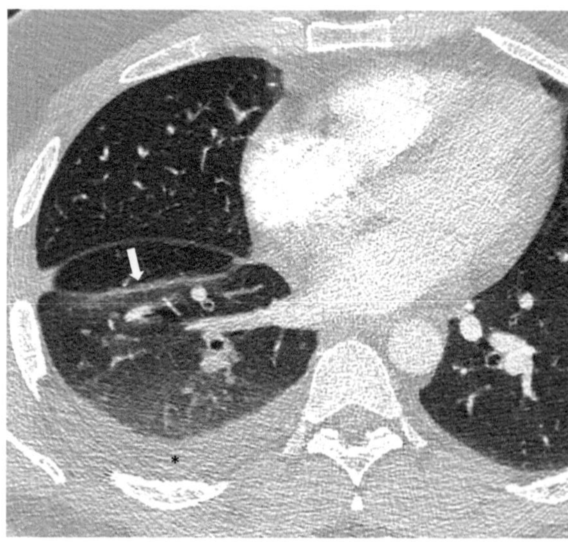

Fig. 20 Parenchymal band. Axial CTPA image in lung window shows a thin linear opacity in the right lower lobe, extending to the visceral pleura (arrow). A small right pleural effusion can also be noted (asterisk)

into the IVC and hepatic veins. The severity of reflux can be graded semi-quantitatively on a scale of 1–6, whereas 1 is no reflux, 3 is significant reflux into the IVC but not into hepatic veins and 6 is reflux into the IVC and up to distal hepatic veins. Contrast material reflux into the IVC may be seen in various cardiac conditions and in pulmonary hypertension [26]. In the context of acute PE, several studies have shown association between significant degrees of contrast material reflux and all-cause mortality and adverse outcomes [21] (Fig. 24).

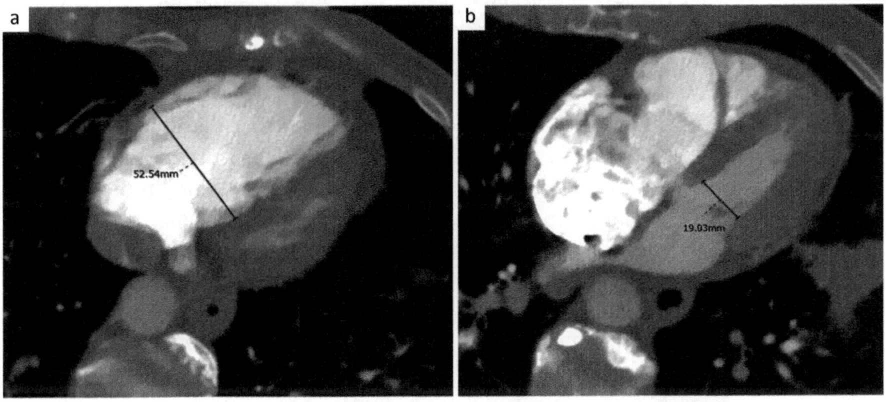

Fig. 21 Increased RV:LV diameter ratio. Axial CTPA images in a patient with extensive bilateral PE (not shown)—(**a**) maximal RV diameter measurement, (**b**) maximal LV diameter measurement. RV:LV diameter ratio is markedly increased at 2.7 in keeping with RV dysfunction

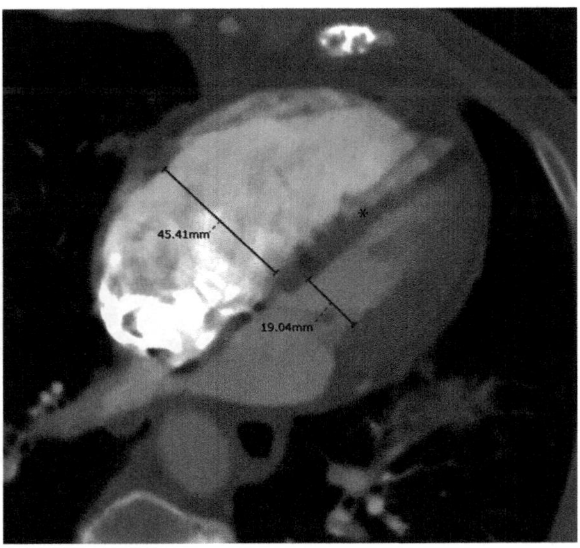

Fig. 22 Increased RV:LV diameter ratio and interventricular septal flattening in a patient with extensive bilateral PE (not shown). Same study as in Fig. 21, here a 4-chamber reconstruction is shown with measurements of maximal RV and LV diameters. RV:LV diameter ratio is markedly increased at 2.3 in keeping with RV dysfunction. Flattening of the interventricular septum (asterisk) indicates RV dysfunction as well

D. **Main pulmonary artery enlargement**

Enlargement of the main pulmonary artery (MPA) may indicate pulmonary hypertension (PHTN) regardless of the etiology. Sensitivity and specificity of this finding for predicting PHTN is related to the method of measurement and the cut-off point used. The two most commonly used methods of measurement are in the transverse diameter—(1) MPA diameter perpendicular to its long axis just proximal to the bifurcation, and (2) ratio between MPA diameter (measured

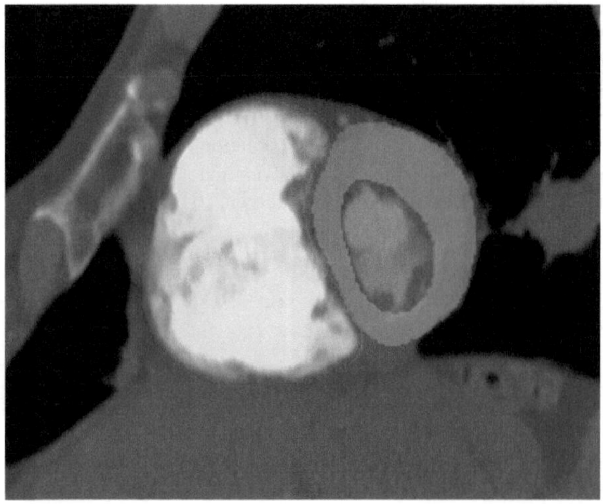

Fig. 23 Increased RV:LV volume ratio. Same study as in Figs. 21 and 22. Here, automated segmentation of cardiac chambers is shown in short axis view, using a dedicated software (Philips Intellispace portal) enabling calculation of cardiac chambers volumes. Calculated RV volume was 132 mL versus 35 mL of LV volume, resulting in a volume ratio of 3.7

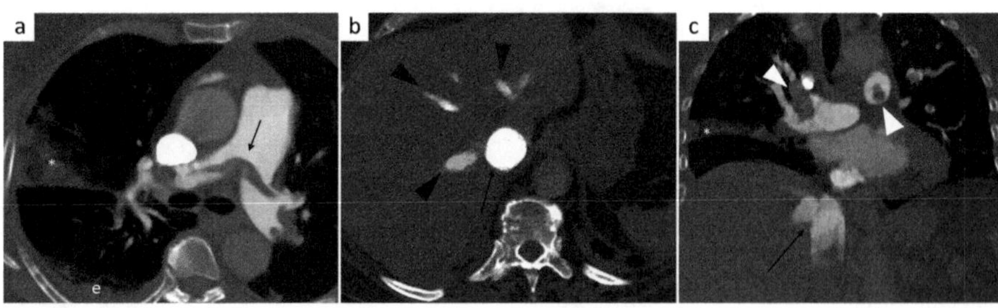

Fig. 24 Significant contrast material reflux into the inferior vena cava (IVC) and hepatic veins in a patient with extensive bilateral PE. **a** CTPA axial image shows a saddle embolus within the main pulmonary artery, extending into the right and left pulmonary arteries. A wedge shaped opacity in the lateral segment of the right middle lobe (RML) (asterisk) consistent with a parenchymal infarct and a small right pleural effusion (e) can also be seen. **b** Axial image from the same study shows significant contrast material reflux into the IVC (black arrow) and hepatic veins (black arrowheads). **c** Coronal reconstruction image from the same study again shows significant contrast material reflux into the IVC (black arrow) and one hepatic vein that is included in this plane. Additionally, several filling defects are seen within the pulmonary arteries (white arrowheads point on a complete filling defect within the trunkus anterior in the right lung and a partial filling defect in the left main pulmonary artery). The RML infarct is again noted (asterisk)

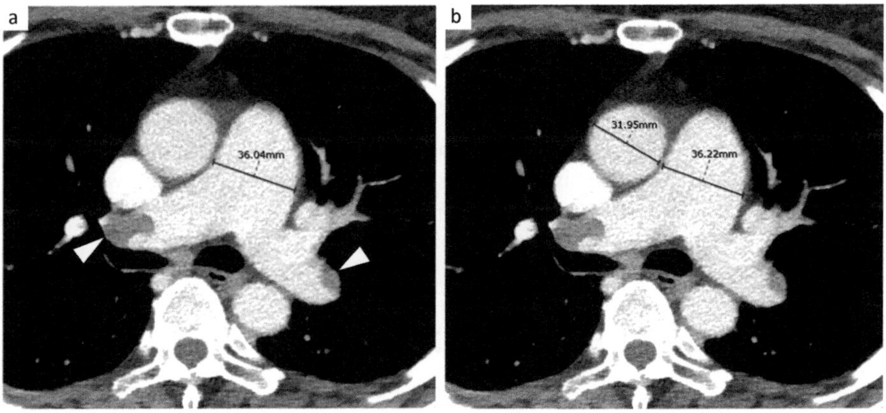

Fig. 25 Main pulmonary artery (MPA) dilatation. Same CTPA axial image in (**a**) and (**b**) demonstrates two methods of measurement. **a** Transverse measurement of the MPA perpendicular to its long axis just proximal to the bifurcation; a diameter greater than 29 mm indicates MPA dilatation. **b** A ratio between the MPA diameter measured as in (**a**) and the ascending aorta diameter measured at the same level. A ratio above 0.9 or 1 indicates MPA dilatation. Here a ratio of 1.13 was calculated. Pulmonary emboli can be noted in the right pulmonary artery and in the left interlobar artery (arrowheads)

at the same way as described earlier) and the ascending aorta at the same level. Cut-off points of 29 mm and 0.9–1 ratio respectively are acceptable [27] (Fig. 25).

E. **Other vascular measurements**

Several publications have shown statistically significant larger dimensions of the superior vena cava, azygos vein and coronary sinus among patients with significant versus non-significant PE [28], among non-survivors versus survivors of acute PE [29] or among patients with higher pulmonary artery systolic pressure [30].

F. **Left atrial size**

In recent years, several publications have shown negative correlation between left atrial size and severity of PE. Evidence, however, is limit to relatively small retrospective cohorts, and further large prospective studies are required to clarify the prognostic value of left atrial size in acute PE, and to establish a cut-off value for area and/or volume for discrimination between high-risk and low-risk patients [31].

G. **Clot burden**

Two main methods for calculating clot burden have been described by Qanadli et al. [32] and Mastora et al. [33], both are taking into consideration clot location and degree of luminal occlusion in determining the clot index. However, calculating clot burden is somewhat cumbersome and has not been commonly adapted in day-to-day clinical practice. Additionally, most publications and two large meta-analyses [21, 34] showed no correlation between clot burden and all-cause mortality, although correlation between clot burden and adverse clinical outcomes has been shown.

H. **Perfusion defects score**
As described below dual-energy CT enables to obtain perfusion maps of lung parenchyma, and to identify perfusion defects analogous to pulmonary scintigraphy. The extent of perfusion defects has been shown to correlate with RV:LV diameter ratio and obstruction score and with adverse clinical outcomes [22].

6 Multienergy CT in PE Imaging

CT images are actually graphic representations of CT numbers expressed in Hounsfield units (the CT number is the material's linear attenuation coefficient normalized by that of water) [35]. The CT number depends on 3 parameters—a material's chemical composition (effective atomic number), its mass density and the effective energy of the X-ray beam used. Thus, for a certain beam energy, different materials may have the same CT number if one has a higher atomic number but the other has a higher mass density, and therefore will not be differentiated on the CT image. Multienergy CT utilizes the fact that these X-ray attenuation characteristics are both material and energy dependent. While the effect of mass density on the CT number is not dependent on the X-ray beam energy, the effect of effective atomic number is very much so. Therefore, by using multiple energies it is possible to "decompose" a tissue and differentiate its various materials [35].

There are two main approaches for acquiring multienergy information—detector based methods and source based methods. In a detector based system a single polychromatic x-ray beam is used and two layers of detectors selectively absorb high or low energy photons, thus creating two spectrally distinct data sets. Source based systems use various methods for generating two separate tube potentials, for example two separate X-ray tubes with two corresponding detector sets offset at an angle of approximately 90 degrees within the gantry [35].

With regards to CTPA, dual energy CT (DECT) has several potential advantages. The ability of material decomposition enables absolute iodine concentration measurement within the lung parenchyma and thus creation of quantitative perfused blood volume images superimposed on the standard grey-scale CT image (Fig. 26). Of note, this is not a time-resolved dynamic perfusion imaging but rather a static image representing lung perfusion at a certain moment, analogous to pulmonary scintigraphy. Several publications have shown DECT perfusion maps to improve detection of small subsegmental PE (Fig. 27). Additionally, the use of perfusion maps may have a prognostic value, as correlation between the extent of perfusion defects on DECT and adverse clinical outcomes has been shown [36, 37] (Fig. 28).

Another advantage of DECT is the ability to generate virtual monoenergetic images. As mentioned above, vascular enhancement increases as x-ray beam energy decreases toward the k-absorption edge of iodine. However, decrease in x-ray beam

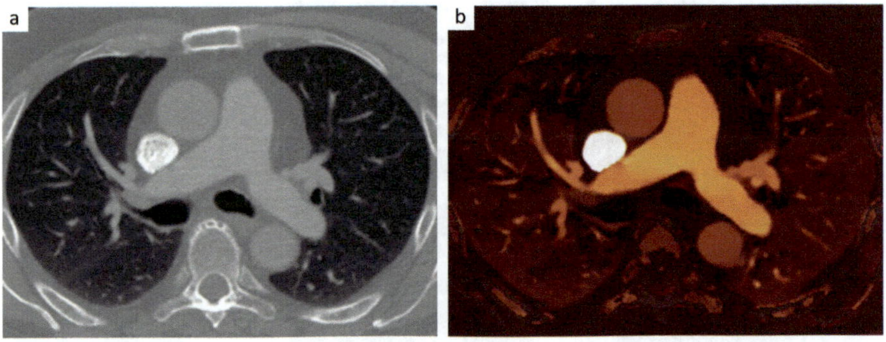

Fig. 26 Iodine density map (perfusion map). Dual energy CT enables material decomposition and thus quantification of perfused iodine within the lung parenchyma. Iodine density or concentration in mg/mL is represented as a color-coded image (**b**) overlaid on the "standard" greyscale CTPA image (**a**)

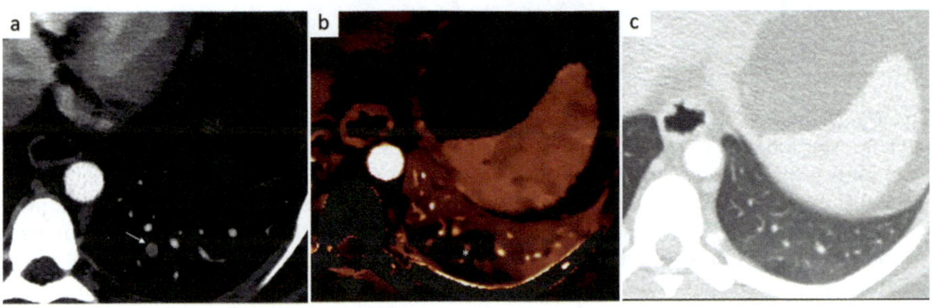

Fig. 27 Perfusion defect in subsegmental PE. **a** Standard greyscale CTPA axial image shows a complete filling defect within a subsegmental artery in the posterior segment of the left lower lobe (LLL). **b** Color coded iodine concentration map (perfusion map) overlaid on the standard greyscale image shows a subpleural wedge shaped perfusion defect (asterisk) in the parenchyma supplied by the corresponding vessel. **c** CTPA axial image in standard greyscale lung window at the same level as in (**b**) does not detect the obvious parenchymal abnormality seen on the perfusion map

energy causes increase in image noise. DECT enables the reader to retrospectively generate images at ultra-low energy levels (i.e. 40–70 keV) with optimal balance between vascular enhancement and image noise. Additionally, iterative reconstruction techniques are applied in DECT as in single energy CT to further reduce image noise and enable the use of ultra-low energy images. Virtual monoenergetic images may salvage studies in which sub-optimal enhancement of the pulmonary arteries has been achieved (Fig. 29), and potentially enable to prospectively reduce injected contrast material volume.

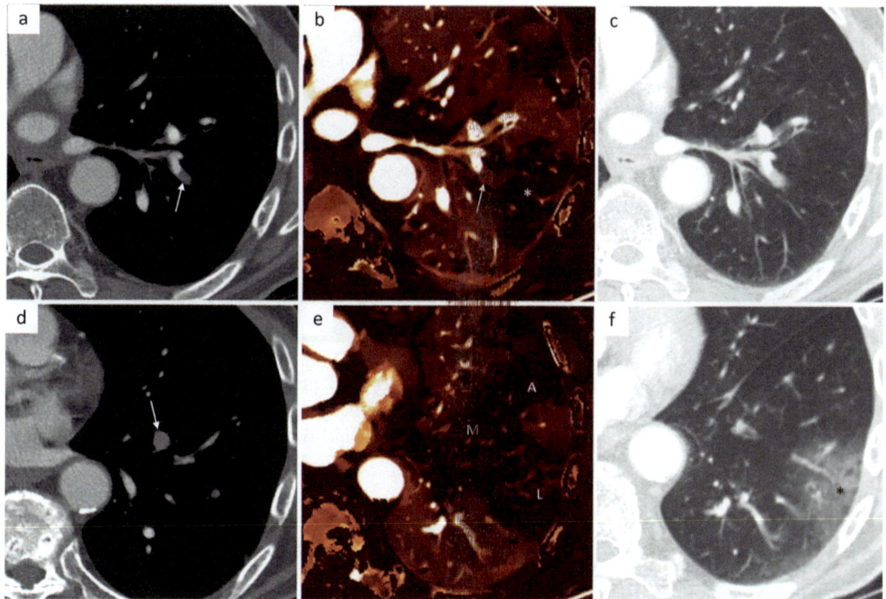

Fig. 28 Multiple perfusion defects. In the left column (**a**, **d**) axial CTPA images at two levels of the left lower lobe (LLL) show complete filling defects in the lateral segmental LLL artery (arrow in **a**) and in the anterior-medial segmental LLL artery (arrow in **d**). In the middle column (**b**, **e**) perfusion maps overlaid on the greyscale images show a segmental perfusion defect in the lateral segment of the LLL (white asterisk in **b**) corresponding to the segmental PE (arrow in figure **a** and **b**), and more caudally confluent large volume perfusion defects involving the lateral and the anterior-medial segments of the LLL (L, A and M respectively in figure **e**) corresponding to the multi-segmental PE. In the right column (**c**, **f**) axial CTPA images in lung windows show only subtle oligemia in the lateral and anterior-medial segments of the LLL, much harder to recognize compared to the obvious defects seen on the perfusion maps. Additionally, a subpleural wedge shaped ground-glass opacity is seen in the lateral LLL segment (black asterisk), consistent with pulmonary infarct, much smaller however than the hypoperfused volume seen on the perfusion maps

7 Computer Assisted Detection

Traditional computer assisted detection (CAD) of pulmonary emboli has been studied over the last two decades with limited clinical use, mostly due to relatively high false positive rates, greatly depending on image quality. However, in recent years various artificial intelligence (AI) algorithms have shown high diagnostic accuracy for PE detection with sensitivity and specificity above 90 percent [38].

AI algorithms can improve inexperienced readers' accuracy for PE detection in an on-call setting for example and can shorten CTPA reading times. Importantly, by automatically screening for PE all contrast enhanced CTs, AI can shorten

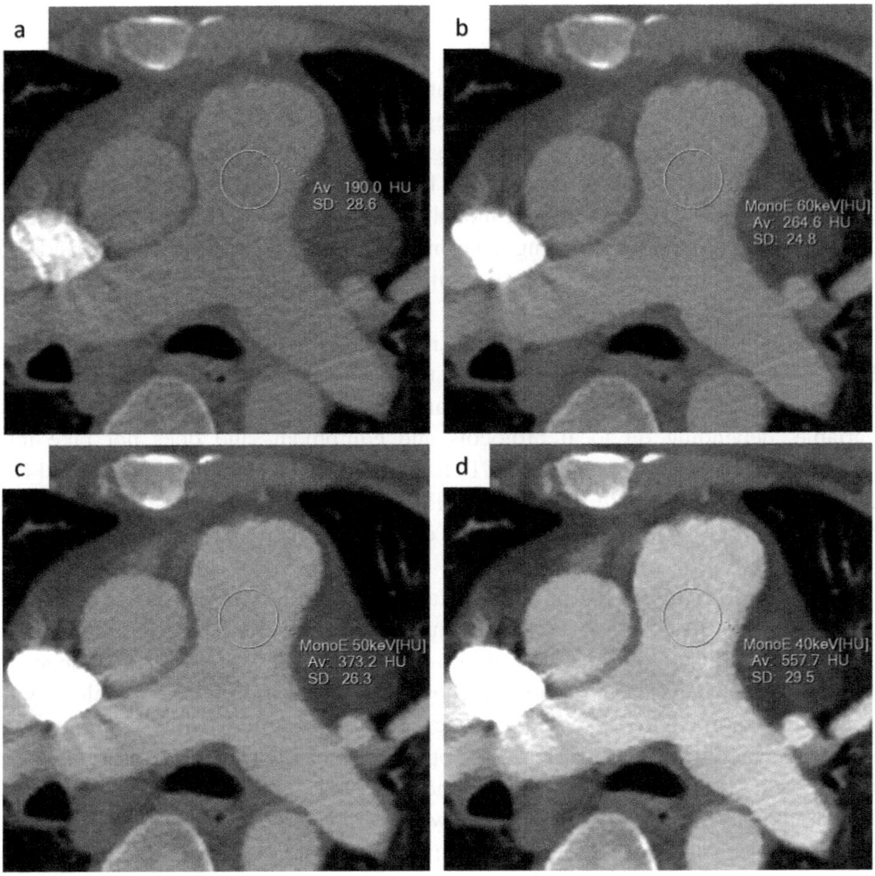

Fig. 29 Virtual monoenergetic images. **a** CTPA axial image at the level of the main pulmonary artery (MPA) bifurcation. Peak arterial enhancement achieved in this study was sub-optimal around 190 Hounsfield units (HU). The following images (**b–d**) show retrospectively generated virtual monoenergetic images with decreasing kilovoltage (60 keV in **b**, 50 keV in **c** and 40 keV in **d**). In each image a circular region of interest (ROI) was placed on the MPA measuring average density in HU and its standard deviation (SD) which directly correlates with image noise. It is easily seen that as keV decreases, arterial enhancement increases up to 557 HU in (**d**), way above the minimal 250 HU required for a diagnostic CTPA. Notice that image noise did not increase

turnaround times of positive studies, including contrast enhanced CTs performed in a non-CTPA protocol for other indications. Such a system is currently used in routine clinical work at our institution. Radiologists get a pop-up notification of every PE detected by the AI algorithm, usually before the study has been read, and thus can prioritize it accordingly.

8 CTPA in pregnancy

Both CTPA and ventilation-perfusion scan are considered safe in pregnant patients [39]. Common concerns that arise regarding CTPA are increased ratio of non-diagnostic studies due to physiologic changes in pregnancy and radiation exposure to maternal breast tissue. As to fetal radiation dose—it is lower in CTPA compared to V/Q scan, and in both modalities well below the reported threshold of 100 milliGray (mGy) for inducing deterministic effects to the fetus, and considered sufficiently low that it does not pose significant increased risk for future childhood malignancy [40].

Maternal breast tissue is thought to be more radiosensitive during pregnancy and lactation. Most publications show CTPA to deliver higher maternal radiation dose, and specifically breast tissue dose, compared to V/Q scan; However, data is highly variable, depending on local protocols and equipment, and does not take into account recent developments in CT technology and imaging protocols [41]. Diagnostic accuracy of V/Q scan and CTPA in pregnant women has been shown to be equivalent [41, 42], with similar rates of indeterminate and non-diagnostic tests [43].

When performing CTPA in pregnant and lactating patients, protocol modifications should be made to minimize maternal and specifically breast tissue radiation dose and to reduce the probability of non-diagnostic scans. Physiologic changes in pregnancy that may lead to a non-diagnostic CTPA include: increased blood volume, tachycardia and increased cardiac output—potentially dilute intraluminal contrast material and thus decrease opacification of the pulmonary arteries; Increased IVC pressure—potentially increases the effect of contrast material interruption by non-opacified blood flow from the IVC into the right heart and pulmonary arteries during deep inspiration; Difficulty in breath holding—may increase respiratory motion artifacts.

Modifications to the CT protocol that may diminish these effects include higher contrast material injection rate (e.g. 5–6 mL/s), higher contrast material concentration (e.g. 370–400 mg/mL) and avoiding deep inspiration breath hold by proper coaching prior to the scan for shallow held inspiration [44, 45]. Radiation dose can be reduced by using low tube potential of 100 kVp or even 80 kVp when possible, which has the additional benefit of increasing contrast enhancement. Reducing tube potential during the bolus tracking phase to 80kVp is recommended as well, as this part of the study has been shown to contribute significantly to breast tissue radiation dose. Scan length should be reduced to the minimum possible, for example from the humeral heads to approximately 2 cm below the lowest dome of the diaphragm [44] or from the aortic arch or approximately 1 cm above it to the diaphragm dome or to the end of the sternum [40, 46]. In addition, commonly used image reconstruction algorithms (i.e. iterative reconstruction) enable to overcome image noise without increasing radiation dose. Auto-modulation of radiation dose further reduces exposure by automatically tailoring beam kV and current (mAs) to patient weight and size and modulating beam energy along the z-axis according to patient's body habitus.

DECT can be particularly useful in the setting of pregnancy or lactation as it achieves higher contrast attenuation and may allow lower radiation dose without significant degradation of image quality [47].

9 CTPA Radiation dose

The radiation dose in CTPA is highly variable, greatly dependent on scanner type and generation, patient characteristics, scan protocol and image reconstruction algorithms. Literature from recent years report CTPA effective dose ranging from as allow as 1.82 mSv (phantom scans on a contemporary 128 slice scanner) [48] or 2.34 mSv (non-obese patients scans on spectral detector CT) [49] to around 9.29 mSv (64 slice scanner with older reconstruction algorithm—filtered back projection). For comparison, the annual average background radiation exposure in the U.S is 3 mSv which is equivalent to 30 chest X-rays [50].

References

1. Stein PD, Fowler SE, Goodman LR, Gottschalk A, Hales CA, Hull RD, Leeper KV Jr, Popovich J Jr, Quinn DA, Sos TA, Sostman HD, Tapson VF, Wakefield TW, Weg JG, Woodard PK; PIOPED II Investigators. Multidetector computed tomography for acute pulmonary embolism. N Engl J Med. 2006;354(22):2317–27. https://doi.org/10.1056/NEJMoa052367. PMID: 16738268.
2. Quiroz R, Kucher N, Zou KH, Kipfmueller F, Costello P, Goldhaber SZ, Schoepf UJ. Clinical validity of a negative computed tomography scan in patients with suspected pulmonary embolism: a systematic review. JAMA. 2005;293(16):2012–7. https://doi.org/10.1001/jama.293.16.2012. PMID: 15855435.
3. Patel P, Patel P, Bhatt M, Braun C, Begum H, Wiercioch W, Varghese J, Wooldridge D, Alturkmani H, Thomas M, Baig M, Bahaj W, Khatib R, Kehar R, Ponnapureddy R, Sethi A, Mustafa A, Lim W, Le Gal G, Bates SM, Haramati LB, Kline J, Lang E, Righini M, Kalot MA, Husainat NM, Jabiri YNA, Schünemann HJ, Mustafa RA. Systematic review and meta-analysis of test accuracy for the diagnosis of suspected pulmonary embolism. Blood Adv. 2020;4(18):4296–311. https://doi.org/10.1182/bloodadvances.2019001052. PMID: 32915980; PMCID: PMC7509887.
4. Wittram C. How I do it: CT pulmonary angiography. AJR Am J Roentgenol. 2007;188(5):1255–61. https://doi.org/10.2214/AJR.06.1104 PMID: 17449768.
5. Bae KT, Tao C, Gürel S, Hong C, Zhu F, Gebke TA, Milite M, Hildebolt CF. Effect of patient weight and scanning duration on contrast enhancement during pulmonary multidetector CT angiography. Radiology. 2007;242(2):582–9. https://doi.org/10.1148/radiol.2422052132 PMID: 17255426.
6. Jones SE, Wittram C. The indeterminate CT pulmonary angiogram: imaging characteristics and patient clinical outcome. Radiology. 2005;237(1):329–37. https://doi.org/10.1148/radiol.2371041520 PMID: 16183940.

7. Cademartiri F, van der Lugt A, Luccichenti G, Pavone P, Krestin GP. Parameters affecting bolus geometry in CTA: a review. J Comput Assist Tomogr. 2002 Jul-Aug;26(4):598–607. doi: https://doi.org/10.1097/00004728-200207000-00022. PMID: 12218827.
8. Saade C, Bourne R, Wilkinson M, Brennan P. Contrast Medium Administration and Parameters Affecting Bolus Geometry in Multidetector Computed Tomography Angiography: An Overview. J Med Imaging Radiat Sci. 2011 Sep;42(3):113-117. doi: https://doi.org/10.1016/j.jmir.2011.05.002. Epub 2011 Jul 27. PMID: 31051857
9. Taslakian B, Latson LA, Truong MT, Aaltonen E, Shiau MC, Girvin F, Alpert JB, Wickstrom M, Ko JP. CT pulmonary angiography of adult pulmonary vascular diseases: Technical considerations and interpretive pitfalls. Eur J Radiol. 2016 Nov;85(11):2049-2063. doi: https://doi.org/10.1016/j.ejrad.2016.09.017. Epub 2016 Sep 16. PMID: 27776659
10. Foti G, Silva R, Faccioli N, Fighera A, Menghini R, Campagnola A, Carbognin G. Identification of pulmonary embolism: diagnostic accuracy of venous-phase dual-energy CT in comparison to pulmonary arteries CT angiography. Eur Radiol. 2021 Apr;31(4):1923-1931. https://doi.org/10.1007/s00330-020-07286-7. Epub 2020 Sep 23. PMID: 32965572
11. Andreou AK, Curtin JJ, Wilde S, Clark A. Does pregnancy affect vascular enhancement in patients undergoing CT pulmonary angiography? Eur Radiol. 2008 Dec;18(12):2716-22. doi: https://doi.org/10.1007/s00330-008-1114-7. Epub 2008 Jul 24. PMID: 18651147
12. Mortimer AM, Singh RK, Hughes J, Greenwood R, Hamilton MC. Use of expiratory CT pulmonary angiography to reduce inspiration and breath-hold associated artefact: contrast dynamics and implications for scan protocol. Clin Radiol. 2011 Dec;66(12):1159-66. doi: https://doi.org/10.1016/j.crad.2011.06.012. Epub 2011 Sep 1. PMID: 21889766
13. Bauer RW, Schell B, Beeres M, Wichmann JL, Bodelle B, Vogl TJ, Kerl JM. High-pitch dual-source computed tomography pulmonary angiography in freely breathing patients. J Thorac Imaging. 2012;27(6):376–81. https://doi.org/10.1097/RTI.0b013e318250067e PMID: 22487993.
14. Shuman WP, Leipsic JA, Busey JM, Green DE, Pipavath SN, Hague CJ, Koprowicz KM. Prospectively ECG gated CT pulmonary angiography versus helical ungated CT pulmonary angiography: impact on cardiac related motion artifacts and patient radiation dose. Eur J Radiol. 2012 Sep;81(9):2444-9. https://doi.org/10.1016/j.ejrad.2011.06.017. Epub 2011 Jun 23. PMID: 21703791
15. Saade C, Bourne R, El-Merhi F, Somanathan A, Chakraborty D, Brennan P. An optimised patient-specific approach to administration of contrast agent for CT pulmonary angiography. Eur Radiol. 2013 Nov;23(11):3205-12. doi: https://doi.org/10.1007/s00330-013-2919-6. Epub 2013 Jun 4. PMID: 23732690
16. Marten K, Engelke C, Funke M, Obenauer S, Baum F, Grabbe E. ECG-gated multislice spiral CT for diagnosis of acute pulmonary embolism Clin Radiol. 2003;58(11):862–8. https://doi.org/10.1016/s0009-9260(03)00348-9 PMID: 14581010.
17. Palacio D, Benveniste MF, Betancourt-Cuellar SL, Gladish GW. Multidetector computed tomography pulmonary angiography pitfalls in the evaluation of pulmonary embolism with emphasis in technique. Semin Roentgenol. 2015 Jul;50(3):217-25. doi: https://doi.org/10.1053/j.ro.2015.01.012. Epub 2015 Feb 3. PMID: 26002242
18. Moore AJE, Wachsmann J, Chamarthy MR, Panjikaran L, Tanabe Y, Rajiah P. Imaging of acute pulmonary embolism: an update. Cardiovasc Diagn Ther. 2018 Jun;8(3):225-243. doi: https://doi.org/10.21037/cdt.2017.12.01. PMID: 30057872; PMCID: PMC6039809
19. Coche EE, Müller NL, Kim KI, Wiggs BR, Mayo JR. Acute pulmonary embolism: ancillary findings at spiral CT. Radiology. 1998;207(3):753–8. https://doi.org/10.1148/radiology.207.3.9609900 PMID: 9609900.
20. Shah AA, Davis SD, Gamsu G, Intriere L. Parenchymal and pleural findings in patients with and patients without acute pulmonary embolism detected at spiral CT. Radiology. 1999;211(1):147–53. https://doi.org/10.1148/radiology.211.1.r99ap03147 PMID: 10189464.
21. Meinel FG, Nance JW Jr, Schoepf UJ, Hoffmann VS, Thierfelder KM, Costello P, Goldhaber SZ, Bamberg F. Predictive Value of Computed Tomography in Acute Pulmonary

Embolism: Systematic Review and Meta-analysis. Am J Med. 2015 Jul;128(7):747-59.e2. doi: https://doi.org/10.1016/j.amjmed.2015.01.023. Epub 2015 Feb 11. PMID: 25680885
22. Albrecht MH, Bickford MW, Nance JW Jr, Zhang L, De Cecco CN, Wichmann JL, Vogl TJ, Schoepf UJ. State-of-the-Art Pulmonary CT Angiography for Acute Pulmonary Embolism. AJR Am J Roentgenol. 2017 Mar;208(3):495-504. doi: https://doi.org/10.2214/AJR.16.17202 . Epub 2016 Nov 29. PMID: 27897042
23. Kang DK, Ramos-Duran L, Schoepf UJ, Armstrong AM, Abro JA, Ravenel JG, Thilo C. Reproducibility of CT signs of right ventricular dysfunction in acute pulmonary embolism AJR Am J Roentgenol. 2010;194(6):1500–6. https://doi.org/10.2214/AJR.09.3717 PMID: 20489089.
24. Ammari Z, Hasnie AA, Ruzieh M, Dasa O, Al-Sarie M, Shastri P, Ashcherkin N, Brewster PS, Cooper CJ, Gupta R. Prognostic Value of Computed Tomography Versus Echocardiography Derived Right to Left Ventricular Diameter Ratio in Acute Pulmonary Embolism. Am J Med Sci. 2021 Apr;361(4):445-450. doi: https://doi.org/10.1016/j.amjms.2020.07.008. Epub 2020 Jul 8. PMID: 32753280
25. Kang DK, Thilo C, Schoepf UJ, Barraza JM Jr, Nance JW Jr, Bastarrika G, Abro JA, Ravenel JG, Costello P, Goldhaber SZ. CT signs of right ventricular dysfunction: prognostic role in acute pulmonary embolism JACC Cardiovasc Imaging. 2011;4(8):841–9. https://doi.org/10.1016/j.jcmg.2011.04.013 PMID: 21835376.
26. Aviram G, Cohen D, Steinvil A, Shmueli H, Keren G, Banai S, Berliner S, Rogowski O. Significance of reflux of contrast medium into the inferior vena cava on computerized tomographic pulmonary angiogram. Am J Cardiol. 2012 Feb 1;109(3):432-7. doi: https://doi.org/10.1016/j.amjcard.2011.09.033. Epub 2011 Nov 9. PMID: 22074991
27. François CJ, Schiebler ML. Imaging of Pulmonary Hypertension. Radiol Clin North Am. 2016 Nov;54(6):1133-1149. doi: https://doi.org/10.1016/j.rcl.2016.05.011. Epub 2016 Aug 13. PMID: 27719980
28. Collomb D, Paramelle PJ, Calaque O, Bosson JL, Vanzetto G, Barnoud D, Pison C, Coulomb M, Ferretti G. Severity assessment of acute pulmonary embolism: evaluation using helical CT. Eur Radiol. 2003 Jul;13(7):1508-14. doi: https://doi.org/10.1007/s00330-002-1804-5. Epub 2003 Feb 7. PMID: 12835961
29. Ghaye B, Ghuysen A, Willems V, Lambermont B, Gerard P, D'Orio V, Gevenois PA, Dondelinger RF. Severe pulmonary embolism:pulmonary artery clot load scores and cardiovascular parameters as predictors of mortality. Radiology. 2006 Jun;239(3):884-91. doi: https://doi.org/10.1148/radiol.2392050075. Epub 2006 Apr 7. PMID: 16603659
30. Staskiewicz G, Czekajska-Chehab E, Przegalinski J, Tomaszewski A, Torres K, Torres A, Trojanowska A, Maciejewski R, Drop A. Widening of coronary sinus in CT pulmonary angiography indicates right ventricular dysfunction in patients with acute pulmonary embolism. Eur Radiol. 2010 Jul;20(7):1615-20. doi: https://doi.org/10.1007/s00330-009-1702-1. Epub 2010 Jan 13. PMID: 20069425
31. Zuin M, Rigatelli G, Turchetta S, Zonzin P, Zuliani G, Roncon L. Left atrial size measured on CT pulmonary angiography: another parameter of pulmonary embolism severity? A systematic review. J Thromb Thrombolysis. 2020 Jul;50(1):181–189. doi: https://doi.org/10.1007/s11239-019-01994-8. PMID: 31754905.
32. Qanadli SD, El Hajjam M, Vieillard-Baron A, Joseph T, Mesurolle B, Oliva VL, Barré O, Bruckert F, Dubourg O, Lacombe P. New CT index to quantify arterial obstruction in pulmonary embolism: comparison with angiographic index and echocardiography. AJR Am J Roentgenol. 2001 Jun;176(6):1415-20. doi: https://doi.org/10.2214/ajr.176.6.1761415. PMID: 11373204
33. Mastora I, Remy-Jardin M, Masson P, Galland E, Delannoy V, Bauchart JJ, Remy J. Severity of acute pulmonary embolism: evaluation of a new spiral CT angiographic score in correlation with echocardiographic data. Eur Radiol. 2003;13(1):29–35. https://doi.org/10.1007/s00330-002-1515-y. Epub 2002 Jun 19. PMID: 12541107
34. Vedovati MC, Germini F, Agnelli G, Becattini C. Prognostic role of embolic burden assessed at computed tomography angiography in patients with acute pulmonary embolism: systematic

review and meta-analysis. J Thromb Haemost. 2013;11(12):2092–102. https://doi.org/10.1111/jth.12429. PMID: 24134450
35. McCollough CH, Boedeker K, Cody D, Duan X, Flohr T, Halliburton SS, Hsieh J, Layman RR, Pelc NJ. Principles and applications of multienergy CT: Report of AAPM Task Group 291. Med Phys. 2020;47(7):e881–912. https://doi.org/10.1002/mp.14157. Epub 2020 May 28. PMID: 32215937.
36. Apfaltrer P, Bachmann V, Meyer M, Henzler T, Barraza JM, Gruettner J, Walter T, Schoepf UJ, Schoenberg SO, Fink C. Prognostic value of perfusion defect volume at dual energy CTA in patients with pulmonary embolism: correlation with CTA obstruction scores, CT parameters of right ventricular dysfunction and adverse clinical outcome. Eur J Radiol. 2012;81(11):3592–7. https://doi.org/10.1016/j.ejrad.2012.02.008. Epub 2012 Apr 9. PMID: 22495202.
37. Bauer RW, Frellesen C, Renker M, Schell B, Lehnert T, Ackermann H, Schoepf UJ, Jacobi V, Vogl TJ, Kerl JM. Dual energy CT pulmonary blood volume assessment in acute pulmonary embolism—correlation with D-dimer level, right heart strain and clinical outcome. Eur Radiol. 2011;21(9):1914-21. https://doi.org/10.1007/s00330-011-2135-1. Epub 2011 Apr 30. PMID: 21533631.
38. Weikert T, Winkel DJ, Bremerich J, Stieltjes B, Parmar V, Sauter AW, Sommer G. Automated detection of pulmonary embolism in CT pulmonary angiograms using an AI-powered algorithm. Eur Radiol. 2020;30(12):6545–53. https://doi.org/10.1007/s00330-020-06998-0. Epub 2020 Jul 3. PMID: 32621243
39. Malhamé I, Tagalakis V, Dayan N. Diagnosing pulmonary embolism in pregnancy: synthesis of current guidelines and new evidence. J Obstet Gynaecol Can. 2020;42(12):1546–9. https://doi.org/10.1016/j.jogc.2020.03.025. Epub 2020 Apr 28. PMID: 32723607.
40. Tester J, Hammerschlag G, Irving L, Pascoe D, Rees M. Investigation and diagnostic imaging of suspected pulmonary embolism during pregnancy and the puerperium: A review of the literature. J Med Imaging Radiat Oncol. 2020;64(4):505–15. https://doi.org/10.1111/1754-9485.13027. Epub 2020 Apr 20. PMID: 32307898.
41. Tromeur C, van der Pol LM, Le Roux PY, Ende-Verhaar Y, Salaun PY, Leroyer C, Couturaud F, Kroft LJM, Huisman MV, Klok FA. Computed tomography pulmonary angiography *versus* ventilation-perfusion lung scanning for diagnosing pulmonary embolism during pregnancy: a systematic review and meta-analysis. Haematologica. 2019;104(1):176–88. https://doi.org/10.3324/haematol.2018.196121. Epub 2018 Aug 16. PMID: 30115658; PMCID: PMC6312023.
42. van Mens TE, Scheres LJ, de Jong PG, Leeflang MM, Nijkeuter M, Middeldorp S. Imaging for the exclusion of pulmonary embolism in pregnancy. Cochrane Database Syst Rev. 2017;1(1):CD011053. https://doi.org/10.1002/14651858.CD011053.pub2. PMID: 28124411; PMCID: PMC6464730.
43. Armstrong L, Gleeson F, Mackillop L, Mutch S, Beale A. Survey of UK imaging practice for the investigation of pulmonary embolism in pregnancy. Clin Radiol. 2017;72(8):696–701. https://doi.org/10.1016/j.crad.2017.03.030. Epub 2017 May 22. PMID: 28545681.
44. Gillespie C, Foley S, Rowan M, Ewins K, NiAinle F, MacMahon P. The OPTICA study (Optimised Computed Tomography Pulmonary Angiography in Pregnancy Quality and Safety study): Rationale and design of a prospective trial assessing the quality and safety of an optimised CTPA protocol in pregnancy. Thromb Res. 2019;177:172–9. https://doi.org/10.1016/j.thromres.2019.03.007. Epub 2019 Mar 13. PMID: 30921536.
45. Ridge CA, Mhuircheartaigh JN, Dodd JD, Skehan SJ. Pulmonary CT angiography protocol adapted to the hemodynamic effects of pregnancy. AJR Am J Roentgenol. 2011;197(5):1058–63. https://doi.org/10.2214/AJR.10.5385. PMID: 22021496.
46. Halpenny D, Park B, Alpert J, Latson L Jr, Kim N, Babb J, Shiau M, Ko J. Low dose computed tomography pulmonary angiography protocol for imaging pregnant patients: Can dose reduction be achieved without reducing image quality? Clin Imaging. 2017;44:101–105. https://doi.org/10.1016/j.clinimag.2017.03.020. Epub 2017 Apr 7. PMID: 28500985.

47. McDermott S, Otrakji A, Flores EJ, Kalra MK, Shepard JO, Digumarthy SR. Should dual-energy computed tomography pulmonary angiography replace single-energy computed tomography pulmonary angiography in pregnant and postpartum patients? J Comput Assist Tomogr. 2018;42(1):25–32. https://doi.org/10.1097/RCT.0000000000000655. PMID: 28786905.
48. Tonkopi E, Manos D, Ross A. Foes the use of contemporary CT scanners alter the radiation dose debate in the imaging work up for pulmonary embolism? Radiat Prot Dosimetry. 2019;187(3):353–60. https://doi.org/10.1093/rpd/ncz174. PMID: 31411698
49. Sauter AP, Shapira N, Kopp FK, Aichele J, Bodden J, Knipfer A, Rummeny EJ, Noël PB. CTPA with a conventional CT at 100 kVp vs. a spectral-detector CT at 120 kVp: Comparison of radiation exposure, diagnostic performance and image quality. Eur J Radiol Open. 2020;7:100234. https://doi.org/10.1016/j.ejro.2020.100234. PMID: 32420413; PMCID: PMC7215101.
50. Jones JG, Mills CN, Mogensen MA, Lee CI. Radiation dose from medical imaging: a primer for emergency physicians. West J Emerg Med. 2012;13(2):202–10. https://doi.org/10.5811/westjem.2011.11.6804. PMID: 22900113; PMCID: PMC3415811.

Ventilation/Perfusion Scintigraphy for the Diagnosis of Pulmonary Embolism and Chronic Thromboembolic Pulmonary Hypertension

Yodphat Krausz, Mahmood Zidan, and Simona Ben-Haim

1 Introduction

Acute pulmonary embolism (PE) interferes with the optimal status of gas exchange in the lungs, affecting both perfusion and ventilation. Early after embolization, within minutes to a few hours, ventilation is diverted from non-perfused to normally perfused lung due to local bronchoconstriction associated with hypocapnia. Within 18–24 hours after embolization, reduced production of surfactant distal to embolization causes shrinkage of the alveolar space in the non-perfused region. This sequence of events is of significance when interpreting the ventilation/perfusion (V/Q) scintigraphy in patients with suspected acute PE, keeping in mind that the clinically overt episode of acute PE is often preceded by clinically occult episodes.

2 DIAGNOSIS of PE

The diagnosis of PE is based on the combination of factors: clinical assessment of symptoms and signs, blood sampling of D-dimer testing, and imaging with either V/Q scintigraphy or pulmonary multidetector computed tomography of the pul-

Y. Krausz · M. Zidan · S. Ben-Haim (✉)
Department of Biophysics and Nuclear Medicine, Hadassah Medical Organization, Jerusalem, Israel
e-mail: simonabh@hadassah.org.il

Y. Krausz · S. Ben-Haim
Faculty of Medicine, Hebrew University of Jerusalem, Jerusalem, Israel

S. Ben-Haim
Institute of Nuclear Medicine, University College London and UCL Hospitals, NHS Trust, London, UK

E. Herzog (ed.), *Pulmonary Embolism*,
https://doi.org/10.1007/978-3-030-87090-4_7

monary arteries (CTPA). CTPA is considered first-line imaging in the daily clinical routine for patients with suspected PE, and has become the most common procedure for the diagnosis of PE or for yielding an alternative diagnosis [1, 2]. When CTPA is contraindicated (i.e., due to radiographic contrast reactions or renal failure) V/Q scintigraphy is recommended.

Diagnosis of PE based on clinical symptoms alone is unreliable. Symptoms and signs such as dyspnea, tachypnea, tachycardia, pleuritic chest pain, cough and hemoptysis are nonspecific and have a poor positive predictive value (PPV) when used alone. Arterial blood gas analysis often reveals hypoxemia and hypocapnia. However, up to 40% of the patients with PE have normal arterial oxygen saturation. D-dimer plasma levels are elevated in the presence of acute thrombosis due to activation of fibrinolysis. The production of fibrin is enhanced also in other conditions such as cancer, inflammation, bleeding, trauma, surgery, and necrosis and therefore the PPV of elevated D-dimer levels is low, but a normal D-dimer level renders the diagnosis of acute PE or venous thromboembolism (VTE) unlikely. Electrocardiographic changes indicative of right ventricle overload are usually observed in the more severe cases of PE. In milder cases the only abnormality may be sinus tachycardia, present in 40% of patients. Atrial arrhythmias, most frequently atrial fibrillation, may also be associated with acute PE. PE rarely occurs in the absence of risk factors. In a retrospective study in more than 2000 patients with suspected PE, there was <1% PE in the absence known risk factors: age >65 years, immobilization (travel, etc.), malignancy, hypercoagulability, elevated estrogen (pregnancy and peripartum, hormone-replacement, oral contraceptives) or previous VTE [3].

Assessment of the clinical probability of acute PE helps clinicians to identify patients with VTE, stratify the risk of morbidity and mortality in patients with VTE, and to choose the most appropriate imaging test for diagnosing or excluding PE [4]. Clinical prediction scores (CPS) were developed to standardize clinical decision-making for both diagnosis and prognosis. The most commonly used are the Wells score [5] and the modified Geneva score [6]. Patients with suspected acute PE are stratified into unlikely/likely and low/intermediate/high risk categories. Patients with a low or intermediate clinical probability and positive D-dimer, and patients with a high or likely clinical probability require further assessment with imaging with either CTPA or V/Q.

3 IMAGING of PE

A preliminary chest X-ray (or preferably a chest CT) is important in all patients suspected of PE for exclusion of alternative conditions (pulmonary edema, pneumonia, trauma, pneumothorax, etc.) and as an aid in the interpretation of subsequent imaging tests. The presence of any abnormality on the initial chest radiograph decreases the utility of scintigraphy. Conversely, a normal chest radiograph strongly indicates that scintigraphy will have a high likelihood of confirming or refuting the diagnosis of PE. Chest imaging may also define the requirement for ventilation scintigraphy and is pivotal in interpretation of the perfusion scintigraphy.

CTPA has become the method of choice for imaging the pulmonary vasculature and for identifying acute pulmonary embolism [7]. CTPA is fast, widely available and may also identify other causes for patients' symptoms. CTPA has also superior sensitivity for the detection of small subsegmental emboli when compared to planar V/Q imaging, although these small emboli are likely reabsorbed with no clinical effect. CTPA confirms the diagnosis of PE in clinically high probability patients (PPV >95%), but is overused in patients with low or intermediate pretest probability of PE [8]. It is not without its risks, however, which include contrast-induced nephropathy, anaphylaxis, and a relatively high radiation dose of 5.4 mSv (compared to 1.2–2 mSv for V/Q) [4, 9]. CTPA delivers a relatively large radiation dose to young females' radiosensitive breast. There are, however, low-dose CT protocols that should be applied.

4 Radionuclide V/Q Scintigraphy

A combined ventilation (V) and perfusion (Q) study is performed to detect acute PE. V/Q scintigraphy exploits the unique pulmonary arterial segmental anatomy (Fig. 1). Occlusive thrombi affecting individual pulmonary arteries produce characteristic lobar, segmental or subsegmental peripheral wedge-shaped defects with the base projecting to the lung periphery.

When perfusion within bronchopulmonary segment(s) is affected by PE, ventilation is usually preserved, a pattern termed V/Q mismatch [2] (Fig. 2). At a later stage, when emboli partly resolve or recanalization occurs, the pattern of V/Q mismatch becomes less distinct. PE are usually multiple, because emboli fragment when passing through the right heart and main pulmonary arteries. PE can be a single event or a recurring process giving rise to multiple emboli over time. V/Q mismatch involving pulmonary lobar, segmental or subsegmental arteries may be caused by other disorders such as congenital pulmonary vascular abnormalities, veno-occlusive disease, vasculitis, lung cancer or tuberculous mediastinal adenopathy. Furthermore, defects in lung perfusion can also be observed in additional conditions, e.g., in prior unresolved PE, compression or invasion of pulmonary vessels by tumors or granulomata, emphysema, bronchiectasis, pneumonic consolidation, atelectasis, and localized bronchial obstruction. Most of these conditions affect primarily ventilation with subsequent reduction of local perfusion. That is due to intrapulmonary adaptation mechanisms that attempt to maximize the efficiency of pulmonary gas exchange by diverting blood flow from under-ventilated to better ventilated areas. These conditions will therefore exhibit matched V/Q defects on lung scintigraphy (Fig. 3).

A baseline V/Q study is suggested in all patients immediately (or within 24 hours of diagnosis), as a reference for subsequent follow-up studies to be performed for assessing recovery of pulmonary perfusion.

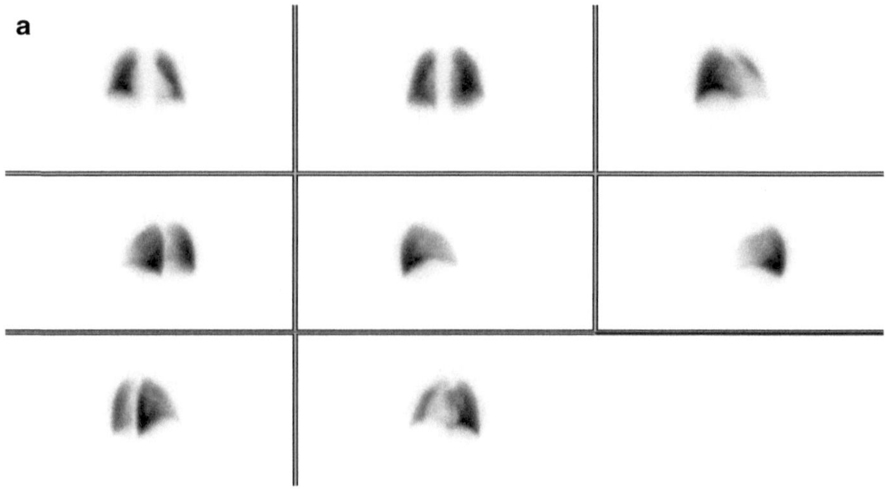

Fig. 1 A 22-year old man with shortness of breath and elevated D-dimer following travel with suspected acute PE was referred for V/Q scintigraphy. Chest X-ray was normal. **a** Planar perfusion study (top row from left: anterior, posterior, RAO views; middle row: LPO, Rt lateral, Lt lateral views; bottom row: RPO and LAO views); **b** SPECT perfusion: serial tomographic axial images from apex (top) to base (bottom) and **c** SPECT ventilation: serial tomographic axial images from apex (top) to base (bottom) showing uniform perfusion and ventilation in both lung fields, excluding acute PE. PE = pulmonary embolism; V/Q = ventilation/perfusion; RAO = right anterior oblique; LPO = left posterior oblique; RPO = right posterior oblique; LAO = left anterior oblique; SPECT = single photon emission tomography

Lung perfusion scintigraphy is based on microembolization. ^{99m}Tc-macroaggregates of albumin (^{99m}Tc-MAA) are intravenously injected, the distribution of which mirrors the distribution of blood flow within the lungs. The adult-administered activity is 111–185-MBq (3–5 mCi), with 200,000–700,000 particles 15–100 μm in size. These particles lodge in the pulmonary capillaries and in the precapillary arterioles, causing microembolization of <1% of the pulmonary capillary bed. In patients with pulmonary hypertension or right-to-left shunt, the number of particles is reduced to 100,000–200,000 without affecting the quality of images.

The ventilation study contributes to assessment of regional distribution of ventilation in various clinical conditions. The presence of under-perfused but normally ventilated areas (V/Q mismatch) is consistent with acute PE, whereas in conditions affecting both perfusion and ventilation PE is unlikely. The ventilation study may precede or may follow the perfusion study. Radiopharmaceuticals for ventilation scintigraphy are administered by inhalation, and are divided into two classes:

(1) Radio-aerosols such as ^{99m}Tc-diethylenetriaminepentacetate (DTPA) or more commonly ^{99m}Tc-technegas are produced by special nebulizers allowing inhalation of the suspended phase containing the radioactive particles. The

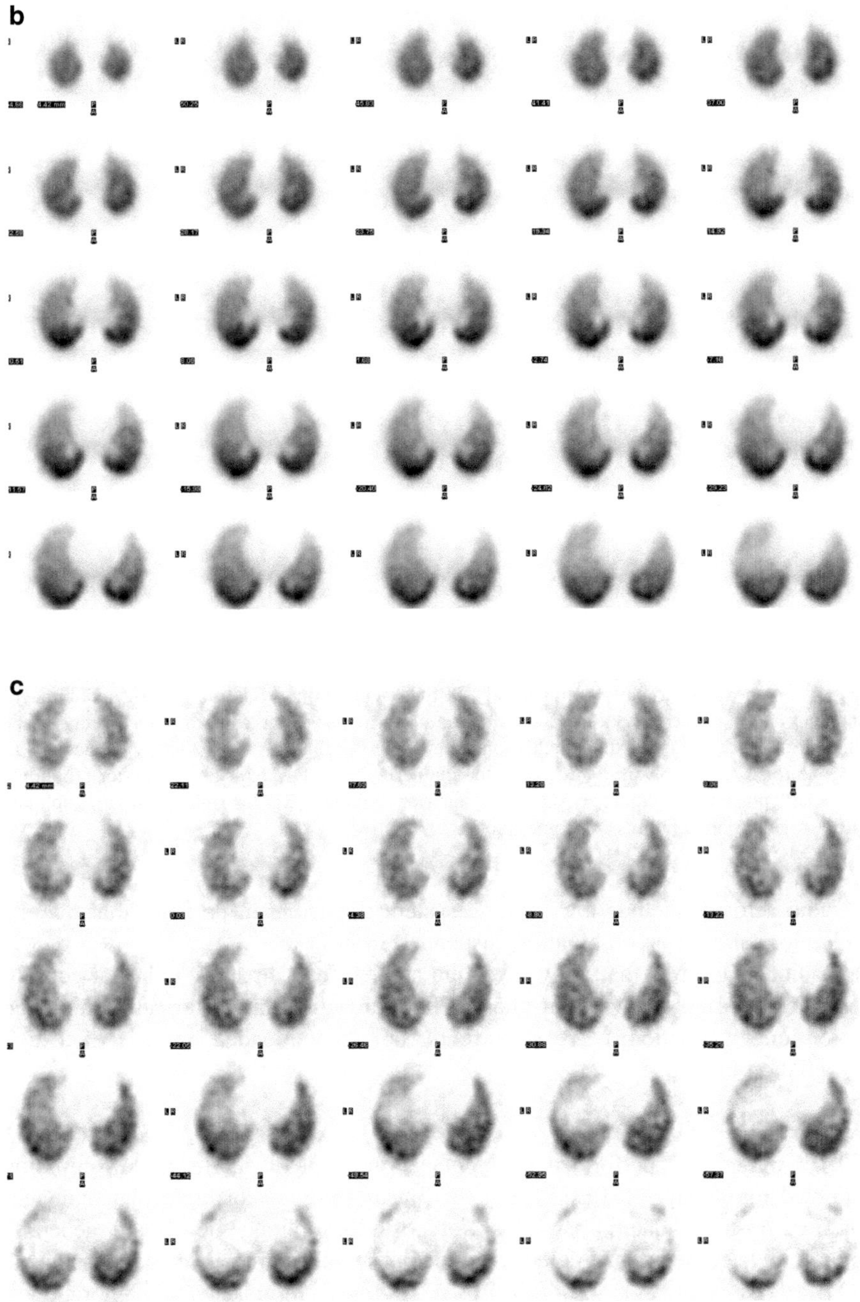

Fig. 1 (continued)

a

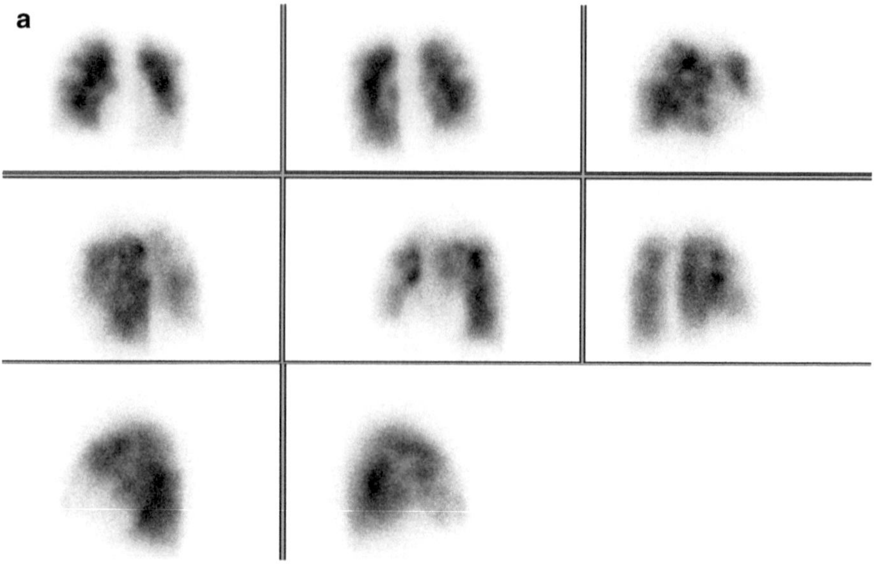

Fig. 2 A 56-year old woman with h/o breast cancer, shortness of breath and elevated D-dimer with suspected acute PE was referred for V/Q scintigraphy. Chest X-ray was normal. **a** Planar perfusion study (top row from left: anterior, posterior, RAO views; middle row: LPO, LAO, RPO views; bottom row: Lt lateral and Rt lateral views); **b** SPECT perfusion: serial tomographic axial images from apex (top) to base (bottom) and **c** SPECT ventilation: serial tomographic axial images from apex (top) to base (bottom) showing non-uniform perfusion with multiple wedge-shape perfusion defects in both lung fields and uniform ventilation, consistent with acute PE. PE = pulmonary embolism; V/Q = ventilation/perfusion; RAO = right anterior oblique; LPO = left posterior oblique; LAO = left anterior oblique; RPO = right posterior oblique; SPECT = single photon emission tomography

radio-aerosols include a two-phase system consisting of particles that may be liquid, solid, or a combination suspended in gas.

(2) Radioactive gases that allow dynamic single-breath imaging either at equilibrium or during the washout phase. The radioactive gas historically employed for lung ventilation ^{133}Xe is currently not recommended because of a high radiation burden.

Imaging Protocols

V/Q scintigraphy is performed using planar imaging or single photon emission computed tomography (SPECT). For the planar study six or eight planar images (anterior, posterior, lateral, anterior and posterior oblique views) are generally required to detect segmental defects, but medial segments may be poorly visualized. V/Q SPECT or preferably hybrid SPECT/CT allows a more accurate exploration of all lung segments and better identification of segmental and subsegmental perfusion defects typical of PE, particularly in the middle lobe and lingula that may be poorly depicted by planar imaging. Tomographic imaging may also reduce the frequency

b

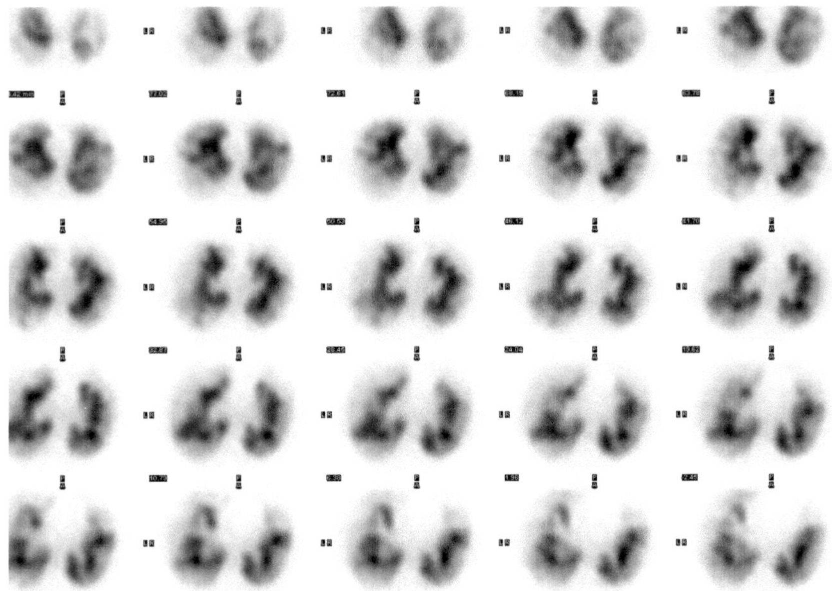

c

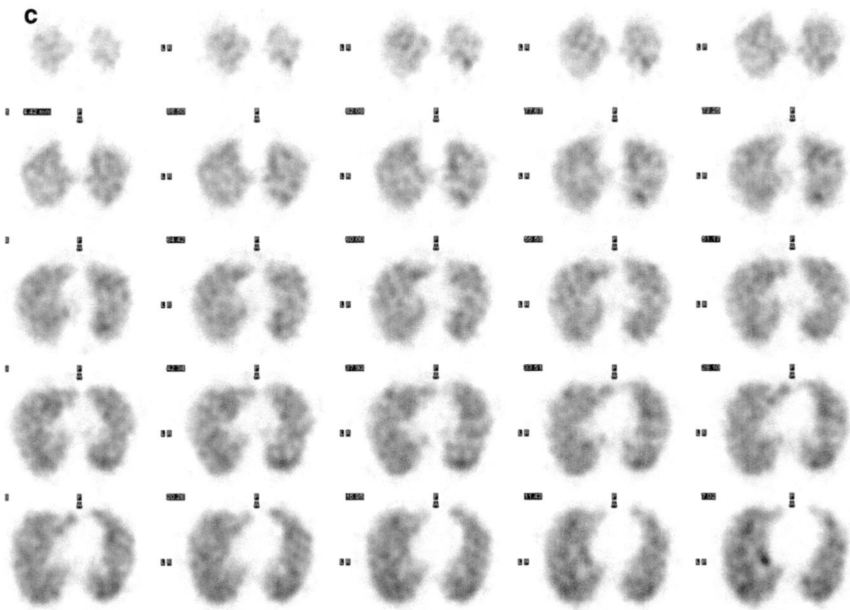

Fig. 2 (continued)

a

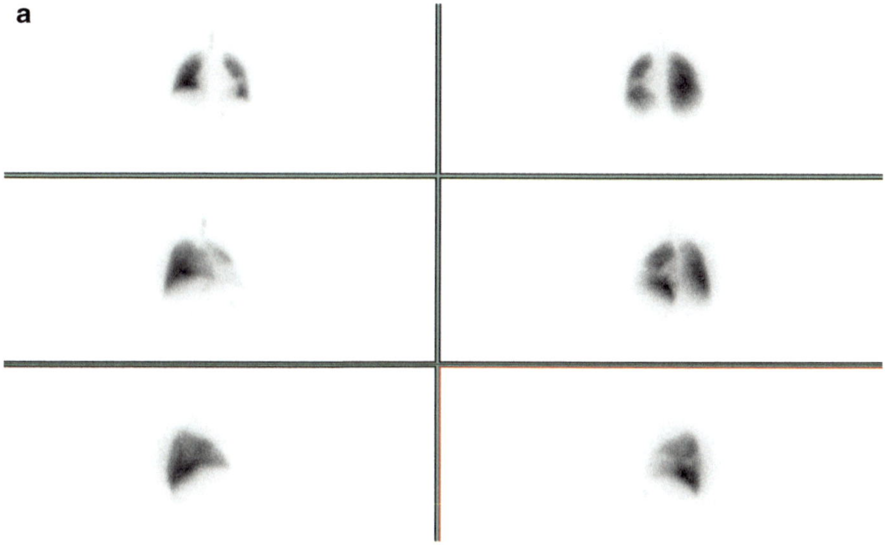

Fig. 3 A 28-years old woman with h/o asthma, shortness of breath and elevated D-dimer with suspected acute PE was referred for V/Q scintigraphy. **a** Planar perfusion study (top row from left: anterior, posterior views; middle row: RAO, LPO views; bottom row: Rt lateral and Lt lateral views); **b** SPECT/CT perfusion: selected axial slice with CT (top left), SPECT (top right), fused SPECT/CT (bottom left) and MIP and **c** SPECT/CT ventilation: selected axial slice with CT (top left), SPECT (top right), fused SPECT/CT (bottom left) and MIP showing a wedge-shaped perfusion defect in the superior segment of LLL (red marker) with reduced ventilation (V/Q match) and matching mosaic-pattern on the corresponding CT slice. Note central airways deposition on the ventilation study, due to turbulence and difficulty breathing. These findings are not consistent with PE and are likely due to the known asthma and COPD. PE = pulmonary embolism; V/Q = ventilation/perfusion; RAO = right anterior oblique; LPO = left posterior oblique; MIP = maximum intensity projection image; SPECT = single photon emission tomography; LLL = left lower lobe; COPD = chronic obstructive pulmonary disease

of non-diagnostic studies and is valuable for monitoring response to treatment and follow-up. V/Q SPECT is also highly diagnostic in patients with suspected PE with other comorbidities such as chronic obstructive pulmonary disease, left heart failure, pneumonia, tumor, etc. [2].

Gutte et al. [10] compared the diagnostic performance of V/Q SPECT with planar V/Q scintigraphy in 36 consecutive patients suspected of acute PE. Eleven patients (31%) were diagnosed with PE. V/Q SPECT had a sensitivity of 100% and specificity of 87%, compared to 64% and 72%, respectively, for planar V/Q scintigraphy. In a more recent study in 84 patients Mazurek et al. [11] reported sensitivity of 73% and specificity of 43% for planar, 88% and 47%, respectively, for SPECT and 100% and 83%, respectively, for SPECT/CT ($p < 0.001$). In a retrospective study in 102 patients V/Q SPECT/CT had 100% sensitivity and 94.4% specificity when compared with CTPA [12].

b

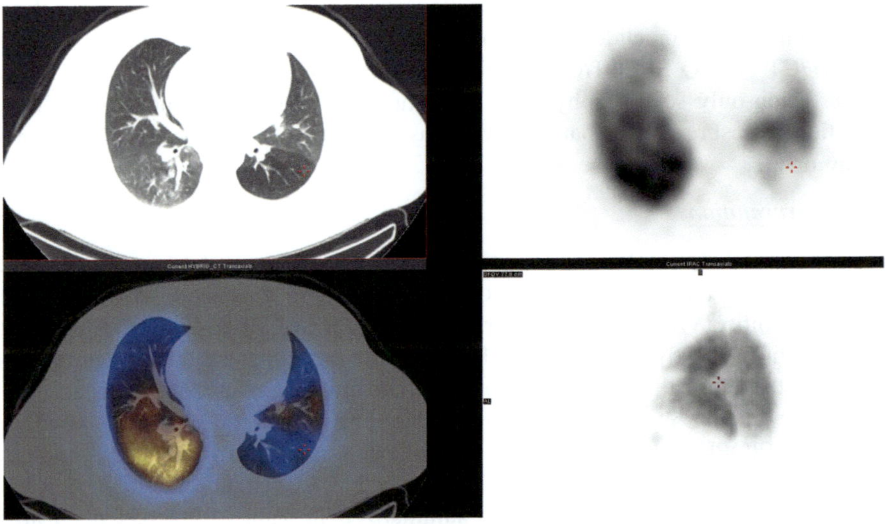

c

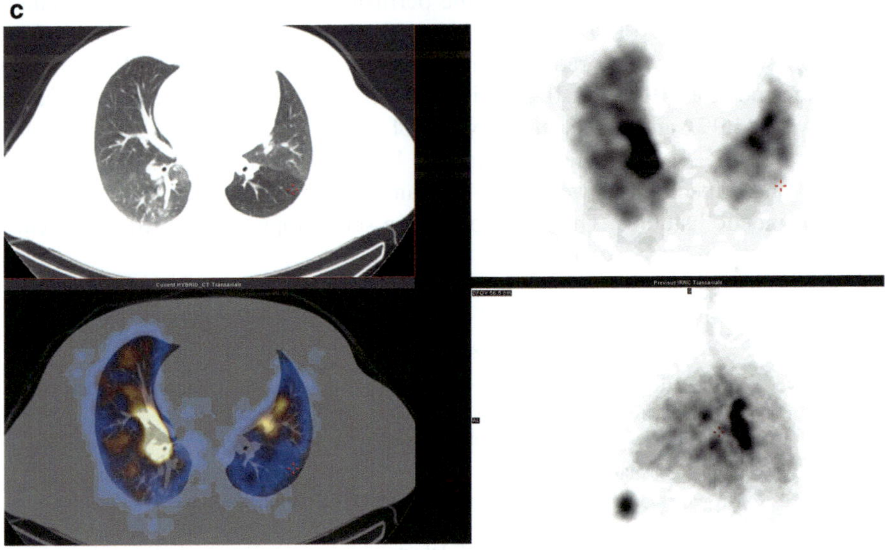

Fig. 3 (continued)

The low-dose CT component of the SPECT/CT study provides data for attenuation correction as well as morphologic information superior to chest X-ray. In 81 patients with suspected PE V/Q SPECT had a sensitivity of 97% and a specificity of 88%. When low-dose CT was added the specificity increased to 100% with no change in sensitivity, whereas CTPA alone had a sensitivity of 68% and a specificity of 100% [13]. The CT component of SPECT/CT (even a low-dose, non-contrast-enhanced study) is particularly useful to identify alternative causes for the symptoms raising the clinical suspicion of PE and/or for the perfusion defects detected in the radionuclide component of the scan [14]. Thus, either perfusion-only SPECT/CT or V/Q SPECT/CT imaging is recommended.

Perfusion-only scintigraphy is recommended in pregnant women to minimize radiation exposure and in patients with suspected massive PE with normal chest X-ray or CT.

V/Q interpretation

Interpretation V/Q scintigraphy is standardized. Findings are frequently classified according to a three-tier classification: a normal V/Q study excludes PE and a high-probability V/Q study in the presence of intermediate-to-high pretest probability confirms it [15] (Figs. 1, 2, 3). In cases with non-diagnostic V/Q scintigraphy or when the clinical pretest likelihood and imaging tests are discrepant, further diagnostic testing is required. Interpretation criteria of V/Q studies based on modified PIOPED II (Prospective Investigative Study of Acute Pulmonary Embolism Diagnosis) and PISAPED (Prospective Investigation Study of Acute Pulmonary Embolism Diagnosis) are summarized in Table 1. In patients with a normal chest X-ray, performing only the perfusion lung scan is acceptable and is the rule for the PISAPED protocol [16, 17]. Sostman et al. [15] assessed the perfusion study and chest radiographs in patients with suspected PE (Table 1). Using the modified PIOPED II criteria, the sensitivity of a PE-positive perfusion study was 84.9% and the specificity of PE-negative study was 92.7%, when excluding 20.6% "non-diagnostic" studies. Using the PISAPED criteria, the sensitivity and specificity were 80.4% and 96.6%, respectively, with no "non-diagnostic" studies. Therefore, perfusion scintigraphy combined with a chest

Table 1 Interpretation of lung scintigraphy by modified PIOPEDII and PISAPED criteria[a]

Finding	Modified PIOPED II [18]	PISAPED [17]
PE-positive	– High probability ($\geq$2 segmental perfusion defects with no corresponding X-ray abnormality)	$\geq$1 wedge-shaped perfusion defect
PE-negative	– Normal perfusion – Very low probability (nonsegmental defects) – 1–3 small subsegmental defects – Perfusion defect < X-ray lesion – Single segment V/Q match in upper or mid lung zone – "Stripe sign" around perfusion defect – Pleural effusion > third of pleural cavity and no other perfusion defect	– Normal perfusion – Non-wedge shaped perfusion defect – Perfusion defect due to enlarged heart, mediastinum or diaphragm
Non-diagnostic	– All other findings	

[a] Modified from Sostman et al. [15]

PIOPED—Prospective Investigative Study of Acute Pulmonary Embolism Diagnosis; PISAPED—Prospective Investigation Study of Acute Pulmonary Embolism Diagnosis

X-ray provides diagnostic accuracy similar to both V/Q scintigraphy and CTPA, with a lower radiation dose. Similar criteria were.

V/Q or CTPA?

V/Q SPECT and CTPA have similar diagnostic accuracies, although CTPA detects PE in smaller vessels. The sensitivity, specificity, PPV and NPV of V/Q were 80.5%, 96.6%, 84.7% and 94.5%, respectively (0% non-diagnostic studies using PISAPED) compared to 83%, 96%, 85.7% and 94.8%, respectively, for CTPA (6% non-diagnostic studies, excluded from analysis) [8, 15]. The radiation dose of V/Q is significantly lower than CTPA, therefore V/Q is preferable in young women and in the follow up of patients with known PE. V/Q is also preferable in patients with moderate to severe renal impairment due to the risk of contrast-induced nephropathy with CTPA. In pregnancy the radiation dose to the maternal breast is significantly less with V/Q, and fetal radiation exposure can also be limited with V/Q to 0.25 mSv, comparable to CTPA [19]. Therefore V/Q is also preferable during pregnancy. Breastfeeding needs to be interrupted for 13 hours after V/Q, but not after CTPA.

Follow-Up Imaging After Acute Pulmonary Embolism

The outcome varies in patients treated for acute PE, ranging from total resolution to permanent vascular occlusion. Recurrent PE can be difficult to diagnose if a baseline perfusion study documenting the state of perfusion following recovery is not available for comparison. Recurring PE can occur within 2 years from an acute episode, with an associated risk of mortality [20].

Lung perfusion scintigraphy is the optimal imaging modality for monitoring recovery of pulmonary perfusion after acute PE, for assessing progression or regression of small and large emboli. It enables monitoring the efficacy of therapy, as well as long-term follow-up. V/Q scintigraphy is more feasible, and is associated with fewer biological risks and lower radiation dosimetry compared to CTPA. It has also proven to mirror improvement in partial pressure of oxygen in arterial blood, which continues up until at least 1 year after the acute episode [21]. Perfusion-only scintigraphy may be performed for monitoring during the initial phase of treatment. Untreated or poorly treated acute PE may also lead to chronic thromboembolic pulmonary hypertension, which is severely debilitating and potentially fatal [22].

Optimal monitoring for the risk of developing chronic thromboembolic pulmonary hypertension is usually performed soon after acute PE (i.e., at 1 and 4 weeks) and then at 3, 6, and 12 months. Lung perfusion also plays a role in diagnostic screening of patients with pulmonary hypertension. Undiagnosed chronic thromboembolic disease is frequently the condition underlying pulmonary hypertension, even in patients with no prior clinically obvious episode of acute PE [21, 23].

5 Chronic Thromboembolic Pulmonary Hypertension (CTEPH)

Chronic thromboembolic pulmonary hypertension (CTEPH) is a rare life-threatening complication of untreated or poorly treated acute PE. CTEPH is classified as group 4 pulmonary hypertension with a mean pulmonary artery pressure ≥ 25 mm Hg and mean pulmonary arterial wedge pressure ≤ 15 mm Hg. The incidence is estimated at 0.4–4.8% among survivors of acute pulmonary embolism (PE) [22, 23], occurring up to 2-y following the acute event. Risk factors for the development of CTEPH include a previous pulmonary embolism, younger age, a large perfusion defect, and idiopathic pulmonary embolism at presentation. Up to 63% of patients diagnosed with CTEPH have no history of documented PE.

There are no effective screening procedures to detect CTEPH after PE [24]. Most cases are diagnosed during investigation of pulmonary hypertension. CTEPH might be a consequence of repeated unrecognized small PEs. The clinical presentation of CTEPH is often insidious. Delayed diagnosis of CTEPH may result in progressive increase in pulmonary vascular resistance and right-sided heart failure with associated increased morbidity. CTEPH carries a poor prognosis when not treated, with a 30% 5-year survival rate in patients with mean pulmonary artery pressure >30 mm Hg. Pulmonary endarterectomy is the definitive treatment for CTEPH, improving hemodynamic parameters and outcome, but the mortality rate associated with this procedure is 4–8%.

Diagnostic Imaging

Identifying CTEPH as the cause of pulmonary hypertension is facilitated by several imaging techniques, including V/Q scintigraphy, CTPA, high-resolution CT (HRCT), pulmonary digital subtraction angiography (DSA), and, more recently, magnetic resonance angiography. Pulmonary function tests, transthoracic echocardiography, right heart catheterization, and pulmonary angiography can also assist in the diagnosis.

Invasive PA was considered in the past the reference standard for diagnosis and operability assessments in CTEPH, but it is gradually being replaced by noninvasive technologies, such as CTPA and ventilation-perfusion (V/Q) scanning. After at least 3 months of effective anticoagulation, V/Q scintigraphy with at least one segmental perfusion defect and pulmonary artery obstruction on CTPA are diagnostic for CTEPH [24]. In most patients V/Q scintigraphy shows multiple moderate and large perfusion defects with V/Q mismatch. Perfusion defects of CTEPH can be different from those of acute PE, as they evolve over time and may be smaller. In the presence of a normal chest radiograph, perfusion-only scan might be sufficient to diagnose or rule out CTEPH [25].

V/Q scintigraphy is more sensitive than CTPA for detecting CTEPH and therefore is recommended for the initial workup of patients with unexplained pulmonary hypertension [23] (Fig. 4). The superior performance of V/Q scintigraphy compared to CTPA for CTEPH has been documented by Tunariu et al. [26],

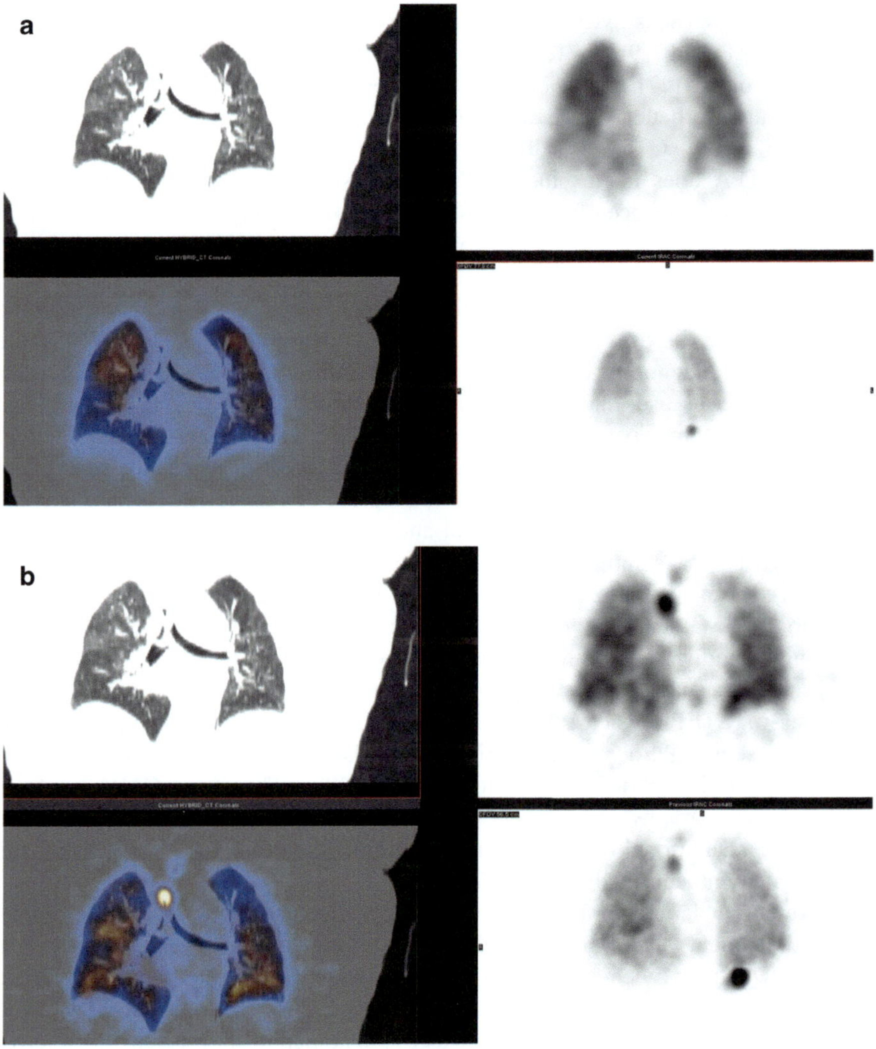

Fig. 4 A 77-years old man with 6 months shortness of breath, pulmonary hypertension, right ventricular failure and suspected CTEPH. V/Q scintigraphy was performed. **a** A selected coronal CT (top left), SPECT (top right), fused SPECT/CT (bottom left) perfusion slice and perfusion MIP (bottom right) and **b** a selected coronal CT (top left), SPECT (top right), fused SPECT/CT (bottom left) ventilation slice and ventilation MIP (bottom right) show perfusion defects in the basal segments of the RLL with preserved ventilation, consistent with CTEPH. Note central airways deposition on the ventilation study, due to turbulence and difficulty breathing and the swallowed activity in the stomach. CTEPH = chronic thromboembolic pulmonary hypertension; V/Q = ventilation/perfusion; SPECT = single photon emission computed tomography; MIP = maximum intensity projection; RLL = right lower lobe

who demonstrated sensitivity 97.4%, specificity 90% and NPV 98.5%, compared to 51.3%, 99.3% and 79.7%, respectively, for CTPA. Similar results were also reported by others [27]. The reason for the superior sensitivity of V/Q scanning has been attributed to better visualization of subsegmental defects compared to CTPA [28]. High quality CTPA is adequate for diagnosis of proximal CTEPH, but a negative CTPA does not exclude CTEPH as distal disease can be missed [29]. Although the significance of the extra sensitivity in detecting subsegmental defects for acute PE is disputed, it is crucial for the diagnosis of CTEPH, also enabling to determine potential operability.

Normal V/Q scintigraphy excludes the presence of surgically accessible chronic thromboembolic disease. High probability V/Q scintigraphy makes CTEPH the most likely diagnosis, although other conditions, including pulmonary veno-occlusive disease, may result in similar findings.

V/Q scintigraphy does not localize the extent of disease anatomically, neither does it correlate with the severity of CTEPH and therefore it cannot be used to determine if the obstruction is amenable to surgery. Perfusion defects may become less prominent over time despite clinical and hemodynamic progression [23]. The advantage of V/Q scintigraphy is the ease of interpretation (either normal or abnormal). It was recommended by the Joint Task Force of the European Society of Cardiology (ESC) and the European Respiratory Society (ERS) for the initial screening of individuals with pulmonary hypertension [24] and became the preferred screening study in the evaluation of patients with pulmonary hypertension for diagnosis of CTEPH. CTPA has a higher specificity than V/Q scintigraphy for identifying segmental obstructions with fewer false positive findings, likely due to direct visualization of intraluminal obstructions [28]. Therefore, CTPA complements V/Q scintigraphy in the preoperative assessment of patients with CTEPH and also provides additional anatomical information of the pulmonary vasculature, the lung parenchyma and mediastinum [29].

Following endarterectomy, reperfused lung segments may appear more prominent and segments that were normally perfused prior to surgery may appear less perfused. This phenomenon is due to reduced pressure and preferential flow in the blood vessels after endarterectomy and relatively reduced flow in the rest of the pulmonary circulation. This "vascular steal" phenomenon may result in the erroneous appearance of a high-probability V/Q study with no clinical evidence of an acute PE. The extent and severity of these "pseudo-defects" decrease within 9–12 months [30]. Familiarity with the patterns of perfusion defects seen during the initial workup of CTEPH and the expected posttreatment changes seen at follow-up imaging is essential for accurate interpretation of V/Q scintigraphy.

6 In Summary

- PE cannot be reliably diagnosed based on clinical data alone.
- Lung perfusion scintigraphy with ^{99m}Tc-MAA is the cornerstone of radionuclide imaging in patients with suspected PE.
- A normal perfusion study excludes the diagnosis of acute PE.
- The addition of ventilation in V/Q scintigraphy increases the specificity of radionuclide imaging for the diagnosis of acute PE.
- V/Q with SPECT/CT and CTPA have comparable diagnostic accuracies, but V/Q is preferable in young women, in pregnant women, in the follow up of patients with known PE and in patients with renal impairment.
- V/Q scintigraphy is the optimal imaging modality for monitoring recovery of pulmonary perfusion after acute PE, to assess the efficacy of therapy, as well as for long-term follow-up.
- Following diagnosis and primary treatment of acute PE, follow-up is important for timely diagnosis of CTEPH, a severely debilitating and potentially fatal condition.
- Undiagnosed chronic thromboembolic disease is frequently underlying pulmonary hypertension.
- Lung perfusion scintigraphy plays an important role in diagnostic screening in patients with pulmonary hypertension.

References

1. Stein PD, Woodard PK, Weg JG, Wakefield TW, Tapson VF, Sostman HD, et al. Diagnostic pathways in acute pulmonary embolism: recommendations of the PIOPED II Investigators. Radiology. 2007;242:15–21.
2. Bajc M, Neilly JB, Miniati M, Schuemichen C, Meignan M, Jonson B. EANM Committee. EANM guidelines for ventilation/perfusion scintigraphy: Part 1. Pulmonary imaging with ventilation/perfusion single photon emission tomography. Eur J Nucl Med Mol Imaging. 2009;36(8):1356–70.
3. Mamlouk MD, vanSonnenberg E, Gosalia R, et al. Pulmonary embolism at CT angiography: implications for appropriateness, cost and radiation exposure in 2003 patients. Radiology. 2010;256:625–32.
4. Bajc M, Neilly JB, Miniati M, Schuemichen C, Meignan M, Jonson B. EANM guidelines for ventilation/perfusion scintigraphy. Part 2. Algorithms and clinical considerations for diagnosis of pulmonary emboli with V/PSPECT and MDCT. Eur J Nucl Med Mol Imaging. 2009;36:1528–38.
5. Wells PS, Anderson DR, Rodgers M, Ginsberg JS, Kearon C, Gent M, et al. Derivation of a simple clinical model to categorize patients' probability of pulmonary embolism: increasing the model's utility with simpliRED D-dimer. Thromb Haemost. 2000;83:416–20.
6. Le Gal G, Righini M, Roy PM, Sanchez O, Aujesky D, Bounameaux H, et al. Prediction of pulmonary embolism in the emergency department: the revised Geneva score. Ann Intern Med. 2006;144:165–71.
7. Konstantinides SV, Torbicki A, Agnelli G, Danchin N, Fitzmaurice D, Galié N, et al. 2014 ESC guidelines on the diagnosis and management of acute pulmonary embolism: the

task force for the diagnosis and management of acute pulmonary embolism of the European Society of Cardiology (ESC) endorsed by the European Respiratory Society (ERS). Eur Heart J. 2014;35:3033–80.

8. Stein PD, Fowler SE, Goodman LR, et al. Multidetector computed tomography for acute pulmonary embolism. N Engl J Med. 2006;354:2317–27.
9. Essien E-O, Rali P, Mathai SC. Pulmonary embolism. Med Clin N Am. 2019;103(3):549–64.
10. Gutte H, Mortensen J, Jensen CV, von der Recke P, Petersen CL, Kristoffersen US, Kjaer A. Comparison of V/Q SPECT and planar V/Q lung scintigraphy in diagnosing acute pulmonary embolism. Nucl Med Commun. 2010;31(1):82–6.
11. Mazurek A, Dziuk M, Witkowska-Patena E, Piszczek S, Gizewska A. The utility of hybrid SPECT/CT lung perfusion scintigraphy in pulmonary embolism diagnosis. Respiration. 2015;90:393–401.
12. Bhatia KD, Ambati C, Dhaliwal R, Paschkewitz R, Hsu E, Ho B, et al. SPECT-CT/VQ versus CTPA for diagnosing pulmonary embolus and other lung pathology: pre-existing lung disease should not be a contraindication. J Med Imaging Radiat Oncol. 2016;60:492–7.
13. Gutte H, Mortensen J, Jensen CV, Johnbeck CB, von der Recke P, Petersen CL, et al. Detection of pulmonary embolism with combined ventilation-perfusion SPECT and low-dose CT: head-to head comparison with multidetector CT angiography. J Nucl Med. 2009;50:1987–92.
14. Simanek M, Koranda P. The benefit of personalized hybrid SPECT/CT pulmonary imaging. Am J Nucl Med Mol Imaging. 2016;6:215–22.
15. Sostman HD, Miniati M, Gottschalk A, et al. Sensitivity and specificity of perfusion scintigraphy combined with chest radiography for acute pulmonary embolism in PIOPED II. J Nucl Med. 2008;49:1741–8.
16. Miniati M, Pistolesi M, Marini C, Di Ricco G, Formichi B, Prediletto R, et al. Value of perfusion lung scan in the diagnosis of pulmonary embolism: results of the Prospective Investigative Study of Acute Pulmonary Embolism Diagnosis (PISA-PED). Am J Respir Crit Care Med. 1996;154:1387–93.
17. Miniati M, Sostman HD, Gottschalk A, Monti S, Pistolesi M. Perfusion lung scintigraphy for the diagnosis of pulmonary embolism: a reappraisal and review of the prospective investigative study of pulmonary embolism diagnosis methods. Semin Nucl Med. 2008;38:450–61.
18. Stein PD, Woodard PK, Weg JG, Wakefield TW, Tapson VF Sostman HD, et!al. Diagnostic pathways in acute pulmonary embolism: recommendations of the PIOPED II investigators. Am J Med. 2006;119:1048–55.
19. Matthews S. Imaging pulmonary embolism in pregnancy: what is the most appropriate imaging protocol? Br J Radiol. 2006;79:441–4.
20. Miniati M, Monti S, Bottai M, Scoscia E, Bauleo C, Tonelli L, et al. Survival and restoration of pulmonary perfusion in a long-term follow-up of patients after acute pulmonary embolism. Medicine (Baltimore). 2006;85:253–62.
21. Reid JH, Coche EE, Inoue T, Kim EE, Dondi M, Watanabe N, et al. Is the lung scan alive and well? Facts and controversies in defining the role of lung scintigraphy for the diagnosis of pulmonary embolism in the era of MDCT. Eur J Nucl Med Mol Imaging. 2009;36:505–21.
22. Pengo V, Lensing AW, Prins MH, Marchiori A, Davidson BL, Tiozzo F, et al. Thromboembolic pulmonary hypertension study group. incidence of chronic pulmonary hypertension after pulmonary embolism. N Engl J Med. 2004;350:2257–64.
23. Moradi F, Morris TA, Hoh CK. Perfusion scintigraphy in diagnosis and management of thromboembolic pulmonary hypertension. Radiographics. 2019;39:169–85.
24. Galiè N, Humbert M, Vachiery JL, et al. 2015 ESC/ERS guidelines for the diagnosis and treatment of pulmonary hypertension: The Joint Task Force for the Diagnosis and Treatment of Pulmonary Hypertension of the European Society of Cardiology (ESC) and the European Respiratory Society (ERS)–endorsed by Association for European Paediatric and Congenital Cardiology (AEPC), International Society for Heart and Lung Transplantation (ISHLT). Eur Heart J. 2016;37(1):67–119.

25. Lang IM, Klepetko W. Update on chronic thromboembolic pulmonary hypertension, a frequently undiagnosed condition. Rev Esp Cardiol. 2009;62(2):120–5.
26. Tunariu N, Gibbs SJR, Win Z, Gin-Sing W, Graham A, Gishen P, et al. Ventilation-perfusion scintigraphy is more sensitive than multidetector CTPA in detecting chronic thromboembolic pulmonary disease as a treatable cause of pulmonary hypertension. J Nucl Med. 2007;48:680–4.
27. Wang M, Wu D, Ma R, Zhang Z, Zhang H, Han K, Xiong C, Wang L, Fang W. Comparison of V/Q SPECT and CT angiography for the diagnosis of chronic thromboembolic pulmonary hypertension. Radiology. 2020;296:420–9.
28. Leblanc M, Narinder P. V/Q SPECT and computed tomographic pulmonary angiography. Semin Nucl Med. 2010;40(6):426–41.
29. Edward JA, Mandras S. An update on the management of chronic thromboembolic pulmonary hypertension. Curr Probl Cardiol. 2017;42:7–38.
30. Moser KM, Metezky ML, Auger WR, Fedullo PF. Resolution of vascular steal after pulmonary thromboendarterectomy Chest. 1993;104(5):1441–4.

Imaging Modalities in Pulmonary Embolism—Pulmonary Angiography

Allan I. Bloom, David Planer, Ronny Alcalai, and Gabby Elbaz-Greener

1 Background

Chest imaging plays an important role in the evaluation and management of acute pulmonary embolism (PE). Computed tomography pulmonary angiography (CTPA) is the current standard of care and provides accurate diagnosis with rapid turnaround time. CTPA also provides information regarding other potential causes of acute chest pain [1].

The advent of CTPA has in recent years led to a dramatic reduction in the use of conventional direct catheter pulmonary angiography (CPA) for the diagnosis of acute pulmonary embolism (PE). As a result, readers may be less familiar with this modality than in the past. In fact, the procedure itself has undergone important technical changes, the most important of which was probably the change from "cut-film" angiography to digital subtraction angiography (DSA) in 1980 [2].

CPA was the reference standard for the diagnosis of PE in the PIOPED I and PIOPED II trials [3, 4]. However, it is an invasive procedure and has a limited role for PE diagnosis in the modern era of multi-detector CTPA. It is now used only when a concomitant endovascular treatment is planned.

The basic requirement for the performance of pulmonary angiography is the ability to safely insert a diagnostic angiographic catheter into the pulmonary arterial tree wherein iodinated contrast is injected directly into the circulation. Rapid

A. I. Bloom (✉)
Department of Medical Imaging, Interventional and Vascular Radiology, Hadassah University Medical Center, Jerusalem, Israel
e-mail: allan@hadassah.org.il

D. Planer · R. Alcalai · G. Elbaz-Greener
Department of Cardiology, Faculty of Medicine, Hadassah University Medical Center, Hebrew University of Jerusalem, Jerusalem, Israel

E. Herzog (ed.), *Pulmonary Embolism*,
https://doi.org/10.1007/978-3-030-87090-4_8

high-resolution filming is required to produce diagnostic images that can both diagnose a variety of pathologies as well as guide catheter directed interventions.

2 Anatomy and Angiography

As with many vascular trees in the human body there are the "common" and the "variant" patterns which are frequently observed. The same is true for the pulmonary arteries. Embryologically, they are derived from the sixth embryonal arches. Part of the main pulmonary artery (MPA), together with the left pulmonary artery (LPA), arise from the ventral left arch, whereas the right pulmonary artery (RPA) arises from the persistent sixth dorsal arch.

The MPA has a straight antero-posterior (AP) course, is approximately 3–5 cm long and is therefore best visualized on a cranio-caudal angulated (AP) or a lateral view angiogram. The RPA is longer than the left, has a more horizontal course and is often more difficult to catheterize than the LPA which is a continuation of the MPA (Fig. 1).

The arterial supply to the lungs follows the lobar anatomy; upper, middle and lower on the right side with upper, lingula and lower on the left (Fig. 1). The division into smaller segmental branches within each lobe together with numerous

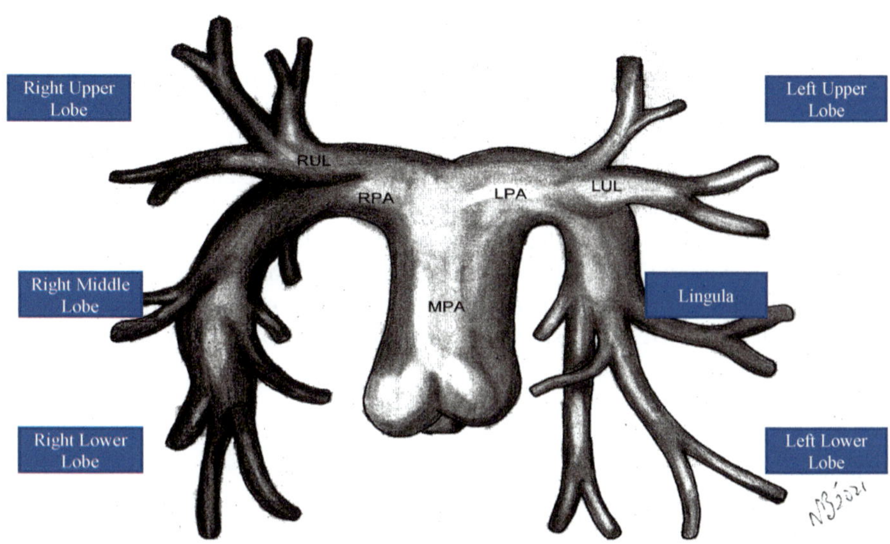

Fig. 1 Pulmonary arterial anatomy schematic. LPA = Left Pulmonary Artery; LUL = Left Upper Lobe; MPA = Main Pulmonary Artery; RPA = Right Pulmonary Artery; RUL = Right Upper Lobe

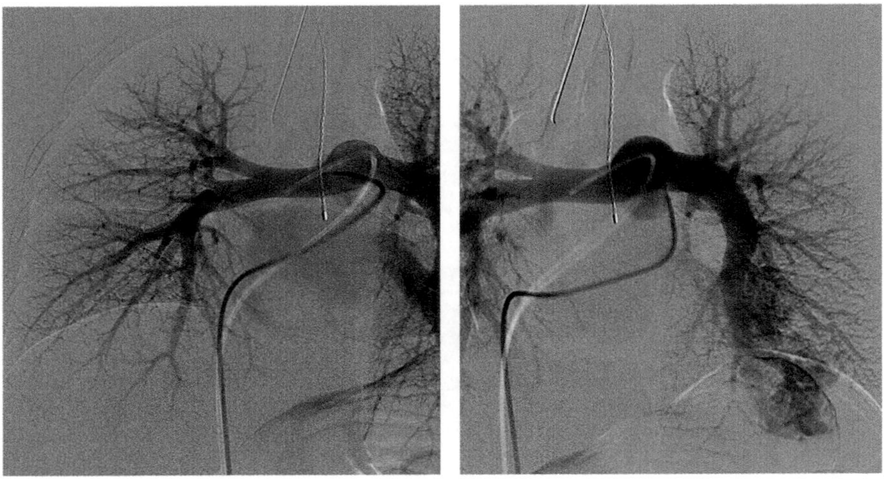

Fig. 2 Pulmonary artery digital subtraction angiography

anatomical variants can be clearly identified at angiography, provided that the patient can comply with breath holding during filming. In the context of pulmonary embolism, the extent of branch vessel involvement is used to quantify both severity and distribution. Several angiographic angulated views are required to optimally elucidate the arterial anatomy of both lungs (Fig. 2).

There are several recognized angiographic findings associated with pulmonary embolism (Table 1). It is important to distinguish between acute and chronic PE, to identify evidence of pulmonary hypertension and right heart failure.

Table 1 Angiographic findings assocaited with acute and chronic pulmonary embolism

Condition	Angiographic findings
Acute pulmonary emboli (Fig. 3)	Intraluminal filling defect Abrupt vessel cutoff Abrupt vessel diameter transition Absent vessel(s) Slow flow Absent venous drainage Parenchymal oligemia Pulmonary hypertension (direct measurement)
Chronic pulmonary emboli	Enlarged central arteries Webs/stenosis Proximal/peripheral pulmonary artery occlusions Pulmonary hypertension (direct measurement)

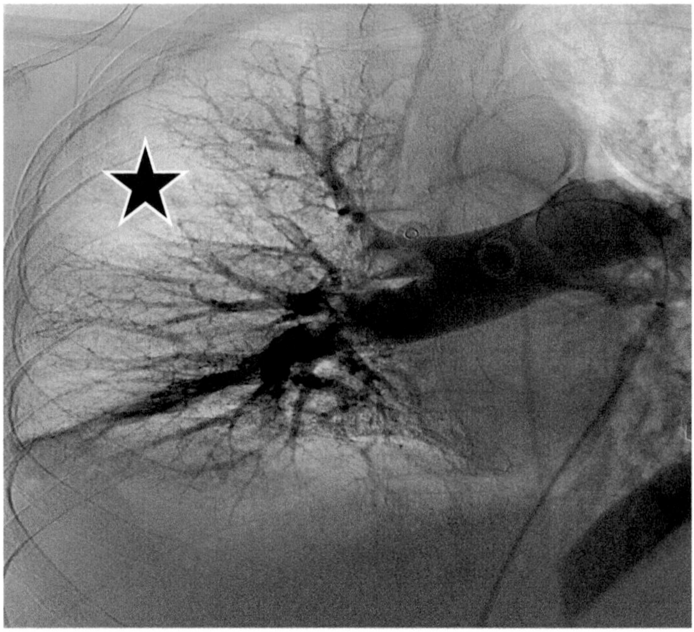

Fig. 3 Digital subtraction pulmonary angiography via a transfemoral approach in a patient with acute sub-massive PE, using a "pigtail" catheter located in the right pulmonary artery. Numerous partially occlusive intra luminal filling defects are seen in both upper and lower lobe arteries together with and area of absent perfusion and vessel occlusion in the upper lobe (star)

3 Indications for Catheter Pulmonary Angiography

A variety of pathological entities involving the pulmonary arteries can be accurately and safely diagnosed using pulmonary angiography. However, with a few notable exceptions, pulmonary angiography is largely reserved for catheter directed intervention or for direct measurement or monitoring of pulmonary arterial parameters.

A detailed list of indications and examples of CPA are outlined in Table 2 and are shown in Figs. 4, 5 and 6.

4 Contraindications (Relative) to Catheter Pulmonary Angiography

First ask two questions:

1. Is the procedure necessary?
2. What is the alternative?

Table 2 Indications for diagnostic pulmonary angiography and intervention

Condition	Indication & examples	Catheter intervention
Acute/chronic PE	Pre-operative evaluation Follow up after intervention	Catheter directed therapy Fibrinolysis, thrombectomy, angioplasty
Pediatric cardiovascular disorders	Congenital heart disease, post-operative (Definition of anatomic/physiological parameters)	Catheter directed therapy
Pulmonary artery tumor	Sarcoma (Fig. 4a, b) Diagnosis/treatment	Direct endovascular tumor biopsy Pulmonary artery stenting
Vasculitis	Takayasu arteritis, Bechet's disease	Angioplasty and stenting Embolization
Pulmonary artery stenosis	Post transplantation, congenital, tumor, fibrosis, vasculitis, others	Angioplasty, stenting
Pseudo-aneurysm/ arteriovenous fistula	Massive hemoptysis (Rasmussen aneurysm), traumatic, mycosis	Embolization
Arteriovenous malformation	HHT, sporadic (Fig. 5) Hemorrhage, paradoxical embolism, deoxygenation	Embolization
Foreign body embolization	Central venous catheter, venous implants (Fig. 6a–c)	Foreign body retrieval
Pulmonary artery aneurysm	Hemorrhage	Embolization

For clinically indicated procedures there are several relative contraindications.

Firstly, left bundle branch block (LBBB) requires temporary pacing in order to prevent possible complete heart block if right bundle branch block (RBBB) occurs during the procedure. Secondly, severe right heart failure, for example in the context of acute massive or sub massive PE, may be exacerbated if large volumes of iodinated contrast agent are directly injected into the pulmonary circulation. In this situation reduction of contrast volumes may allow safe angiography whilst obtaining images of diagnostic quality.

Thirdly, life threatening hypersensitivity to iodine-based contrast material and lastly severe pulmonary hypertension are also considered to be contraindications.

However, when the procedure is deemed to be necessary, appropriate patient preparation and intra procedural monitoring, in the presence of an anesthesiology team, is mandatory.

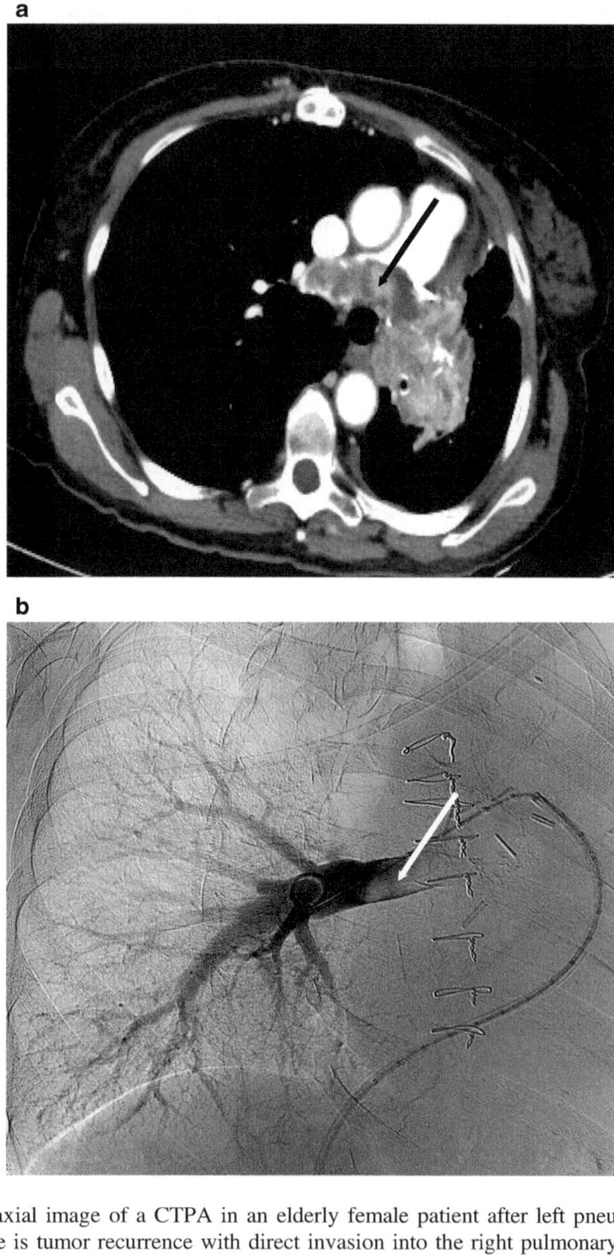

Fig. 4 **a** An axial image of a CTPA in an elderly female patient after left pneumonectomy for sarcoma. There is tumor recurrence with direct invasion into the right pulmonary artery (arrow). **b** Pulmonary angiography in the same patient shows a large filling defect (recurrent sarcoma) in the right pulmonary artery (arrow). During the procedure the pressure gradient across the lesion (proximal and distal vessel) was measured, before and after stent insertion to improve pulmonary artery perfusion

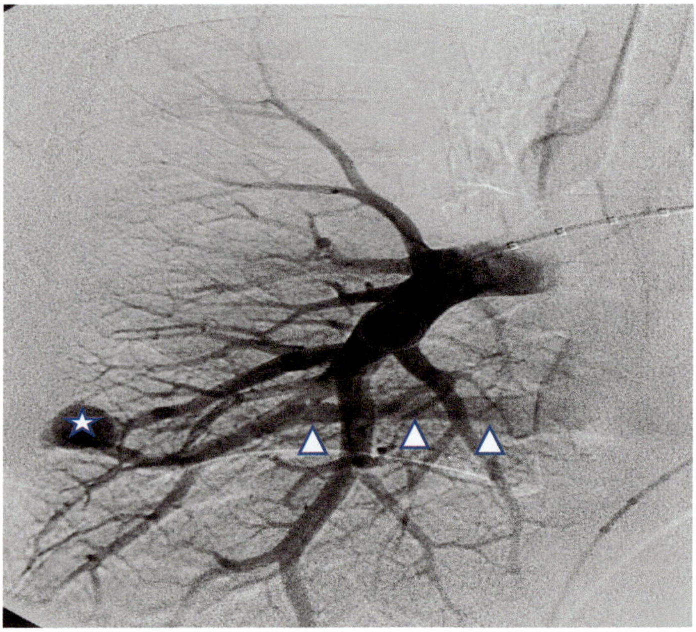

Fig. 5 Digital subtraction angiography of the right lower lobe pulmonary artery via a transfemoral approach, using a "pigtail" catheter. A pulmonary arteriovenous malformation is seen with a feeding artery, aneurysmal dilatation (star) and an early draining vein (arrow heads). Selective embolization was performed

5 Patient Preparation and Technique

As with any intervention it is crucial to explain to the patient (together with family members if relevant) why the procedure is being performed, what to expect during the procedure and what is the expected outcome?

5.1 Flow Chart

1. Review the medical history and existing imaging (CTA/MRI etc.)
2. Patient preparation:
    a. Fasting (conscious sedation or general anesthesia may be required)
    b. IV hydration especially if renal failure is present
    c. Pre-medication if iodinated contrast sensitivity is known or suspected
    d. Written informed consent with appropriate documentation in the patient record.

a

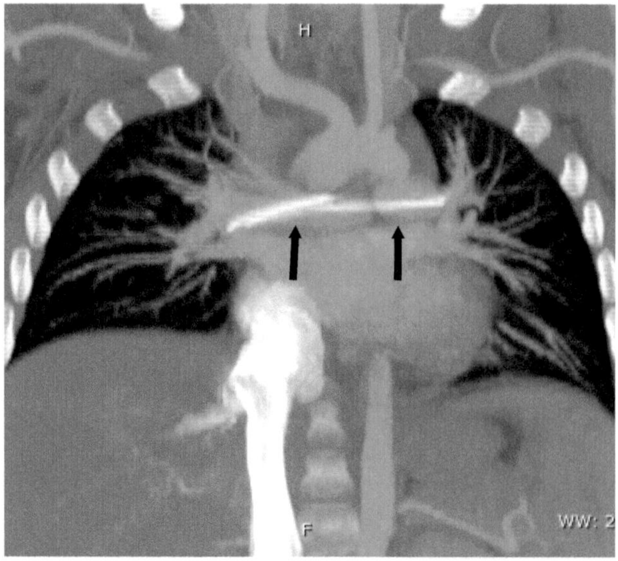

b

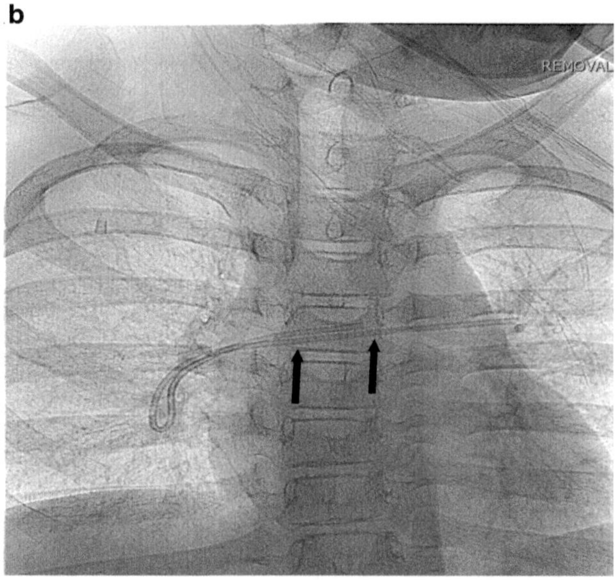

Fig. 6 **a** Coronal reconstructed CTPA shows a foreign body (detached central venous catheter) located across the left and right pulmonary arteries (arrows). **b** Fluoroscopic image of the chest acquired prior to direct pulmonary angiography showing the catheter (foreign body) location (arrows). **c** Foreign body retrieval shows the detached catheter (arrow), together with a guiding catheter inserted via a transfemoral venous approach crossing the right atrium,ventricle and main pulmonary artery, with it's tip located in the proximal right pulmonary artery . The foreign body was removed using a snare device

c

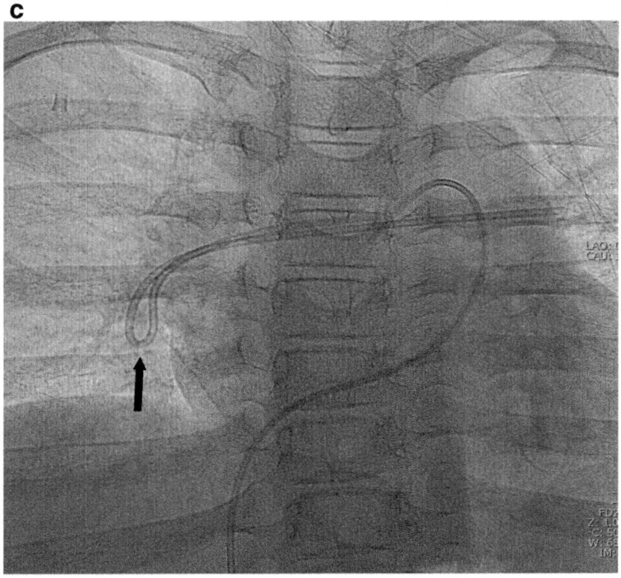

Fig. 6 (continued)

3. Planning venous access: there are three commonly used alternatives for access, trans-femoral (most common), trans-jugular or via an upper arm vein (basilica/ brachial/cephalic). The common femoral vein is often preferred due to its' size, compressibility and "straight line" approach to the MPA.
4. Procedural considerations: continuous monitoring of vital signs, ECG and pulmonary artery pressure measurement are required to safely perform the procedure.
   Selection of an appropriate angulated angiographic catheter will facilitate rapid, safe placement in the MPA. A specialized catheter of at least 6-French diameter is required. It should have multiple distal side holes so that high volume, high pressure contrast injection can be safely performed. Additional catheters may be required to selectively catheterize right or left pulmonary arteries, or lobar/ segmental branches as indicated.
5. Contrast agents: It is important to use non-ionic iodinated contrast with an adequate iodine concentration (350 mgl/ml) in order to both acquire diagnostic images as well reducing the risk of contrast reaction and right heart failure.
6. Pulmonary arterial pressure measurement: normal PA pressure ranges between 15 and 30 mmHg. Severe hypertension (≥ 70 mmHG) is considered to be a contraindication for high volume contrast injection. Reduction in pulmonary arterial hypertension is direct physiological evidence of effective treatment of pulmonary embolism.

7. Imaging requirements: High quality angiographic machines with digital subtraction and non-subtracted imaging, rapid film rates (4–6/second or higher) together with power injectors that can administer 20–30 ml/s of contrast are necessary. Image post processing capability may be very helpful in elucidating areas of uncertainty. Additional angulated, selected or magnified views of specific regions may be required to confirm findings.

6 Complications and Anticipated Outcome of Catheter Pulmonary Angiography

The risks of CPA were shown to be sufficiently low in prior publications [5–7] in order to justify it as a diagnostic tool in the appropriate clinical setting. Serious complications from this procedure are rare. Mortality occurred in 0.3–2%. Non-fatal major complications such as respiratory distress (CPR or intubation), renal failure requiring dialysis, access site complications requiring transfusion of at least two units blood, wire/catheter complications (perforation) have been reported in 5%. Minor complications including nausea, vomiting, narcotic overdose, arrhythmia with spontaneous conversion or prompt response to drug therapy, urticaria, itching or periorbital edema, renal dysfunction/hypotension/pulmonary congestion responding to medications/fluids and minor access site hematoma are reported in 5% [5]. Overall the complication rate of CPA is higher in patients with marked pulmonary hypertension (≥ 60 mmHg) when compared to patients with moderate pulmonary hypertension [6].

In experienced hands, the technical success rate of diagnostic CPA approaches 100%.

References

1. Moore AJE, Wachsmann J, Chamarthy MR, Panjikaran L, Tanabe Y, Rajiah P. Imaging of acute pulmonary embolism: an update. Cardiovasc Diagn Ther. 2018;8:225–43.
2. Crummy AB, Strother CM, Mistretta CA. The history of digital subtraction angiography. J Vasc Interv Radiol. 2018;29:1138–41.
3. PIOPED Investigators. Value of the ventilation/perfusion scan in acute pulmonary embolism. Results of the prospective investigation of pulmonary embolism diagnosis (PIOPED). JAMA. 1990;263:2753–9.
4. Stein PD, Fowler SE, Goodman LR, Gottschalk A, Hales CA, Hull RD, Leeper KV Jr, Popovich J Jr, Quinn DA, Sos TA, Sostman HD, Tapson VF, Wakefield TW, Weg JG, Woodard PK, Investigators PI. Multidetector computed tomography for acute pulmonary embolism. N Engl J Med. 2006;354:2317–27.
5. Stein PD, Athanasoulis C, Alavi A, Greenspan RH, Hales CA, Saltzman HA, Vreim CE, Terrin ML, Weg JG. Complications and validity of pulmonary angiography in acute pulmonary embolism. Circulation. 1992;85:462–8.

6. Hofmann LV, Lee DS, Gupta A, Arepally A, Sood S, Girgis R, Eng J. Safety and hemodynamic effects of pulmonary angiography in patients with pulmonary hypertension: 10-year single-center experience. AJR Am J Roentgenol. 2004;183:779–86.
7. Nicod P, Peterson K, Levine M, Dittrich H, Buchbinder M, Chappuis F, Moser K. Pulmonary angiography in severe chronic pulmonary hypertension. Ann Intern Med. 1987;107:565–8.

Integrating Clinical, Laboratory and Imaging Tests in the Diagnosis of Pulmonary Embolism

Neville Berkman

A diagnosis of an acute venous thromboembolic event (VTE) requires evaluation of risk factors and integration of clinical and laboratory tests.

1 Clinical Presentation

Clinical presentation of acute pulmonary embolism (PE) is usually non-specific and depends on extent of PE and the presence of preexisting cardiac and respiratory disease. Acute PE is not infrequently identified coincidentally, particularly when distal or sub-segmental. In a series of 1880 cases of confirmed PE, the most common symptoms were dyspnea (50%), pleuritic chest pain (39%), signs of DVT (unilateral extremity swelling) (24%), cough (23%), substernal chest pain (15%), fever (10%), hemoptysis (8%), syncope (6%) and unilateral leg pain (6%) [1, 2]). Hypotension or shock is a relatively infrequent presentation of acute PE and suggests more severe disease. 17.3% of patients presenting to the emergency room with syncope had PE [3], although a subsequent meta-analysis found this number to be much lower [4].

Findings on physical examination are also non-specific and, like presenting symptoms, vary according to extent of PE. Tachycardia, tachypnea (>20 breaths per minute) are frequent. Their presence predicts severity of PE and their absence reduces the likelihood of this diagnosis. Signs of acute pulmonary hypertension, including tricuspid incompetence, accentuated P2 and signs of right ventricular failure suggest more severe PE. Findings over the lungs are variable, and may be normal. There may be reduced air entry, crackles or wheezes.

N. Berkman (✉)
Institute of Pulmonary Medicine, Hadassah-Hebrew University Medical Center, Jerusalem, Israel
e-mail: neville@hadassah.org.il

E. Herzog (ed.), *Pulmonary Embolism*,
https://doi.org/10.1007/978-3-030-87090-4_9

Hypoxemia is frequent, but normal arterial oxygen saturation (SaO_2) is not unusual (40%) [5]. Hypocapnia, respiratory alkalosis and widened alveolar-arterial gradient are also often present.

Findings on standard chest X-ray are non-specific, and may show the presence of consolidation, pleural effusion, enlarged pulmonary arteries, elevated hemi-diaphragm, atelectasis, focal oligemia or cardiomegaly. More specific finding include a normal chest x-ray, presence of a peripheral wedge shaped infiltrate and Hampton's hump (dome shaped pleural-based pulmonary opacification) [6].

Electrocardiographic changes are common, especially T wave inversion and ST segment abnormalities. Signs of right ventricular strain, such as right axis deviation and right bundle branch block may be present. The classical S1Q3T3 pattern is uncommon and non-specific. Atrial fibrillation is the most common arrhythmia, atrial or ventricular premature beats are common.

2 Evaluation of Clinical Probability

The first essential step in all algorithms for the diagnosis of acute PE is assessment of clinical probability for this diagnosis. This step involves evaluation of risk factors for VTE, clinical history, physical examination and evaluation of basic (and non-specific) tests.

Several prediction scores are widely used in clinical practice, however empirical clinical judgement, although less reproducible and quantifiable, is probably as good as prediction scores [7]. Likelihood for VTE increases with an increase in the number of risk factors; nevertheless, no identifiable predisposing factor is present in a large minority of patients with acute VTE (40%).

The most widely used prediction scores are the Wells, simplified Wells criteria and the revised Geneva scores [8–10] (Table 1). The latter has been further simplified with each criteria given a score of 1. The relative frequency of PE for each subgroup (low, intermediate, high) is similar in all the prediction scores: 8–10% for low likelihood, 30% in the intermediate or moderate probability groups an 65–75% in the high probability groups. Several studies have validated these prediction scores and comparative studies have found them to have similar accuracy [7].

More recent publications have made attempts to better identify patients in whom PE can be excluded with a high level of confidence and without the need to perform CT. Using the "Pulmonary embolism Rule-out criteria (PERC)" was found to be non-inferior to standard approaches in ruling out PE, but reduced the number of CTs performed from 23 to 13%. PERC criteria include 8 variables: age < 50, pulse rate < 100, oxygen saturation $> 94\%$, absence of leg swelling, hemoptysis, recent trauma or surgery, previous VTE, oral hormone use [11].

Table 1 Prediction scores for acute pulmonary embolism

Wells Criteria		Clinical probability		
Clinical symptoms of DVT (leg swelling, pain on palpation)	3.0	**Wells criteria**		
Other diagnosis less likely than PE	3.0	High	>6.0	
Heart rate > 100	1.5	Moderate	2.0–6.0	
Immobilization ($\geq$3 days) or recent surgery (last 4 weeks)	1.5	Low	<2	
Previous DVT or PE	1.5			
Hemoptysis	1.0	**Modified wells criteria**		
Malignancy	1.0	PE likely	>4.0	
		PE unlikely	$\leq$4.0	
Geneva Score		**Revised Geneva score**		**Simplified Geneva**
Previous DVT or PE	2	Age > 65	1	1
Heart rate > 100	1	Previous DVT or PE	3	1
Recent surgery	3	Recent surgery or fracture (one month)	2	1
Age		Active malignancy	2	1
60–79	1	Unilateral lower limb pain	3	1
$\geq$ 80	2	Hemoptysis	2	1
Arterial blood gases		Heart rate:		
CO_2 (kPa)		75–94	3	1
<4.8	2	$\geq$95	5	2
4.8–5.19	1	Pain on lower limb palpation and unilateral edema	4	1
O2 (kPa)				
<6.5	4			
6.5–7.99	3			
8- 9.49	2			
9.5–10.99	1			
Chest x-ray				
Atelectasis	1			
Elevated hemi diaphragm	1			
Clinical probability		**Clinical probability**		
Three—level score		**Three—level score**		
Low	0–4	Low	0–3	0–1
Intermediate	2–6	Intermediate	4–10	2–4

(continued)

Table 1 (continued)

Wells Criteria		Clinical probability		
High	≥ 9	High	≥ 11	≥ 5
		Two—level scores		
		PE-unlikely	0–5	0–2
		PE- likely	≥ 6	≥ 3

3 D-Dimer Testing

D-dimer is a simple and widely available blood test that has a high sensitivity but low specificity for PE. Cumulative sensitivity is 97% and specificity is 39%. It is thus useful to exclude but not to diagnose PE. D-dimer testing is of little value in hospitalized patients or patients post-surgery where the false positivity for the test is expected to be high.

Use of a highly sensitive D-dimer assay is recommended. Several quantitative ELISA (enzyme-linked immunosorbent assay) assays are commercially available and have a diagnostic sensitivity of >95%. "On-the-spot" D-dimer tests are available, but are less sensitive [12] (88%) and therefore suitable for clinical settings where pretest probability for PE is expected to be low.

D-dimer should not be used alone to diagnose PE and a positive test should be followed by imaging. D-dimer testing is not recommended in patients with high clinical probability for PE as a negative test is not enough to rule out this diagnosis.

An age-adjusted approach for determining the upper limit of normal for D-dimer is now standard practice. D-dimer tends to increase with age resulting in progressively lower specificity for this test when a fixed cut-off approach is used. In the "ADJUST-PE" study, the upper limit for D-dimer was adjusted for age: 500ug/L in patients younger than 50 years of age and age multiplied by 10 for older patients. Patients with age adjusted normal D-dimer and non-high or low clinical probability were followed for three months without undergoing CTPA or receiving anticoagulants. Of 2898 patients with a non-high or unlikely clinical probability for PE, 337 patients had D-dimer over 500 but below age-adjusted cut off normal values. Only one failure (PE) was observed (0.3%). Using this method in patients over age 75, PE was excluded in 29.7% of cases as compared to only 6.4% of cases for a fixed cutoff of 500 ug/L [13].

4 Computerised Tomography Pulmonary Angiography (CTPA) and Ventilation-Perfusion Scintigraphy

CTPA and ventilation-perfusion scintigraphy are the most important diagnostic tests for acute PE. The diagnostic value, advantages and indications for each depends on the clinical circumstances as detailed below (see "Integration")

5 Further Investigations

Additional diagnostic studies that have a role in the diagnosis of acute PE include echocardiography, MRI and ultrasound duplex of the lower limbs. Pulmonary angiography is no longer recommended for the diagnosis of PE, but is frequently performed prior to balloon angioplasty and when catheter directed thrombolysis is considered [14].

5.1 Lower Limb Ultrasonography

This is the study of choice in suspected deep vein thrombosis (DVT) but for patients with suspected PE, lower limb ultrasonography has low diagnostic sensitivity (41%) and is therefore reserved for cases in which CTPA cannot be performed [15]. This test has a place in pregnant patients with suspected PE and in patients with clinical signs suggestive of DVT.

5.2 Magnetic Resonance Imaging

The diagnostic value of MRI for the diagnosis of acute PE is limited by a relatively low sensitivity. In a meta-analysis of 1170 patients, sensitivity was 80.9% with a specificity of 96.4% [16].

5.3 Echocardiography

Bedside transthoracic echocardiography is recommended in patients with suspected acute PE and hemodynamic instability. Echocardiography is essential for the diagnosis of chronic thromboembolic pulmonary hypertension. For acute PE, echocardiography has sensitivity of only 29–52% and specificity of 86–97%. Specificity is reduced in patients with comorbidities. The presence of the '60/60' sign (pulmonary ejection acceleration time measured in the RV outflow tract <60 ms together with a peak systolic tricuspid valve gradient <60 mmHg) or with McConnell sign (reduced contractility of the right ventricular free wall compared to the apex) is suggestive of PE but has low sensitivity for this diagnosis. Echocardiography in suspected acute PE is of use in patients who cannot undergo CTPA or VQ scan, especially in an intensive care setting. It is an important modality to assess severity and to help decide on treatment, particularly in intermediate-high risk patients. Enlarged and impaired RV function, particularly RV/LV ratio $\geq$ 1 and TAPSE < 1.6 predict severity and mortality in PE [17].

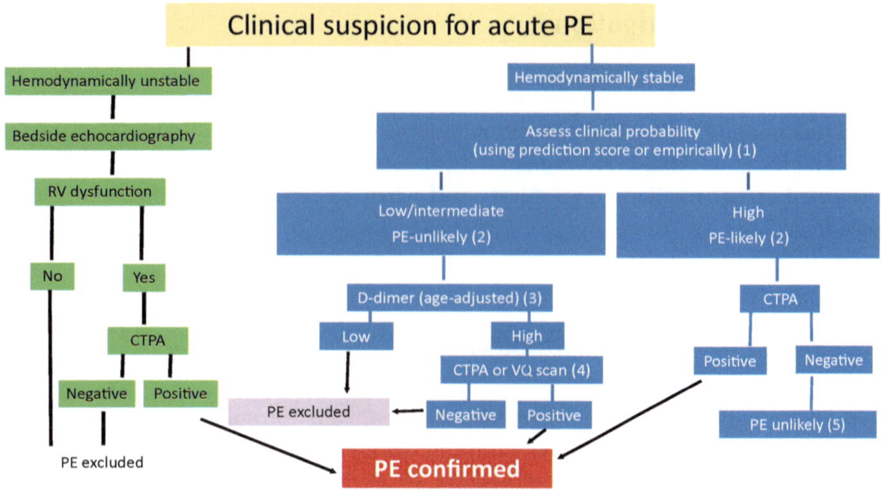

Fig. 1 Flow chart for the diagnosis of acute pulmonary embolism. (1) Assessment of clinical probability according to prediction scores, most commonly simplified Wells criteria or revised or simplified Geneva scores or by empiric clinical assessment. (2) Low or intermediate when low, intermediate and high probability scores are used, PE-likely or unlikely when dichotomous scores are used. PERC criteria may be used in low prevalence groups. (3) Different D-dimer cut-offs may be used according to clinical criteria. (4) CTPA is usually preferred (unless there is renal dysfunction, iodine sensitivity, pregnancy), Ventilation-perfusion scintigraphy is an alternative in patients with low clinical suspicion for PE. SPECT scintigraphy is preferred to planar radionuclide imaging. (5) Additional imaging may be considered when CTPA is negative in patients with high clinical probability

6 Integration (Fig. 1)

The first consideration in all diagnostic algorithms for acute suspected PE is whether the patient is hemodynamically stable. Unstable patients require bedside echocardiography, and if there is evidence of right ventricular dysfunction, CTPA should be performed.

For hemodynamically stable patients, clinical probability evaluation is assessed using a prediction score as detailed above. Validity of scores needs to take the population being evaluated into account. For example, PERC rule out is only valid in a patient cohort with low incidence or likelihood of PE (<5%). The clinical probability assessment is used to decide whether to proceed to testing for D-dimers or to proceed directly to chest imaging. Current recommendations are that patients with low and intermediate clinical probability with a three-level prediction score and PE-unlikely score for two-level scores should perform D-dimer testing. High probability / PE-likely patients should not perform D-dimer testing but should be referred directly for an imaging study [18–22]. For dichotomous cut-off prediction scores (PE-unlikely vs. PE-likely), patients with PE-unlikely scores have a likelihood of around 12% for PE, while those who are PE-likely have a probability of PE of 30%. This work-scheme results in a high number of patients without PE who will undergo imaging.

In an attempt to reduce the number of unnecessary CTs performed for diagnosis of PE, several recent studies have attempted to use variable D-dimer cut-off values, depending on clinical probability parameters. In the YEARS study, 3465 patients were evaluated for pulmonary embolism. Management was based on assessment of the YEARS clinical decision rule (three items: clinical signs of DVT, hemoptysis and whether PE is the most likely diagnosis) and D-dimer concentration. Patients with no YEARS criteria and D-dimer <1000 ng/ml and those with one or more YEARS criteria and D-dimer <500 ng/ml were followed without performing CTPA. CTPA was performed in all other patients. At three months follow-up, this approach was found to be safe with 0.61% occurrence of VTE. This algorithm resulted in a reduction of 14% in the number of CT scans performed at diagnosis (48% did not undergo CT with the YEARS approach vs. 34% who would have not undergone CT with standard diagnostic approach) [23].

In another study performed in outpatients in Canada, 2017 patients with suspected PE were managed according to clinical pretest probability: for low probability, D-dimer cut off was 1000 ng/ml, for moderate probability, a cut-off of 500 ng/ml was used. This approach reduced the number of CT scans performed to 34.3% (vs. an estimate of 51.9% if a uniform cutoff of 500 ng/ml had been applied) [24].

Patients undergoing diagnostic evaluation for PE, with "high" or "PE-likely" clinical probability and those with elevated D-dimer values should perform imaging. The European Society of Cardiology/ European Respiratory Society (ESC/ ERS) guidelines recommends that the imaging study of choice is computerized tomography with pulmonary angiography (CTPA) with a sensitivity of at least 83% and specificity of 96% for the diagnosis of PE. In selected cases, perfusion lung scan may be used as an alternative (allergy to contrast dye, abnormal renal function) [14]. The American Society of Hematology recommends VQ scan as the preferred initial imaging test in population with positive initial D-dimer test and low (<5%) and intermediate (20%) pretest probability/prevalence for PE (<5%). This recommendation is "to limit radiation exposure for patients likely to have a diagnostic scan". This is relevant in centers where VQ testing is available and have expertise for test interpretation [18]. SPECT is the preferred imaging technique for perfusion scanning. In a meta-analysis of 5923 patients from 19 studies, ventilation/perfusion SPECT and CTPA were found to have similar performance, and both were superior to planar VQ imaging [25].

ESC/ERS guidelines give a high grade recommendation (IA) that a normal CTPA can be used to rule out a diagnosis of PE in low or intermediate probability patients and that a segmental or proximal filling defect can be considered diagnostic for PE in patients with intermediate or high clinical probability (IB). There is lack of clarity as to whether patients with isolated subsegmental defects need further evaluation. There is also doubt as to whether patients in whom clinical probability and imaging are discordant should be sent for further imaging tests, specifically high clinical probability with normal CTPA [14].

In summary, a diagnosis of acute pulmonary embolism requires integration of clinical, laboratory and imaging tests and consideration of risk factors for thromboembolic disease. Clinical probability prediction scores, such as modified Wells or revised Geneva scores are widely used. D-dimer testing is recommended in patients with low or intermediate clinical probability, but should not be performed in high probability patients. Age adjusted D-dimer and variable D-dimer cut-off values according to presence of risk factors are recommended as they reduce the number of unnecessary imaging tests. High clinical probability patients and those with elevated D-dimer values should perform an imaging study, usually computerized tomography pulmonary angiography (CTPA) or a radionuclide ventilation/perfusion scan.

References

1. Pollack CV, Schreiber D, Goldhaber SZ, Slattery D, Fanikos J, O'Neil BJ, Thompson JR, Hiestand B, Briese BA, Pendleton RC, Miller CD, Kline JA. Clinical characteristics, management, and outcomes of patients diagnosed with acute pulmonary embolism in the emergency department: initial report of EMPEROR (Multicenter Emergency Medicine Pulmonary Embolism in the Real World Registry). J Am Coll Cardiol. 2011;57:700–6.
2. Miniati M, Prediletto R, Formichi B, Marini C, Di Ricco G, Tonelli L, Allescia G, Pistolesi M. Accuracy of clinical assessment in the diagnosis of pulmonary embolism. Am J Respir Crit Care Med. 1999;159:864–71.
3. Prandoni P, Lensing AWA, Prins MH, Ciammaichella M, Perlati M, Mumoli N, Bucherini E, Visona A, Bova C, Imberti D, Campostrini S, Barbar S. Prevalence of pulmonary embolism among patients hospitalized for syncope. N Engl J Med. 2016;375:1524–31.
4. Oqab Z, Ganshorn H, Sheldon R. Prevalence of pulmonary embolism in patients presenting with syncope. A systematic review and meta-analysis. Am J Emerg Med. 2018;36(4):551–5.
5. Rodger MA, Carrier M, Jones GN, Rasuli P, Raymond F, Djunaedi H, Wells PS. Diagnostic value of arterial blood gas measurement in suspected pulmonary embolism. Am J Respir Crit Care Med. 2000;162:2105–8.
6. Elliott CG, Goldhaber SZ, Visani L, DeRosa M. Chest radiographs in acute pulmonary embolism. Results from the International Cooperative Pulmonary Embolism Registry. Chest. 2000;118:33–8.
7. Penaloza A, Verschuren F, Meyer G, Quentin-Georget S, Soulie C, Thys F, Roy PM. Comparison of the unstructured clinician gestalt, the wells score, and the revised Geneva score to estimate pretest probability for suspected pulmonary embolism. Ann Emerg Med. 2013;62:117–24.
8. Wells PS, Anderson DR, Rodger M, Ginsberg JS, Kearon C, Gent M, Turpie AG, Bormanis J, Weitz J, Chamberlain M, Bowie D, Barnes D, Hirsh J. Derivation of a simple clinical model to categorize patients' probability of pulmonary embolism: increasing the models utility with the SimpliRED D-dimer. Thromb Haemost. 2000;83:416–20.
9. Douma RA, Gibson NS, Gerdes VE, Buller HR, Wells PS, Perrier A, Le Gal G. Validity and clinical utility of the simplified Wells rule for assessing clinical probability for the exclusion of pulmonary embolism. Thromb Haemost. 2009;101:197–200.
10. Douma RA, Mos IC, Erkens PM, Nizet TA, Durian MF, Hovens MM, van Houten AA, Hofstee HM, Klok FA, ten Cate H, Ullmann EF, Bu¨ller HR, Kamphuisen PW, Huisman MV; Prometheus Study Group. Performance of 4 clinical decision rules in the diagnostic

management of acute pulmonary embolism: a prospective cohort study. Ann Intern Med. 2011;154:709–18.
11. Freund Y, Cachanado M, Aubry A, Orsini C, Raynal PA, Feral Pierssens AL, Charpentier S, Dumas F, Baarir N, Truchot J, Desmettre T, Tazarourte K, Beaume S, Leleu A, Khellaf M, Wargon M, Bloom B, Rousseau A, Simon T, Riou B. Effect of the pulmonary embolism rule out criteria on subsequent thromboembolic events among low risk emergency department patients. JAMA. 2018;319:559–66.
12. Geersing GJ, Janssen KJ, Oudega R, Bax L, Hoes AW, Reitsma JB, Moons KG. Excluding venous thromboembolism using point of care D-dimer tests in outpatients: a diagnostic meta-analysis. BMJ. 2009;339:2990.
13. Righini M, Van Es J, Den Exter PL, Roy PM, Verschuren F, Ghuysen A, Rutschmann OT, Sanchez O, Jaffrelot M, Trinh-Duc A, Le Gal C, Moustafa F, Principe A, Van Housten AA, Ten Wolde M, Douma RA, Hazelaar G, Erkens MG, Van Kralingen KW, Grootenboers MJJH, Durian MF, Cheung W, Meyer G, Bounameaux H, Huisman MV, Kamphuisen PW, Le Gal G. Age-adjusted D-Dimer cutoff levels to rule out pulmonary embolism. JAMA. 2014;311:1117–24.
14. Konstantinides SV, Meyer G, Becattini C, Bueno H, Geersing G-J, Harjola V-P, Huisman MV, Humbert M, Sian Jennings C, Jimenez D, Kucher N, Marthe Lang I, Lankeit M, Lorusso R, Mazzolai L, Meneveau N, Ni F, Prandoni P, Pruszczyk P, Righini M, Torbicki A, Van Belle E, Luis ZJ. 2019 ESC guidelines for the diagnosis and management of acute pulmonary embolism, developed in collaboration with the European respiratory society. Eur Heart J. 2019;00:1–61.
15. Da Costa Rodriues J, Alzuphar S, Combescure C, Le Gal G, Perrier A. Diagnostic characteristics of lower limb venous compression ultrasonography in suspected pulmonary embolism: a meta-analysis. J Thromb Haemost. 2016;14:1765–72.
16. Squizzato A, Pomero F, Allione A, Priotto R, Riva N, Huisman MV, Klok FA, Stein PD, Guasti L, Fenogliob L, Dentali F, Ageno W. Diagnostic accuracy of magnetic resonance imaging in patients with suspected pulmonary embolism: a bivariate meta-analysis. Thromb Res. 2017;154:64–72.
17. Kurnicka K, Lichodziejewska B, Goliszek S, Dzikowska-Diduch O, Zdonczyk O, Kozlowska M, Kostrubiec M, Ciurzynski M, Palczewski P, Grudzka K, Krupa M, Koc M, Pruszczyk P. Echocardiographic pattern of acute pulmonary embolism: analysis of 511 consecutive patients. J Am Soc Echocardiogr. 2016;29:907–13.
18. Patel P, Patel P, Bhatt M, Braun C, Begum H, Wiercioch W, Varghese J, Wooldridge D, Alturkmani H, Thomas M, Baig M, Bahaj W, Khatib R, Kehar R, Ponnapureddy R, Sethi A, Mustafa A, Lim W, Le Gal G, Bates SM, Haramati LB, Kline J, Lang E, Righini M, Kalot MA, Husainat NM, Al Jabiri YN, Schunemann HJ, Mustafa RA. Systematic review and meta analysis of test accuracy for the diagnosis suspected pulmonary embolism. Blood Adv. 2020;4:4296–310.
19. Simon MA, Tan C, Hilden P, Gesner L, Julius B, Effectiveness of clinical decision tools in predicting pulmonary embolism. Pulm Med. 2021;Article 8880893:1–5.
20. Kline JA, Diagnosis and exclusion of pulmonary embolism. Thromb Res. 2018;163:207–20.
21. Herzog E, Elbaz-Greener G, Planer D, Koren T, Amir O, Shapiro J, Kalish Y, Pathway for the diagnosis management of pulmonary embolism. Crit Pathw Cardiol. 2021;20:57–62.
22. Tritschler T, Kraaijpoel N, Le Gal G, Wells PS. Venous thromboembolism Advances in diagnosis and treatment. JAMA. 2018;320:1583–94.
23. Van der Hulle T, Cheung WY, Kooij S, Beenrn L FM, Van Bemmel T, Van Es J, Faber LM, Hazelaar GM, Heringhaus C, Hofstee H, Hovens M MC, Kaasjager K AH, Van klink R CJ, Kruip M JHA, Loeffen RF, Mairuhun A TA, Middeldorp S, Nijkeuter M, Van der pol LM, Schol-Gelok S, Wolde MT, Klok FA, Huisman MV. Simplified diagnostic management of suspected pulmonary embolism (the YEARS study): a prospective, multicenter, cohort study. Lancet. 2017;390:289–97.
24. Kearon C, De Wit Cerstin, Parpia s, Schulman S, Afilado M, Hirsch A, Spencer FA, Sharma S, Daragon F, Deshaies JF, Le Gal G, Lazo-Langner A, Wu C, Rudd-Scott L,

Bates SM, Julian JM, Math M, Diagnosis of pulmonary embolism with D–Dimer adjusted to clinical probability. N Engl J Med. 2019;381:2125–34.

25. Phillips JJ, Straitonb J, Staff RT. Planar and SPECT ventilation/perfusion imaging and computed tomography for the diagnosis of pulmonary embolism: a systematic review and meta-analysis of the literature, and cost and dose comparison. Eur J Radiol. 2015;84:1392–400.

Management of the High-Risk Pulmonary Embolism in the Acute Phase—Respiratory, Hemodynamic and Mechanical Support

Asaf Schwartz, Marc Romain, Eyal Herzog, and Sigal Sviri

1 Introduction

Venous thromboembolism (VTE), the combined syndrome of Deep Venous Thrombosis (DVT) and Pulmonary Embolism (PE), is the third most common cause of cardiovascular syndrome encountered in the acute care setting, following acute myocardial ischemia and stroke [1]. It is estimated that VTE is responsible for nearly 1.2 million cases in the United States every year, with 370,000 cases being Pulmonary Embolism (PE) [2]. The patient presenting with high-risk PE (formerly called massive PE) poses difficult challenges to the caretaker. By definition, these patients suffer from hemodynamic instability and require hemodynamic support while planning and executing care designed to prevent end organ damage. Additionally, high-risk PE also creates a severe ventilation/perfusion mismatch, causing hypoxemia, and further exacerbating the severe hemodynamic compromise caused by hypoxic vasoconstriction. While plans are being made to manage these patients with systemic thrombolysis or catheter directed therapy, and while care is being delivered, it is the intensivist's role to maintain the basic life functions of the patient.

The definition of high-risk PE requires the presence of hemodynamic instability. This instability can be manifested in several ways [1]—presentation with cardiac arrest, the presence of obstructive shock (systolic BP of less than 90 mmHg, or the need for vasopressors to maintain systolic BP over 90 mmHg, in face of adequate fluid loading) or persistent hypotension (Systolic BP less than 90 mmHg or systolic BP drop over 40 mmHg, lasting longer than 15 min and not caused by new-onset

A. Schwartz · M. Romain · S. Sviri (✉)
Medical Intensive Care Unit, Division of Medicine, Hadassah Ein Kerem University Hospital, Jerusalem, Israel
e-mail: sigals@hadassah.org.il

E. Herzog
Department of Cardiology, Hadassah Ein Kerem University Hospital, Jerusalem, Israel

E. Herzog (ed.), *Pulmonary Embolism*,
https://doi.org/10.1007/978-3-030-87090-4_10

arrhythmia, hypovolemia, or sepsis) [1]. The main pathophysiology of the hemodynamic compromise in high-risk PE involves a vicious cycle demonstrated in Fig. 1 [3]. Briefly, the increase in pulmonary vascular resistance causes an increase in right ventricular end—diastolic pressure (RVEDP), with septal deviation to the left, along with a decrease in right ventricular stroke volume (caused by ventricular interdependence). Together, these changes cause a decrease in the left ventricular end—diastolic volume (LVEDV) and subsequent decreased stroke volume and mean arterial pressure. Since the right ventricle is being perfused through the coronary arteries during both systole and diastole, the decreased systemic blood pressure, along with the increase in RVEDP, cause ongoing right ventricular ischemia, which causes an additional increase in RVEDP, thus creating a self-perpetuating vicious cycle, with severe progressive shock. In the following sections, we will review the ways in which the intensivist can try to attenuate this process in order to buy time for definitive care to take effect.

2 Respiratory Support

Patients with high-risk PE might present with severe hypoxemia, caused mainly by ventilation perfusion mismatch [4]. In addition to the danger caused by severe hypoxemia and tissue hypoxia, hypoxemia worsens the hemodynamic profile of high-risk PE due to hypoxic vasoconstriction. Although pulmonary embolism is usually accompanied by increased minute ventilation causing hypocapnia, sometimes decreased cardiac output causing increased physiologic dead space can induce hypercapnia, which also worsens Pulmonary Vascular Resistance (PVR). For this reason, aggressive management of hypoxemia and hypercapnia is critical in the management of these patients.

In addition to the conventional methods of oxygen supplementation (through nasal cannula or face mask), during the last few years a new tool for oxygenation was introduced—the High Flow Nasal Cannula (HFNC, Fig. 2) [5]. HFNC allows administration of extremely high flow (up to 60 L/min) of warm and humidified air, together with a high concentration of oxygen (up to 95%) to patients. This provides a non-invasive method of administering high oxygen concentration and flows, thus improving hypoxemia and decreasing the patient's work of breathing, an indirect way of improving the underlying shock.

Although many patients with high-risk PE are in severe extremis, with decreased level of consciousness and impaired gas exchange, the use of endotracheal intubation (ETI) and positive pressure ventilation (PPV) in these patients is problematic. ETI can cause a decrease in cardiac output and mean arterial pressure secondary to administration of induction agents, and PPV can further increase PVR, both of them can worsen the high-risk PE vicious cycle described above. This process was demonstrated in a series of 52 patients undergoing emergent pulmonary embolectomy for high-risk PE [6], 19% of them developing refractory hemodynamic collapse leading to CPR and need for emergent cardiopulmonary

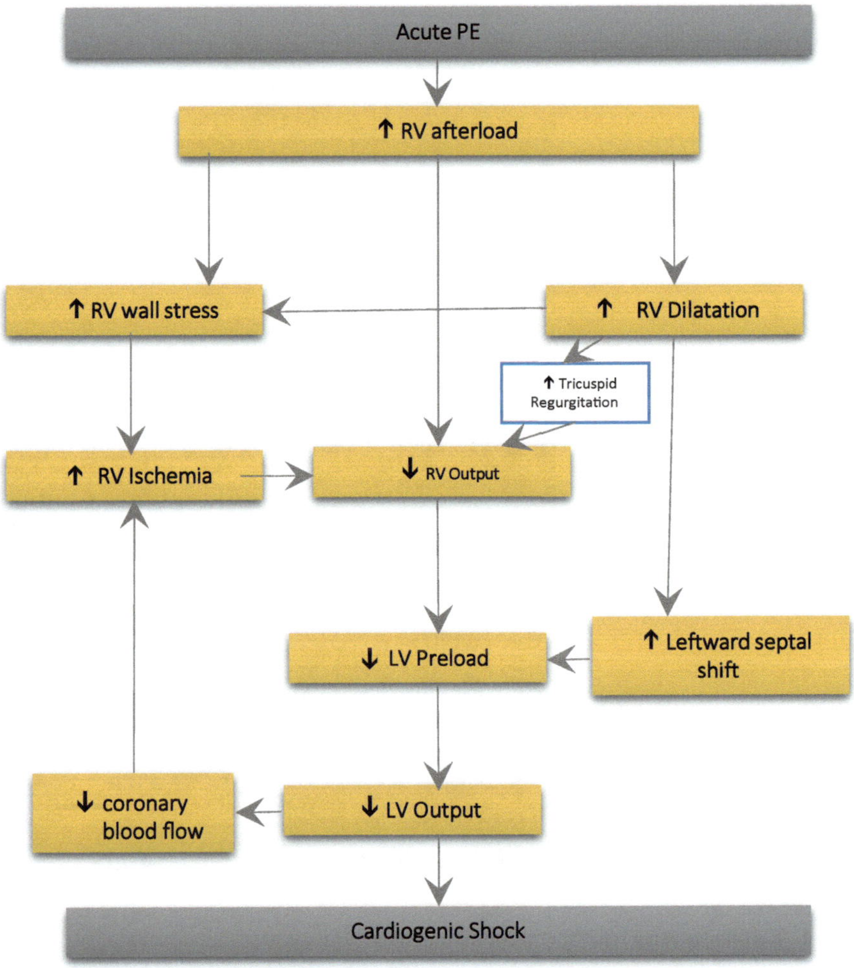

Fig. 1 Right ventricular failure vicious cycle

bypass initiation. The risk for deterioration was not increased by patient's risk factors, hemodynamic status prior to induction, choice of induction agents or location of the blood clot within the pulmonary vascular tree and/or the presence of intra-cardiac blood clots. A series of patients with severe pulmonary hypertension (not necessarily secondary to high-risk PE) demonstrated good outcomes with awake fiberoptic intubation [7], although attempting this in patients with high-risk PE can sometimes be impossible due to diminished consciousness and lack of cooperation. In conclusion, it is recommended to focus on the following principles when intubating high-risk PE patients (Table 1) [3].

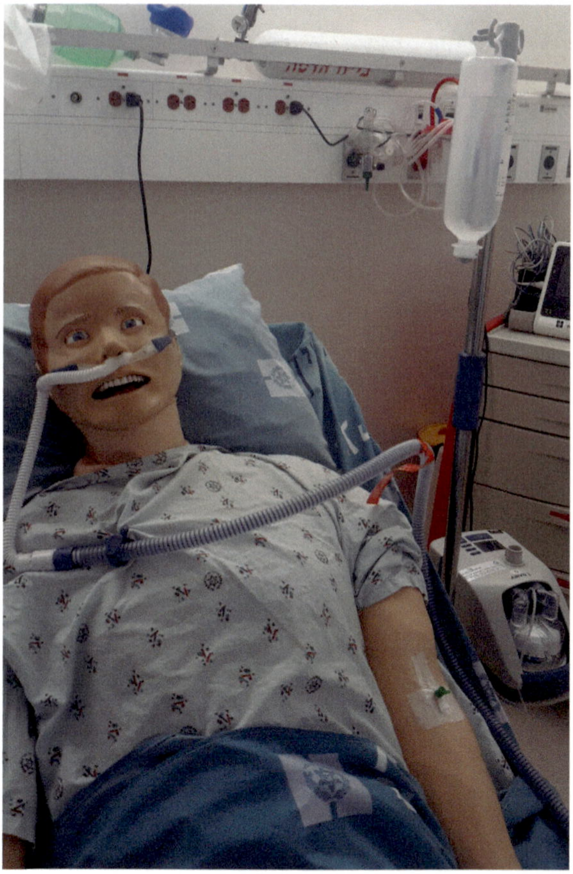

Fig. 2 High flow nasal canula

Table 1 Recommendations for Intubation in high-risk PE patients

Pitfalls	How to overcome the pitfalls
Preventing Systemic Hypotension During Induction	Choosing Etomidate or Ketamine as induction agents
	Optimizing blood pressure with vasopressors before induction
Minimizing hypoxemia during intubation	Using Apneic Oxygenation, performance of intubation by the most skilled provider
Preventing abrupt increases in PVR during positive pressure ventilation	Maintaining normal PaO_2 and $PaCO_2$, using the lowest possible PEEP, using tidal volumes of 6–8 ml/kg to prevent atelectasis and overdistention

1. Use of induction agents with minimal cardioinhibitory or vasoplegic effects (i.e., etomidate and ketamine)
2. Optimize systemic blood pressure prior to induction, with use of vasopressors (i.e., noradrenaline, phenylephrine)
3. Optimize oxygenation and ventilation as possible prior to induction—use of HFNC for apneic oxygenation, minimize apneic pauses during induction of anesthesia
4. The practice of lung protective ventilation—avoiding both excessive and diminished tidal volumes in order to prevent overdistention or atelectasis respectively, and the use of the lowest possible PEEP that maintains proper oxygenation without compromising hemodynamics.

3 Hemodynamic Support

As mentioned earlier, the definition of high-risk PE entails hemodynamic instability [1]. Classically, the management of the patient in profound shock was based on three pillars—judicious fluid resuscitation, inotrope/vasopressor support and correction of the underlying cause. In recent years, a new modality was added to the intensivist's tool box—Extra—Corporeal Life Support, which encompasses the use of Extra—Corporeal Membranous Oxygenation (ECMO) and Mechanical Circulatory Support (MCS), with their different modes of utilization.

3.1 Fluid Management

The administration of fluids for the resuscitation of patients in shock is common and prevalent, especially since it is the most available tool for the clinician at the bedside. In a study by Mercat et al., the use of fluids in patients with high-risk PE was studied in 13 patients with angiographically proven PE with low cardiac index [8]. 400 ml of colloids were infused over 20 min to each patient, with ongoing invasive measurement of hemodynamic parameters. It was shown that fluid loading caused an increase in right ventricular end—diastolic volume index and cardiac index, with no change in right ventricular ejection fraction and pulmonary vascular resistance. The increase in cardiac index was inversely correlated with baseline right ventricular end—diastolic volume index. These findings are in contrast to a previous study done on canines, showing that in a model simulating an acute increase in pulmonary vascular resistance, the infusion of fluids was associated with a decrease in stroke volume and mean blood pressure [9]. This decrease was in contrast with the effect of noradrenaline administration to the dogs. As described earlier, part of the vicious cycle of acute RV failure includes a shift of the inter-ventricular septum to the left, as a result of increased right ventricular afterload, and as can be inferred, the excessive administration of fluids can worsen the cycle. It is therefore accepted today that modest amounts (100–250 ml) of fluid should be administered to patients with low right ventricular filling pressures as a stabilizing measure. Since the direct measurement of right atrial pressure is not feasible in the absence of a central venous catheter, the use of bedside echocardiography is of paramount importance, with evaluation of fluid responsiveness through assessment of cardiac output response to Passive Leg Raise (PLR) test or assessment of IVC diameter (in non-ventilated patients), prior to fluids administration [10].

3.2 Pharmacological Support—Vasopressor and Inotrope support

An important part of the vicious cycle of RV failure is RV ischemia, caused by an increase in RVEDP and PAP relative to mean arterial pressure (MAP). Therefore, increasing the SVR/PVR ratio can counteract this process, and help breaking the cycle. The main way in which this can be reached with the use of vasopressors. Inotropic support can be used to enhance RV contractility, and thus improve LV filling [3]. In this section, we will discuss the ways in which pharmacological support can help the intensivist to stabilize the high-risk PE patient.

3.2.1 Vasopressors

The purpose of vasopressors in high-risk PE is to increase SVR and eventually MAP and prevent RV ischemia. Noradrenaline is the main vasopressor recommended for use in patients with high-risk PE [1, 3], and its use has been demonstrated to be efficacious in several animal models [9, 11–13]. Although the use of noradrenaline is associated with an increase in PVR as well as SVR, the effect on the systemic circulation is more pronounced, thus causing a net increase in SVR/PVR ratio. Noradrenaline's mild beta-adrenergic effect might also improve RV function, and that effect was also demonstrated in a case report of a patient supported with adrenaline infusion for shock caused by high-risk PE [13]. The use of phenylephrine was also suggested as a vasopressor, although the pure alpha agonist nature of this medication is associated with decreased cardiac output [11, 13]. The use of vasopressin is also potentially beneficial in high-risk PE, as vasopressin causes a net increase in SVR, with no effect over the PVR, albeit little experience exists regarding its use in high-risk PE, and the absence of inotropic effect might also cause a decrease in cardiac output eventually [14].

3.2.2 Inotropes

The use of inotropes for management of shock in patients with high-risk PE is secondary to the use of vasopressors, and is mainly aimed at resolving a low cardiac output state, after blood pressure had been stabilized [3]. As mentioned above, adrenaline can be used for stabilization of patients thanks to its combined vaso-pressor and inotropic effects. Experience with the use of dopamine as an inotrope had shown a positive effect over cardiac output, however, its use was limited by high prevalence of tachyarrhythmias present with its use [13]. The main inotrope used for cardiac output support in patients with high-risk PE is dobutamine [1, 3]. Dobutamine was shown to improve right ventricular—pulmonary artery coupling and to decrease PVR in addition to improvement of cardiac output [15]. Due to dobutamine's mild beta 2—adrenergic effect, its use may cause systemic hypotension, however, using it in addition to noradrenaline usually prevents this unwanted side effect. The use of dobutamine was associated with a decrease in PaO_2, probably due to abolished pulmonary hypoxic vasoconstriction, nevertheless, oxygen delivery was shown to improve, probably secondary to the improvement in cardiac output [15]. In addition to the previously described agents, novel agents that are aimed at improving cardiac output while simultaneously decreasing vascular resistance (so called 'inodilators') were also considered in high-risk PE, although present guidelines do not recommend using them. Milrinone, a Phosphodiesterase inhibitor, and Levosimendan, a calcium-sensitizing agent, were shown to improve cardiac output and decrease PVR with relative mild effect over SVR, with relative low occurrence of arrhythmias compared to other inotropic agents [16, 17]. It is important to remember that the use of catecholamines for hemodynamic support is frequently accompanied by worsening tachycardia, and a high potential for developing atrial fibrillation, with loss of right atrial—right ventricular synchrony and loss of the atrial kick. These undesired phenomena are deleterious to right ventricular systolic function, and can additionally worsen RV ischemia due to unwanted tachycardia and increased oxygen demand [3, 18].

3.2.3 Pulmonary Vasodilators

Although it was shown already that the most effective way of reducing PVR in high-risk PE patients is to decrease the clot burden, the option of reducing PVR pharmacologically was studied as well in order to relieve the failing right ventricle. Since the increase in PVR is not solely due to the clot burden, but also due to release of vasoactive agents from platelets, such as serotonin and thromboxane [3], it is the entire pulmonary vascular bed that causes an increased resistance, and not just the part occluded by a clot. Most studies that tried to use vasodilators had failed, mostly due to a greater effect over the SVR compared with PVR (with isoproterenol as the most widely studied agent) [13]. Later, attempts were made to try to assess vasodilators that possess higher affinity to the pulmonary circulation. A single study that tested the use of intravenous Epoprostenol had failed to demonstrate a

Table 2 Recommendations for hemodynamic support in high-risk PE patients

Hemodynamic goal	Intervention and key points
Maintaining normal filling pressure	Judicious fluid resuscitation, avoiding pressure overload that would cause decreased LV stroke volume
Maintaining normal systemic blood pressures	Using noradrenaline mainly to maintain adequate systemic blood pressures and prevent RV ischemia
Improving cardiac output	Using dobutamine in addition to noradrenaline to maintain cardiac output and prevent systemic hypoperfusion
Reducing PVR	Using iNO in ventilated patients to decrease PVR and assist weaning of pressors

significant effect over usual treatment in patients with PE [19]. The most appealing agent aimed at selective reduction of PVR is inhaled nitric oxide (iNO). NO is an endogenous vasodilator, working through enhancement of Guanylate Cyclase activity, and an increase in levels of cGMP. This increase causes protein kinase activation, with subsequent decrease in intra—cellular calcium levels, and de—phosphorylation of myosin light chains, causing arterial relaxation. The use of iNO, which has a very short half—life, is also beneficial by causing a correction of ventilation—perfusion mismatch in patients. Finally, NO also has anti platelet aggregation activity, further attenuating the inflammatory reaction caused by platelet activation [20, 21]. The use of iNO was described in several case reports as an adjunct in the care of patients with high-risk PE, when administered to intubated patients [20, 21]. Unfortunately, no large-scale study has been conducted thus far in patients with high-risk PE showing improvement with the use of iNO. The essentials of hemodynamic support for high-risk PE patients are summarized in Table 2.

4 Extracorporeal Membrane Oxygenation (ECMO) and Mechanical Circulatory Support (MCS)

In the past few years, a new and exciting tool was added to the intensivist's toolkit for the stabilization of shock caused by high-risk PE. Extracorporeal Membrane Oxygenation (ECMO), a tool originally developed for the support of neonates with respiratory distress syndrome, has emerged as a new way of stabilizing high-risk PE patients, which is being increasingly used. Mechanical Circulatory Support (MCS), a general name for both percutaneously and surgically inserted devices for the support of the right and/or left ventricle, also gains favor for the support of high-risk PE patients, while definitive treatment for the underlying problem is pursued.

4.1 ECMO

The use of ECMO in patients with high-risk PE is meant to allow off-loading of the failing right ventricle and provide adequate perfusion regardless of LV function. The vast majority of ECMO are done on high-risk PE patients used Veno—Arterial ECMO (VA—ECMO, Fig. 3). Although several case series published had shown a benefit for the use of ECMO in high-risk PE patients, no prospective trial testing its effectiveness has thus far been published [1]. Most of the information available to us is from case reports and case series only. An early systematic review of 78 patients had shown a favorable prognosis for patients with high-risk PE undergoing ECMO, with 70% overall survival, with most patients undergoing systemic thrombolysis in addition to ECMO. No correlation between the adjunct therapy used for high-risk PE and increased risk of death was shown. Fifty percent of the patients had undergone ECMO as part of cardio—pulmonary resuscitation (CPR) efforts, with 50% survival in these patients [22]. In a large retrospective study from France that looked at 52 patients undergoing VA—ECMO for high-risk PE, 25% had VA—ECMO initiated for refractory cardiogenic shock, and 75% had VA—ECMO initiated after cardiac arrest, almost half of them were initiated as part ECMO CPR (eCPR) [23]. Adjunct interventions for high-risk PE included systemic fibrinolysis (38% of patients), surgical embolectomy (27% of patients) and anti—coagulation only (35% of patients). They were compared to 128 patients who did not undergo ECMO for high-risk PE. In spite of ECMO patients being younger, and less likely to present with cardiac arrest, 30 days mortality in the ECMO group was higher (61.5% vs. 43% in the no ECMO group), and so was the risk of 90 days bleeding (38.5% vs. 6.3%). Only 19 patients (36.5%) were successfully weaned from ECMO. Among the ECMO group, the best outcome was seen in patients undergoing ECMO as part of a strategy that included surgical embolectomy (with no difference between patients undergoing ECMO prior to, or after surgery)—30-day mortality of 29.4% versus 76.5% and 77.7% in patients undergoing thrombolysis and anticoagulation only, respectively. The worst outcome was seen in patients undergoing ECMO alone during CPR, with 30 days mortality of 91%. Due to the retrospective nature of the study, it is obvious that the ECMO group consisted of highly selected patients, with severe disease on presentation and poor outcome. Most of them were recruited after failed thrombolysis and therefore suffered a significant amount of bleeding complications. The authors conclude that VA—ECMO is best utilized as part of a reperfusion strategy that includes surgical embolectomy, and recommend against using VA—ECMO as a stand—alone treatment for high-risk PE. This study showed higher risk of bleeding among those undergoing VA—ECMO along with surgical embolectomy or thrombolysis compared to VA—ECMO alone, although no statistical significance was found. It is important to note that this study did not include patients undergoing catheter directed therapy (CDT), a treatment that is gaining popularity and involves lower doses of fibrinolytics agents, with decreased risk of bleeding. A recent single center case series from Massachusetts General Hospital [24] included 13 patients, with a

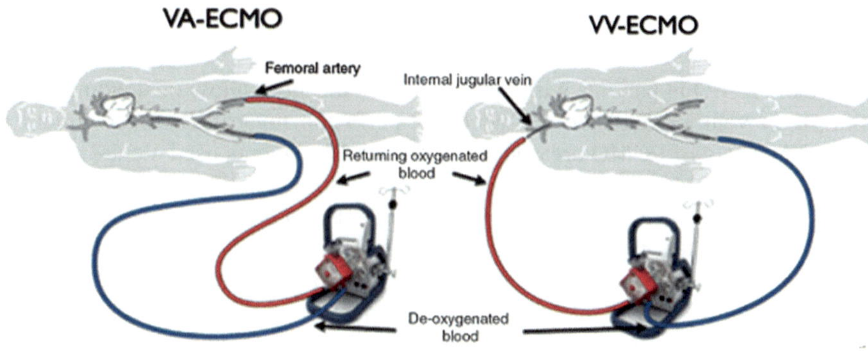

Fig. 3 Veno—arterial extracorporeal membrane oxygenation

mean age of 49. All patients had presented with cardiac arrest, and all of them received VA—ECMO, with 3 of them undergoing central VA—ECMO. Eleven (11) patients had undergone thrombolysis, 8 of them undergoing systemic thrombolysis, and 3 undergoing catheter directed thrombolysis. Four (4) patients had undergone surgical embolectomy, with half of them undergoing this as a rescue procedure after failed systemic thrombolysis. At 30 days, there was 31% mortality, with this number growing to 54% at 1 year. Echocardiogram done at 30 days had shown significant improvement in RV function in 77% of patients. The decision to go on ECMO was made by a PE Response Team (PERT) in all cases, a trend that is gradually evolving around the world for the management of high- and intermediate-risk PE. Once again, the most common complication seen was major bleeding, occurring in 54% of patients. In conclusion, it seems that ECMO is a viable option as bridge therapy for patients with high-risk PE, either before or after a definitive treatment aimed at reducing clot burden. The use of ECMO is accompanied by high risk for major bleeding, and is not recommended as a stand—alone therapy for high-risk PE. ECMO is a treatment option for patients with high-risk PE who have undergone cardiac arrest, and need support after return of spontaneous circulation, or those who are undergoing ECMO cannulation during CPR, in centers capable of doing so.

4.2 MCS

MCS, both surgically and percutaneously implanted, has recently offered clinicians an additional tool in the management of cardiogenic shock, in order to buy the patient time, while definitive care is being administered. In this section, we will focus on the use of percutaneously implanted MCS. The use of MCS in patients with high-risk PE is anecdotal at this point, and is based on case reports only. The use of Impella RP, which is capable of delivering flow of up to 4 L/min is described in three patients in the literature [25, 26]. In the described cases, Impella RP was inserted through the femoral vein, and the inflow segment was located at the proximal inferior vena cava, with a flexible cannula traversing the right atrium, tricuspid valve, and right ventricle, to reach the outflow segment that is placed under fluoroscopic guidance in the pulmonary artery. Impella RP was used in addition to catheter directed thrombolysis in the cases mentioned, and was in place for 2–5 days. All three patients had shown hemodynamic improvement during the use of the device, and recovered from the initial event. Another case report [27] describes the use of Tandem Heart for the support of cardiogenic shock in a patient with high-risk PE that failed initial attempt of care with systemic thrombolysis. For rescue, an intake cannula was inserted through the femoral vein into the inferior vena cava—right atrium junction, and the outflow cannula was inserted through the contralateral femoral vein into the pulmonary artery. Catheter directed thrombolysis was initiated in order to dissolve the remaining clots. Support was given for 6 days, after which the device was removed, and due to findings of DVT in both legs, an inferior vena cava filter was placed. The patient survived without any sequela. Unlike ECMO, the use of MCS is capable of delivering support to the right ventricle directly, and at a reduced risk of bleeding, due to the use of venous access only. Due to the approach via the femoral veins, the presence of deep vein thrombosis has to be taken into account when considering these devices. In conclusion, percutaneously inserted MCS is a reasonable option for hemodynamic support in patients with high-risk PE, and should be seriously considered in patients with high-risk PE and high bleeding risk.

5 Cardiac Arrest Management

High-risk PE patients may present initially as survivors of cardiac arrest. The recent guidelines for the management of cardiac arrest in patients with suspected/proven high-risk PE do not differ from other patients [1]. In patients with cardiac arrest due to pulmonary embolism, the most useful initial test is bedside transthoracic echocardiography (TTE). The bedside TTE will show evidence of significant acute RV dysfunction if acute PE is the cause of the patient's cardiac arrest. In a highly unstable patient, who cannot be mobilized to CT angiography, TTE evidence of RV dysfunction is sufficient to prompt initiation of anticoagulation with heparin and initiation of reperfusion strategy without further testing. In centers where computed tomography pulmonary angiogram (CTPA) is immediately available and feasible, a diagnosis of PE should be confirmed before proceeding to a reperfusion strategy. Management of these patients should take place in an intensive care unit (ICU) setting.

Several issues should be noted in these cases: (1) Primary reperfusion is the treatment of choice for patients with high-risk PE and can be achieved by thrombolysis and/or embolectomy. Thrombolysis can be achieved by a systemic treatment or preferably by a catheter directed therapy. In patients undergoing CPR, the use of systemic thrombolysis should be considered, with the administration of a bolus of 0.6 mg/kg of tPA intravenously over 15 min, to a maximal dose of 50 mg. After the administration of tPA, it is recommended to continue CPR for at least 60 min, in order to allow the medication to work and alleviate the clot burden. (2) The use of ECMO during or after CPR while definitive therapy is given, for hemodynamic support is an option for patients during or after cardiac arrest [22, 23]. (3) Following the reperfusion treatment or preferably during the therapy, the patient should be started on therapeutic hypothermia, nowadays termed "Targeted temperature management" (TTM). The use of this technology was somewhat refrained from in high-risk PE patients, mainly due to concerns regarding bleeding complications [28]. However, several brief case reports have shown that the use of TTM in cardiac arrest survivors with high-risk PE is not associated with

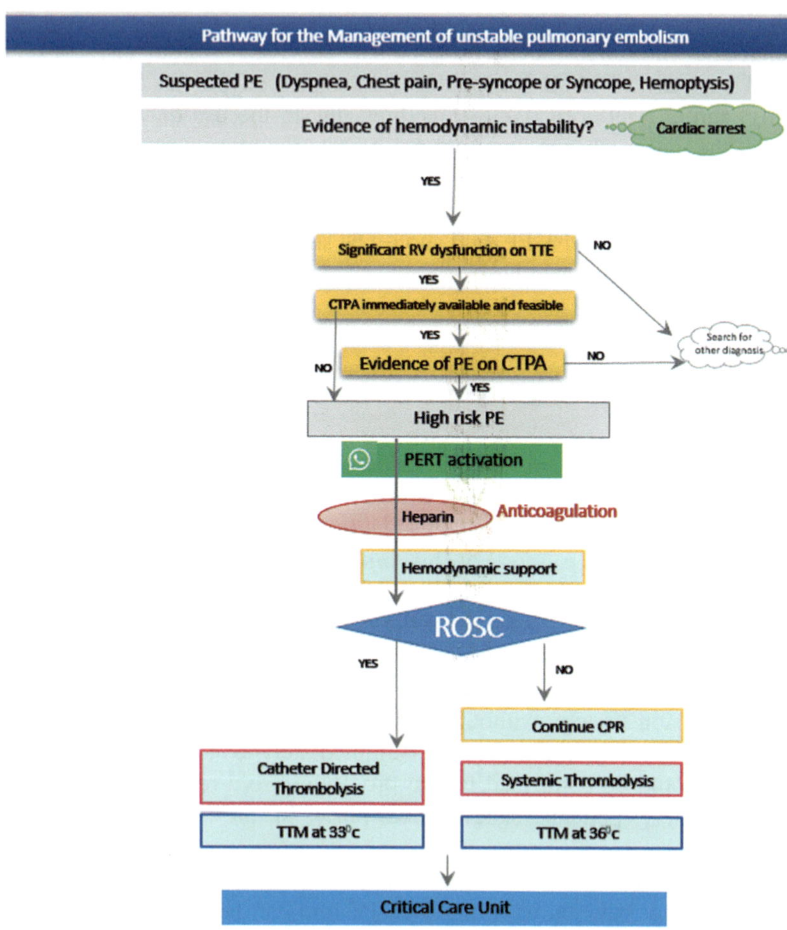

Fig. 4 Clinical pathway for managing the unstable high-risk PE patient

more bleeding events [29, 30], and should be considered in selected cases. A cooling protocol of target temperature of 32–36 °C should be initiated for a cooling duration time of 24 h and a slow rewarming protocol to 37 °C. A maintenance phase at 37 °C should then be taken for additional 24–48 h. The key question regarding the mode of reperfusion and the temperature dose of TTM is the "Restoration of spontaneous circulation". For patients in whom we were not able to restore spontaneous circulation, we recommend to continue CPR and to treat the patient with systemic thrombolysis. The TTM dose with restoration of spontaneous circulation should be at 36 °C to prevent bleeding complications. For patients in whom spontaneous circulation was restored, we recommend using low dose thrombolysis by catheter directed therapy, and the TTM dose should be at 33 °C.

A suggested clinical pathway for managing the unstable high-risk PE patient is shown in Fig. 4.

References

1. Konstantinides SV, Meyer G. 2019 ESC Guidelines for the diagnosis and management of acute pulmonary developed in collaboration with the European Respiratory Society (ERS). Eur Heart J. 2020;41:543–603.
2. Virani SS, et al. Heart Disease and stroke statistics—2021 update a report from the American Heart Association. Circulation. 2021;143:e00–e00.
3. Zhao S, Friedman O. Management of right ventricular failure in pulmonary embolism. Crit Care Clin. 2020;36:505–15.
4. Santolicandro A, Prediletto R, Fornai E, Formichi B, Begliomini E, Giannella-Neto A, Giuntini C. Mechanisms of hypoxemia and hypocapnia in pulmonary embolism. Am J Respir Crit Care Med. 1995;152(1):336–47.
5. Lacroix G, Pons F, D'Aranda E, Legodec J, Romanat PE, Goutorbe P. High-flow oxygen, a therapeutic bridge while awaiting thrombolysis in pulmonary embolism? Am J Emerg Med. 2013;31:463.e1–463.e2.
6. Rosenberger P, Shernan SK, Shekar PS, Tuli JK, Weissmüller T, Aranki SF, Eltzschig HK. Acute hemodynamic collapse after induction of general anesthesia for emergent pulmonary. Anesth Analg. 2006;102:1311–5.
7. Johannes J, Berlin DA, Patel P, Schenck EJ, West FM, Saggar R, Barjaktarevic IZ. A technique of awake bronchoscopic endotracheal intubation for respiratory failure in patients with right heart failure and pulmonary hypertension. Crit Care Med. 2017;45(9):e980–4.
8. Mercat A, Diehl JL, Meyer G, Teboul JL, Sors H. Hemodynamic effects of fluid loading in acute massive pulmonary embolism. Crit Care Med. 1999;27(3):540–4.
9. Ghignone M, Girling L, Prewitt RM. Volume expansion versus norepinephrine in treatment of a low cardiac output complicating an acute increase in right ventricular afterload in dogs. Anesthesiology. 1984;60(2):132–5.
10. Vieillard-Baron A, Naeije R, Haddad F, Bogaard HJ, Bull TM, Fletcher N, Lahm T, Magder S, Orde S, Schmidt G, Pinsky MR. Diagnostic workup, etiologies and management of acute right ventricle failure. Intensive Care Med. 2018;44:774–90.
11. Hirsch LJ, Rooney MW, Wat SS, Kleinmann B, Mathru M. Norepinephrine and phenylephrine effects on right ventricular function in experimental canine pulmonary embolism. Chest. 1991;100(3):796–801.
12. Molloy WD, Lee KY, Girling L, Schick U, Prewitt RM. Treatment of shock in a canine model of pulmonary embolism. Am Rev Respir Dis. 1984;130(5):870–4.

13. Layish DT, Tapson VF. Pharmacologic hemodynamic support in massive pulmonary embolism. Chest. 1997;111(1):218–24.
14. Gordon AC, Wang N, Walley KR, Ashby D, Russell JA. The cardiopulmonary effects of vasopressin compared with norepinephrine in septic shock. Chest. 2012;142(3):593–605.
15. Manier G, Castaing Y. Influence of cardiac output on oxygen exchange in acute pulmonary embolism. Am Rev Respir Dis. 1992;145:130–6.
16. Ventetuolo CE, Klinger JR. Management of acute right ventricular failure in the intensive care unit. Ann Am Thorac Soc. 2014;11(5):811–22.
17. Kerbaul F, Gariboldi V, Giorgi R, Mekkaoui C, Guieu R, Fesler P, Gouin F, Brimioulle S, Collart F. Effects of levosimendan on acute pulmonary embolism-induced right ventricular failure. Crit Care Med. 2007;35:1948–54.
18. Goldstein JA, Harada A, Yagi Y, Barzilai B, Cox JL. Hemodynamic importance of systolic ventricular interaction, augmented right atrial contractility and atrioventricular synchrony in acute right ventricular dysfunction. J Am coll cardiol. 1990;16:181–9.
19. Kooter AJ, Ijzerman RG, Kamp O, Boonstra AB, Smulders YM. No effect of epoprostenol on right ventricular diameter in patients with acute pulmonary embolism: a randomized controlled trial. BMC Pulm Med 2010;10.
20. Szold O, Khoury W, Biderman P, Klausner JM, Halpern P, Weinbroum AA. Inhaled nitric oxide improves pulmonary functions following massive pulmonary embolism: a report of four patients and review of the literature. Lung. 2006;184:1–5.
21. Summerfield DT, Desai H, Levitov A, Grooms DA, Marik PE. Inhaled nitric oxide as salvage therapy in massive pulmonary embolism: a case series. Respir Care. 2012;57:444–8.
22. O'Malley TJ, Choi JH, Maynes EJ, Wood CT, D'Antonio ND, Mellado M, West FM, Galanis T, Gonsalves CF, Marhefka GD, Awsare BK, Merli GJ, Tchantchaleishvili V. Extracorporeal membrane oxygenation in acute massive pulmonary embolism: a systematic review. Perfusion. 2015;30(8):611–6.
23. Meneveau N, Guillon B, Planquette B, Piton G, Kimmoun A, Gaide-Chevronnay L, Aissaoui N, Neuschwander A, Zogheib E, Dupont H, Pili-Floury S, Ecarnot F, Schiele F, Deye N, de Prost N, Favory R, Girard P, Cristinar M, Ferré A, Meyer G, Capellier G, Sanchez O. Outcomes after extracorporeal membrane oxygenation for the treatment of high-risk pulmonary embolism: a multicentre series of 52 cases. Eur Heart J. 2018;39:4196–204.
24. Al-Bawardy R, Rosenfield K, Borges J, Young MN, Albaghdadi M, Rosovsky R, Kabrhel C. Extracorporeal membrane oxygenation in acute massive pulmonary embolism: a case series and review of the literature. Perfusion. 2019;34(1):22–8.
25. Shokr M, Rashed A, Mostafa A, Mohamad T, Schreiber T, Elder M, Kaki A. Impella RP support and catheter-directed thrombolysis. Tex Heart Inst J. 2018;45(3):182–5.
26. Kumar Bhatia N, Dickert NW, Samady H, Babaliaros V. The use of hemodynamic support in massive pulmonary embolism. Catheter Cardiovasc Interv. 2017;90:516–20.
27. Geller BJ, Morrow DA, Sobieszczyk P. Percutaneous right ventricular assist device for massive pulmonary embolism. Circ Cardiovasc Interv. 2012;5:e74–5.
28. Ko E, Lee JH, Chae MK, Lee TR, Sim MS, Shin TG, Cha WC, Jo IJ, Song KJ, Rhee JE, Jeong YK. Successful fibrinolytic and therapeutic hypothermic management of cardiac arrest following massive pulmonary embolism. Clin Exp Emerg Med. 2015;2(3):193–6.
29. Çoner A, Birtay T. Concomitant usage of thrombolytic therapy and therapeutic hypothermia in a case of sudden cardiac arrest due to massive pulmonary embolism. Turk Kardiyol Dern Ars. 2019;47(6):512–5.
30. Oami T, Oshima T, Oku R, Nakanishi K. Successful treatment of pulmonary embolism-induced cardiac arrest by thrombolysis and targeted temperature management during pregnancy. Acute Med Surg. 2018;5:292–5.

Pharmacologic Treatment of Pulmonary Embolism

Bruria Hirsh Raccah, Yosef Kalish, Refat Jabara, Eyal Herzog, and Batia Roth Jelinek

1 Introduction

Acute pulmonary embolism (PE) is a life-threatening condition with a 30 day mortality of 9–11%, and 3 months mortality of 9–17% [1].

After the initial evaluation of the clinical status of a patient with acute PE, the choice of the appropriate management depends on the estimated risk for adverse outcomes. The Pulmonary Embolism Severity Index (PESI) and simplified-PESI (sPESI) are most widely used in clinical settings and in guidelines [2–4].

During the past decade there have seen significant advances in the management of patients, including a wide variety of drugs. Different treatment choices should be individualized according to risk stratification, local protocols and local experience and expertise [2, 3].

A suggested plan for the management of a patient diagnosed with acute pulmonary embolism is presented in Chap. 1.

The timeline for treatment of PE consists of 3 stages:

1. The initial phase where the patient is evaluated for hemodynamic instability. The risk level for adverse outcome and the need for hospitalization and the initial treatment is decided accordingly: going for aggressive measures such as thrombolysis or thrombectomy or starting parenteral or oral anticoagulation.
2. The second phase usually lasts 3–6 months and consists of anticoagulation.

B. H. Raccah (✉)
Faculty of Medicine, School of Pharmacy, Institute for Drug Research, The Hebrew University of Jerusalem, Jerusalem, Israel
e-mail: Bruria.hirsh@mail.huji.ac.il

B. H. Raccah · R. Jabara · E. Herzog
Department of Cardiology, Hadassah University Hospital, Jerusalem, Israel

Y. Kalish · B. R. Jelinek
Department of Hematology, Hadassah-Hebrew University Medical Center, Jerusalem, Israel

E. Herzog (ed.), *Pulmonary Embolism*,
https://doi.org/10.1007/978-3-030-87090-4_11

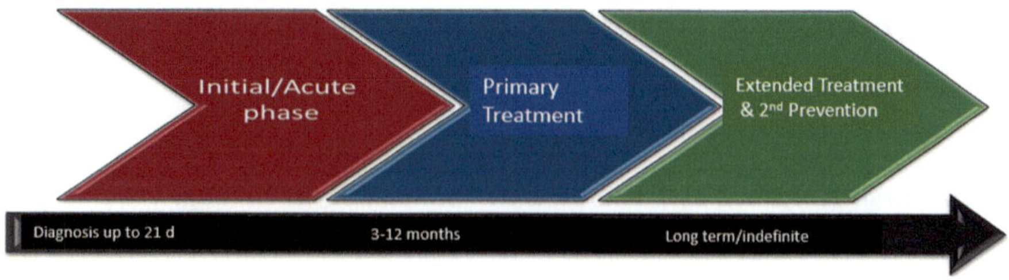

Fig. 1 Timeline of treatment of pulmonary embolism

3. After the primary treatment is completed a decision should be taken about the safety of stopping anticoagulation compared to continuing it for an extended or indefinite duration (Fig. 1).

2 Initial Treatment for Pulmonary Embolism:

Reperfusion treatment by thrombolysis:

2.1 *Systemic thrombolysis for Acute Pulmonary Embolism*

Thrombolytic therapy, either systemic or directed by a catheter into the pulmonary arteries, is a cornerstone treatment for patients with high risk PE or Intermediate high-risk PE.

Thrombolytic therapy causes rapid thrombus lysis by catalyzing the formation of plasmin. The serine protease plasmin is cleaved from the plasminogen, the insoluble fibrin is depredated by plasmin to soluble fibrinogen monomers and clot dissolution. The conversion from plasminogen to active plasmin is increased by thrombolytic agents [5].

Thrombolytic therapies are classified according to their generation and specificity to fibrin. Fibrin specific activates fibrin-bound plasminogen by binding to fibrin on the surface of the clot, whereas non-fibrin specific prompts the alteration of inactive plasminogen to active plasmin regardless the present of fibrin [5].

- First generation agents: streptokinase and urokinase.
  Streptokinase is a single chain polypeptide and not an enzyme. The protein is bounding with the proactivator plasminogen. The complex converts inactive plasminogen to active plasmin and, thus, enhances proteolytic activity. Plasminogen is concentrated in the thrombus or on its surface. Hence the action of Streptokinase occurs within the thrombus as well as on its surface.

Streptokinase is generated by h-hemolytic streptococci. Antibodies to streptokinase are common as human exposure to streptococci is prevalent. Those antibodies are responsible to the inactivation of the complex plasminogen-Streptokinase and the "fast" half-life (approximately 23 minutes) of the drug.
To overcome the presence of the antibodies, a loading dose of streptokinase is required to neutralize these antibodies.
The streptokinase antibodies also increase the risk of resistance in long treatment (above 5 days) or if second treatment is required 12 months after the first treatment. Likewise, the effect may be reduced in patients with recent streptococcal infections such as acute rheumatic fever, streptococcal pharyngitis or acute glomerulonephritis due to a streptococcal infection [6].
urokinase obtained from human neonatal kidney cells grown in tissue culture. There are two forms of urokinase differing in molecular weight but having similar clinical effects [7].

- Second generation:
Tissue plasminogen activator (tPA), manufacture by recombinant DNA technology. Alteplase is a serine protease responsible for the conversion between plasminogen to plasmin. In contrast to Streptokinase, Alteplase is "fibrin specific". Fibrin is a cofactor requires for the activation of plasminogen. Thus the activity of Alteplase is enhancing in the presence of fibrin [8]. Among the fibrin specific agents only Alteplase approved by the FDA for systemic thrombolysis in acute pulmonary embolism [8].
- Third generation:
Tenecteplase (TNK-tPA) and Reteplase are also fibrin specific agents produced by recombinant DNA technology. Both drugs undergo modification to enable them longer half-life and convenience administration. Reteplase is given in two bolus and Tenecteplase is given in a single bolus. TNK-tPA is more fibrin specific than other tPA and relative resistance to plasminogen inhibitor [5].

Tables 1, 2 and 3 outlines the current available agents worldwide.

A meta-analysis compared systemic thrombolytic therapy plus anticoagulation to anticoagulation alone in patients with acute PE. Thrombolytic therapy was associated with a significant reduction in mortality included: PE-related mortality, the combined endpoint of death or treatment escalation and overall mortality (especially in high risk PE) [9]. Thrombolytic therapy was also associated with a significant reduction in PE recurrence. This was achieved with a 9.9% rate of severe bleeding in patients allocated to thrombolytic therapy compare to 3.6% of the control group and a 1.7% rate of intracranial hemorrhage compare to 0.3% of the control group [9]. Contraindication to thrombolysis are present in Table 4 [6].

Table.1 Systemic Thrombolytic regimens type and doses

Type	Regimen	Accelerated regimen[b]	Low-dose regimen[c]	Parenteralanticoagulation	Other
Streptokinase[2,6]	250 000 IU as a loading dose over 30 min, followed by 100 000 IU/h over 12–24 h	1.5 million IU over 2 h		Continuous intravenous infusion of UFH without a loading dose, aPTT should be less than twice the normal control value before thrombolytic therapy is started	Maintenance infusion time should be extended to 72 h if concurrentdeep vein thrombosisis suspected. Administration of Streptokinase will cause marked decreases in plasminogen and fibrinogen levels and increases in TT, APTT, and PT, which usually normalize within 12–24 h. Monitor CBC, TT, aPTT, PT; at baseline, 4 h after therapy initiation
Urokinase[3,7]	4400 IU/kg as a loading dose over 10 min, followed by 4400 IU/kg/h over 12–24 h (see Table 2)	3 million IU over 2 h		Continuous intravenous infusion of UFH without a loading dose, aPTT should be less than twice the normal control value before thrombolytic therapy is started	A decrease in plasma levels of fibrinogen and plasminogen and an increase in the amount of circulating fibrin and fibrinogen degradation products may persist for 12–24 h
Alteplase [3,8]	100 mg over 2 h	0.6 mg/kg over 15 min (maximum dose 50 mg)	50 mg IV infused over 2 h	aPTT should be less than twice the normal control value before thrombolytic therapy is started. Initiate UFH immediately or near the end of alteplase infusion	Following administration of 100 mg Alteplase, there is a decrease (16–36%) in circulating fibrinogen
Retaplase[3] [a]	Double bolus (10 units each bolus, 30 min apart)			UFH 70 IU/kg bolus followed by 15 IU/kg/hr infusion for at least 48 h	Monitor CBC, TT, aPTT, PT, and fibrinogen levels at 4 and 24 h afterthrombolysis

(continued)

Table.1 (continued)

Type	Regimen	Accelerated regimen[b]	Low-dose regimen[c]	Parenteralanticoagulation	Other
Tenecteplase[3a]	A single weight-based intravenous Bolus given over a period of 5–10 s (see Table 3)			UFH infusion rate should be adjusted to achieve aPTT that will be 2.0–2.5 times the upper limit of the normal range	

aPTT activated partial thromboplastin time, *TT* thrombin time, *PT* prothrombin time, *UFH* unfractionated heparin, *CBC* complete blood count
[a]not approved by FDA
[b]not approved by FDA, can be consider in in extreme haemodynamic instability such ascardiac arrest
[c]for selected patients including those with massivePEand high-risk of bleeding (eg, body weight less than 65 kg)

Table.2 Urokinase: weight-based intravenous dosing

Patient weight (Kg)	Total dose in units (loading and continuous infusion)
37–40	2,250,000
41–45	2,500,000
46–50	2,750,000
51–54	3,000,000
55–59	3,250,000
60–64	3,500,000
65–68	3,750,000
69–73	4,000,000
74–77	4,250,000
78–82	4,500,000
83–86	4,750,000
87–91	5,000,000
92–95	5,250,000
96–100	5,500,000
101–104	5,750,000
105–109	6,000,000
110–114	6,250,000

Table.3 Tenecteplase: weight-based intravenous dosing regimen

Weight (kg)	Tenecteplase dose (mg)
<60	30
≥ 60 to <70	35
≥ 70 to <80	40
≥ 80 to <90	45
≥ 90	50

Table.4 Thrombolysis absolute and relative contraindications

Absolute contraindication
– Active or recent internal bleeding
– Recent (within 2 months) cerebrovascular accident, intracranial or intraspinal surgery
– Intracranial neoplasm
– Uncontrollable hypertension with systolic values above 200 mm Hg and/or diastolic values above 100 mm Hg, or hypertensive retinal changes Grades III/IV
– All forms of reduced blood coagulability in particular spontaneous fibrinolysis and extensive clotting disorders
– Recent head trauma
– Known neoplasm with risk of hemorrhage
– Acute pancreatitis
Streptokinase should not be administered to patients having experienced severe allergic reaction to the product
Relative contraindication
– Recent (within 10 days) major surgery
– Recent delivery, abortion
– Recent organ biopsy, previous puncture of non-compressible vessels, intramuscular injections or intubation
– Recent (within 10 days) serious gastrointestinal bleeding
– Recent (within 10 days) trauma including cardiopulmonary resuscitation
– High likelihood of left heart thrombus, e.g., mitral stenosis with atrial fibrillation

(continued)

Table.4 (continued)

– Subacute bacterial endocarditis or pericarditis; isolated cases of a pericarditis, misdiagnosed as acute myocardial infarction and treated with Streptase®, have resulted in pericardial effusions including tamponade – Hemostatic defects including those secondary to severe hepatic or renal disease – Pregnancy – Cerebrovascular disease – Pulmonary diseases with cavitation (e.g., open tuberculosis) or severe bronchitis – Severe diabetes mellitus – Diabetic hemorrhagic retinopathy – Diseases of the urogenital tract with potential sources of bleeding – Septic thrombophlebitis or occluded AV cannula at seriously infected site – Suspicion of severe artherosclerotic degeneration – Any other condition in which bleeding constitutes a significant hazard or would be particularly difficult to manage because of its location

2.2 Local Thrombolysis

The catheters directed therapy (CDT) are used for local thrombolysis treatment as well as for mechanical or ultrasound fragmentation and thrombus aspiration, with in situ reduced-dose thrombolysis.

Randomized control trial (RCT) compared ultrasound-assisted catheter-directed thrombolysis to anticoagulation with unfractionated heparin in fifty-nine patients with intermediate-risk PE. The study demonstrated that ultrasound assisted

Table.5 Alteplase in CDT regimens and doses

Regimen	parenteral anticoagulation
1 mg/hr intraarterially for 24 h (single catheter) or 1 mg/hr/catheter for 12 h (bilateral catheters)[a]	Concomitant systemic heparin was administered with a target aPTT of 60–80 s

[a]consider bolus dose of 0–5 mg/strand
aPTT activated partial thromboplastin time

thrombolysis was associated with a larger decrease in the RV/LV diameter ratio at 24 h, without an increased risk of bleeding [10].

The total dose of CDT is less than 30 mg of tPA. A bolus dose of 0–5 mg/strand followed by an infusion dose can be considered [11, 12]. At our institution we use a loading dose of 3 mg of tPA followed by 1 mg/hour during 12–15 h. With total dose of 18 mg of tPA.

Table 5 outlines Alteplase dose in CDT.

In a systematic review and network meta-analysis CDT was associated with the lower probability of major bleeding and mortality compare to full-dose thrombolysis [13].

Although local thrombolysis by CDT seems promising, these results should be interpreted with caution, considering the relatively small numbers of patients treated the lack of large studies directly comparing catheter directed with systemic thrombolytic therapy, and the lack of data from RCTs on clinical efficacy outcomes.

3 Anticoagulation in Treatment of Pulmonary Embolism

The choice of anticoagulants.

The available anticoagulants are targeted against one or more coagulation factor and belong to several pharmacological groups:

1. Heparins including unfractionated heparin (UFH), low molecular weight heparins (LMWH) and pentasaccharides
2. Vitamin K antagonists
3. Direct oral anticoagulants (DOACs).

3.1 The Heparins

The heparins are naturally occurring glycosaminoglycans that appears as a heparan sulfate on endothelial cells. The pharmacological agent derived from this tissue is a mixture of a variety of heparins with a wide range of molecular weight, up to 30,000 daltons.

Table.6 Characteristics of different preparations of LMWH

Preparation	Mean molecular weight	Anti-Xa: anti IIa ratio	Therapeutic dose	Prophylactic dose
Tinzaparin	4500	1.9	175 IU/kg/d	4500 IU/d
Dalteparin	6000	2.7	100 IU/kg/BID (max. dose 18000 units)	2500–5000 IU/d
Reviparin	4000	1.9	100 IU/kg/BID	
Nadroparin	4500	3.6	90 IU/kg/BID Or 180 IU/kg/d	2850 IU/d
Enoxaparin	4200	3.8	1 mg/kg/BID or 1.5 mg/kg/OD	30–40 mg/d
Bemiparin	3600	8	115 IU/kg/d	2,500–3,500 IU/d

Adapted from NEJM(5) and manufacturer's instructions

In order to improve the bioavailability and stability of the unfractionated heparin, the low molecular weight heparins (LMWH) were extracted from the naturally occurring heparins, by different methods of depolymerization. This group of medications consists of several agents with a molecular weight around 5,000 daltons.

These different preparations vary pharmacokinetically, and result in different ratios of factor Xa versus thrombin (factor II) inhibition (Table 6).

The main effect of the heparins is to inhibit the action of factor Xa by binding to antithrombin and causing a conformational change [5].

The longer the polysaccharide chain, the agent is capable to bind both thrombin and antithrombin, as is the case with unfractionated heparin (UFH). Most LMWH do not have sufficient length to bind to both antithrombin and thrombin, so their main effect will be anti-Xa, and not anti-thrombin, as can be seen in Table 6

Dose adjustment and anti-Xa monitoring is required/advised if:

- estimated creatinine clearance (eCrCl) < 30 mL/min
- Overweight or underweight (BMI $\geq$ 40 kg/m^2 or weight < 50kg)
- Age > 80 years
- Increased bleeding risk (e.g. thrombocytopenia)
- Major drug interaction suspected
- During pregnancy.

Fondaparinux is a synthetic analog of the pentasaccharide that constitutes the binding site of heparin to antithrombin.

Since it is an exceedingly small molecule, its effect is solely anti-Xa.

The main pharmacological properties of the differ heparins are presented in Table 7 [14]. UFH dose and dose adjustment can be seen in Table 8.

Table.7 Pharma cological properties of the heparins

Property	Unfractionated Heparin (UFH)	Low Molecular Weight Heparin (LMWH)	Fondaparinux
Molecular weight (Daltons)	3,000–30,000	1,000–10,000	1728
Monosaccaride units	40–50	13–22	5
antiXa/antiIIa	1:1	2:1–4:1	Anti-Xa only
Interaction with plasma proteins and cells	Yes (albumin, endothel, etc.)	No	No
Biological availability	30–90%	90%	100%
Excretion	Cellular/renal	Renal	Renal
T1/2	0.5–4 h dose dependent	3-6 h	17–21 h
Monitoring	PTT	FXa	FXa
Antidote	Protamin sulfate	Protamin sulphate (Partial effect)	Protamin sulphate (Partial effect)

Table.8 Adjustment of unfractionated heparin dosage

Bolus: 80 units/kg IV bolus maximum 10000 units, or fixed dosing of 5000 units IV
Maintanance: 18 units/kg/h infusion or 1000 units/h
Target therapeutics range: PTT between 50 and 80 s
Consider monitor PTT every 6 h to achieve target PTT

Activated PTT[a]	Change of dosage
<40 s	80 U/kg bolus, increase infusion rate by 3 U/kg/h
40–50 s	40 U/kg bolus, increase infusion rate by 2 U/kg/h
50–80 s	No change
81–100 s	Stop infusion for 1 h, then reduce infusion rate by 2 U/kg/h
>100	Stop infusion for 1 h, then reduce infusion rate by 3 U/kg/h

[a] *PTT* partial thromboplastin time

Adverse effects of heparins:

i. **Bleeding**

The overall risk of bleeding during treatment with heparin is estimated to be 1–4%, with about 9% hematomas at the injection site. Major bleeding according to the International Society on Thrombosis and Hemostasis (ISTH) is defined as an intracranial, gastro-intestinal, intra-ocular, retroperitoneal, or any other bleeding in a critical area or organ or potentially life-threatening bleeding [15]. Among 12,934 unselected patients from a major anticoagulation clinic, the cumulative incidence of major bleeding was 2.5 per 1000 patients (95% confidence interval [CI], 1.7–3.5) [16].

The sort of heparin used (UFH vs. LMWH), dose and treatment duration can affect the risk of bleeding. Patient related factors includes advanced age

(>65years), a previous history of bleeding tendency, renal or liver dysfunction, or concomitant use of anti-aggregating agents [16].

ii. **Heparin induced thrombocytopenia (HIT)**

HIT is an immune prothrombotic disorder caused by antibodies that recognize complexes between platelet factor 4 (PF4) and polyanions such as heparin. Platelet factor 4-heparin-IgG complexes bind to platelet receptors, leading to platelet activation and aggregation, acceleration of soluble clotting reactions, monocyte and endothelial cell procoagulant activity, that may lead to clinical presentation of thrombocytopenia and thrombosis [17]. The diagnosis of HIT is often challenging, since thrombocytopenia is common among hospitalized patients. The diagnostic approach to HIT would be based on clinical elements, including the timely appearance of a drop of > 50% in platelet count, ruling out any other etiology for thrombocytopenia, a new thrombotic event (the thrombotic risk is 17–53% over a 30-day period) and a specialized laboratory evaluation [17]

HIT is more common when UFH is used, compared to LMWH and with a longer duration of heparin use. It is more common in surgical patients, compared to medically ill or obstetric population and more common in females compared to male gender [17].

Although there is consensus among experts that patients with isolated HIT should be treated in the short-term with alternative anticoagulants, there is no firm consensus on the intensity or duration of anticoagulation for this patient population. critically ill patients with thrombosis should be treated with a parenteral direct thrombin inhibitor such as argatroban or bivalirudin. Other patients can be treated with fondaparinux [17]. The direct oral anticoagulants are emerging as the new attractive option for the treatment of HIT, during the acute phase and as a long term therapy, when needed [18].

iii. **Osteoporosis**

The mechanism by which heparins induce osteoporosis is not fully understood, but the postulated hypothesis is that heparin causes increased bone resorption by stimulating osteoclasts and suppressing osteoblast function, leading to decreased bone mass. It has been estimated that bone loss occurs after 6 months of UFH with daily doses of >15,000 units. Data about the effect of LMWH on bone mineral density or as a risk factor for fractures are more controversial. Most studies confirm the prominent role played by UFH in changes in bone metabolism and a lower risk of fractures in patients with long-term LMWH treatment. Fondaparinux showed no effect on osteoblast differentiation or function [19].

iv. **Skin reactions**

Heparin hypersensitivity can present as a mild erythema with little infiltration at the injection site, to a more severe form of eczematous plaques with papulo-vesicles located on an infiltrated erythematous plaque. a generalized eczema or exanthema may also occur. The hypersensitivity reaction appears typically after 7–10 days of treatment and is more common in over-weight women. The local reaction should be differentiated from hematomas, local infections, and eczema caused by skin disinfectants [20].

v. **Elevated liver enzymes**

Hyper-transaminemia: Alanine transaminase (ALT) or Aspartate Aminotransferase (AST) up to 3X the upper limit of normal rang) associated with LMWH was reported in about 4% of cases treated with these agents [21]. This phenomenon has a hepatocellular pattern of injury, short latency (days to weeks), rarely causes symptoms and is usually self-limiting and usually does not necessitate stopping the medication, but close follow up is recommended.

3.2 *Vitamin K Antagonist (VKA)*

Vitamin K antagonists also called coumarins are time honored oral anticoagulants, used in a wide range of clinical settings. The most used preparation is the WARFARIN named after the Wisconsin Alumni Research Foundation that funded Karl Link's research. That led to the discovery of the active compound Dicoumarol that developed to a therapeutic anticoagulant and was approved by the FDA for use in humans in 1954, under the name Coumadin.

Other VKA's that are used as anticoagulants in humans are acenocoumarol (mostly marketed under the brand name Sintrom®), and phenprocoumon (Flathron®, Fenprocoumon® etc). Warfarin is mostly known as Coumadin®.

Vitamin K antagonists act as anticoagulants by inhibiting the enzyme reductase Vitamin K epOxide Reductase Complex (VKORC). When this enzyme is inhibited, vitamin K quinol (KH_2) is not sufficiently regenerated. Vitamin K in its active form is essential for the gamma-carboxylation of coagulation factors II, VII, IX, X involved in the coagulation cascade, and thus, VKAs result in the depletion of these factors within 72–96 h.

The natural anticoagulants protein C and protein S are also affected (Fig. 2) [22].

Genetic polymorphisms in the hepatic cytochrome,

P450 (CYP) 2C9, that metabolizes VKAs, can affect the doses needed to achieve anticoagulation. Warfarin given to patients with CYP2C9*2 or CYP2C9*3 variants will be metabolized less efficiently (by 30% and 90% respectively), the drug will remain in circulation longer, so lower warfarin doses will be needed to achieve anticoagulation.

There are several VKORC1 polymormisms that may affect the dosage of VKA.

The management of anticoagulation with VKA is further complicated by the wide range of drug and food interactions. Food product containing various amounts of vitamin K will affect the level of anticoagulation, so a strict diet containing stable amount of vitamin K is crucial for achieving stable anticoagulation. Antibiotics can change the gut flora, thus changing the amount of absorbed vitamin K [23].

VKAs inhibit several coagulation factors, and some natural anticoagulants, as shown in Fig. 2. Since the half-life of Protein C in considerably shorter than some

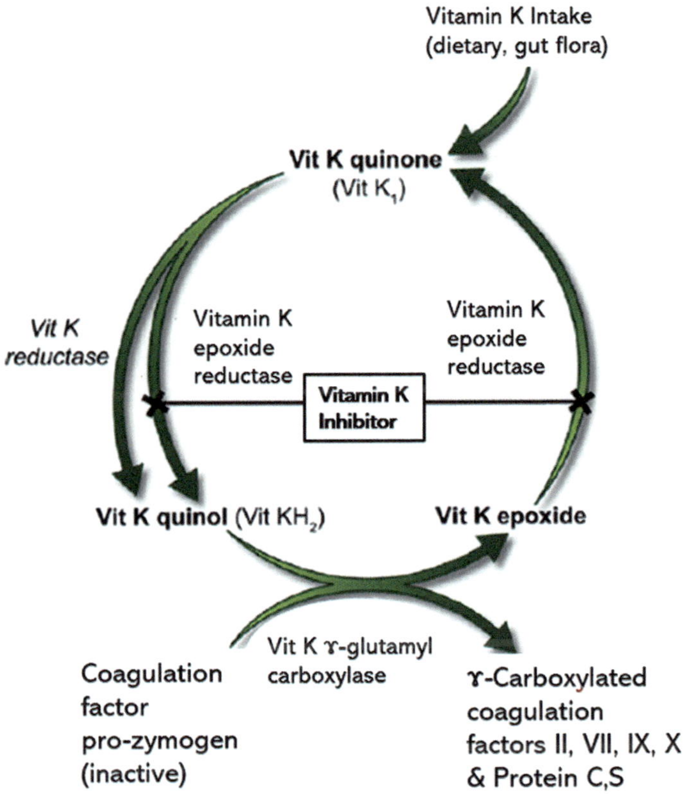

Fig. 2 The effect of vitamin K inhibitors on the coagulation factors

of these coagulation factors, starting treatment with a drug from this group, such as warfarin, can cause a hypercoagulable state. Overlap with a heparin is until the chosen VKA reaches the therapeutic range (international normalized ratio, INR $\geq$ 2.0 for 2 consecutive days) is necessary to avoid thrombotic complications.

During the initial period, the INR should be checked every 2–4 days.

A suggested scheme to start treatment with warfarin is presented in Table 9.

Further dosing should be re-adjusted once a week, aiming to keep the INR in the therapeutic range, 2.0–3.0.

A suggested scheme to maintain the INR in the desired range is presented in Fig. 3.

Once a stable INR was achieved and maintained for a least 4 weekly measurements, monitoring of INR can be gradually reduced to once every 4 weeks, but if a dose-adjustment is required, returning to a weekly monitoring is recommended.

VKA drug interactions:

Many drug-interactions affecting warfarin, involve inhibition of the activity of CYP450 enzymes involved in VKA metabolism. The concomitant use of

Table.9 Dose adjustments during the initial treatment with VKA

Treatment day	INR	Dose adjustment (warfarin)
Day 1	1.0–1.4	2.5–5 mg/d (According to bleeding risk/high sensitivity phenotype)
Day 3	≤ 1.5	Increase dose by 20%
	1.5–1.9	Increase dose by 5–10%
	≥ 2.0	Repeat same dose, Recheck INR next day
Day 4	≥ 2.0	Go to dose adjustment chart (Fig. 3)
Day 4–7	≤ 1.5	Increase dose by 20%
	1.5–1.9	Increase dose by 5–10%
	≥ 2.0	Repeat same dose, Recheck INR next day
	>3.5	Decrease dose by 5–20%
	≥ 2.0	Rechecked: go to dose adjustment chart (Fig. 3)
Day > 7	>2.0	Continue according to dose adjustment chart (Fig. 3)

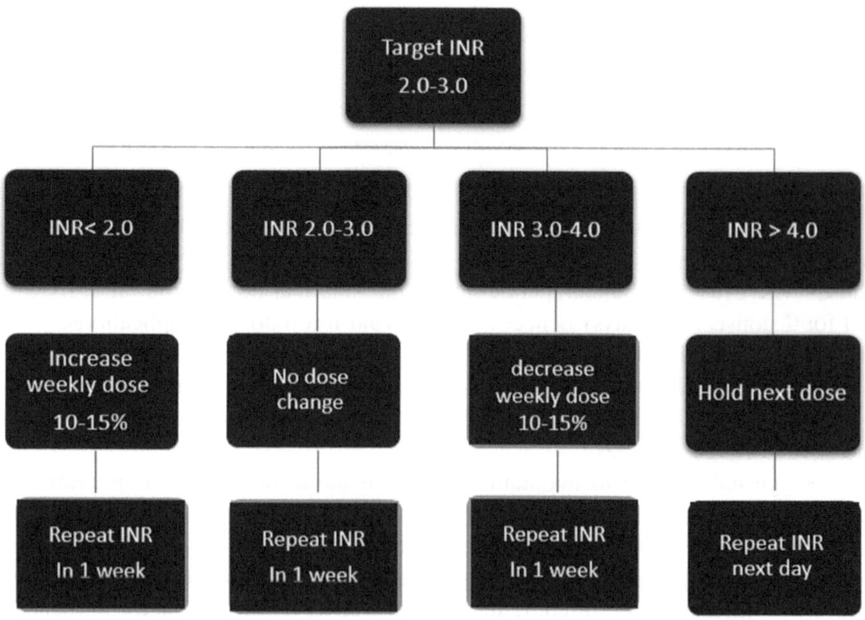

Fig. 3 Dose adjustments during treatment with VKA

medications that induce CYP2C9 such as rifampin, carbamazepine, mercaptopurine, raloxifene and others, results in increased clearance of warfarin and thus less anticoagulation. On the other hand, Amiodarone is a moderate inhibitor of CYP2C9 isoenzymes, thus they may alter warfarin and other VKAs metabolism, and increase PT-INR.

Close INR monitoring is required in any change (adding or stopping) of chronic medication known to inhibit or induce warfarin metabolism.

Some anti-retroviral agents commonly used in HIV patients, and some anti-fungal medications have the same effect on PT-INR. Among them, fluconazole is a potent CYP2C9 inhibitor. Adding fluconazole to chronic treatment with warfarin can cause rapid elevation in INR. Consider 20–70% warfarin dose reduction in combination with fluconazole (especially with high fluconazole dose) and close monitoring. Antibiotic therapy may affect the degree of INR balance in stable patients due to changes in the gut flora: many antibiotics have been found to have INR values above 5, among them: metronidazole, trimethoprim-sulfamethoxazole and quinolones. Other antibiotics such as penicillin, azithromycin, and doxycycline may have also some impact on bleeding risk. Other possible causes of increased INR in disease states without antibiotic treatment include a decrease in vitamin K intake from food and the effect of drugs aimed to reduce fever and pain [24].

Other drugs can also affect warfarin elimination, and decreased efficacy of anti-coagulation. Some herbal food supplements and even food products can have a significant effect on PT-INR. For example, high doses (but probably not moderate consumption) of green tea can lower the INR significantly, and the same effect was observed with long-term consumption of St. John's wort [25].

Over-the-counter medications such as NSAIDs, concomitant use of anti-aggregating agents such as aspirin or P2Y12 inhibitors should be carefully considered due to increased risk of bleeding. The use of alcohol should be avoided, due to enhanced bleeding risk.

Liver dysfunction, lower creatinine clearance and uncompensated congestive heart failure, may contribute to the bleeding risk.

The risk of bleeding rises also with advanced age.

Another major risk factor for an adverse event (thrombosis or hemorrhage) is a labile INR [26].

The risk for thrombosis or bleeding is higher the more the INR moves away from the desired range.

In VTE patients, subtherapeutic INRs were found to be present during 58% of recurrent VTEs, while 48% of major hemorrhagic events occurred at an INR >3.0 [26, 27].

In the pivotal studies comparing the efficacy and safety of DOACs to warfarin in patients with symptomatic deep vein thrombosis/pulmonary embolus, the time in therapeutic range (TTR) was 56.9–63.5% [28]. Whereas in a meta-analysis of 53 studies, 59% (95%CI: 54–64%) of INRs measured and 61% (95%CI: 59–63%) of the time patients were treated were spent outside the therapeutic range [26].

The estimated risk of thrombosis or bleeding is continuous. It was shown that for every 1% increase in TTR, recurrent thromboembolic events may be reduced by 0.46% per year and major hemorrhagic events reduced by 0.30% [26].

The importance of a tight control of INR was demonstrated in a study that examined the outcome of almost 15,000 patients (including 3,326 patients with VTE) treated with VKA and had one episode of extreme anticoagulation [27]. These patients had already a suboptimal INR 90 days before the episode of extreme anticoagulation, TTR was decreased during 90 days after the clinical event. During the time before and after an event of extreme INR (above 8.0), the hazard ratio (HR) for bleeding was 2.1 (CI 1.4–3.2), for thrombosis HR 5.7 (CI 1.5–22.2), and the HR for VKA-related death was 17.0 (CI 2.1–138) [27]. For many patients with pulmonary embolism secondary prevention with VKAs is not extended beyond 6 months, as risk of recurrence may be outweighed by the risk of major bleeding: RR 3.44, 95% CI 1.22–9.74 for bleeding versus RR 0.20, 95% CI 0.11–0.38 for recurrent thrombosis, independent of the period elapsed since the index thromboembolic event [29].

Due to the narrow therapeutic range, the wide variety of food products and medication that can influence the quality of anticoagulation and given the significant risk for bleeding or thrombosis outside the therapeutic range, patients receiving VKA should be followed regularly in a designated anticoagulation clinic, with frequent monitoring of INR. Special attention should be given to any (prescribed or OTC) new medication, or a change in diet (such as during or after hospitalization).

Although self-management of INR can be achieved in selected patients, a proactive schedule, confirming, and tracking appointments and INR results and to maintaining patient communication is crucial for the safety and compliance.

VKA adverse effects:

Warfarin was found to be the most common cause for emergency hospitalization for adverse drug events in the older American population, mostly due to high INR or bleeding [30].

i. **Bleeding:**

   The incidence rate of severe bleeding among a large cohort of adult patients treated with warfarin was 37 per 1000 person-years [31], with higher bleeding risk for men (compared to women), age > 75years, comorbidities such as hypertension, diabetes, renal or hepatic dysfunction, previous TIA/CVA, alcohol use, concomitant treatment with anti-aggregating agents or cancer [31, 32]

   The most devastating hemorrhage being an intracranial bleeding, occurring in 0.70–0.85% of warfarin users, mostly (in about 65% of cases) with INR within the therapeutic range [33]

ii. **Warfarin skin necrosis:**

   Warfarin-induced skin necrosis is a rare side effect, occurring in 0.01–0.1% of patients taking the drug, typically appears during the early 10 days of therapy and affects mostly fat tissue such as breasts, buttocks, and thighs. This adverse effect is mostly attributed to the inhibition of the natural anticoagulant, protein C, before inhibition of factors with longer half-life such as factors IX and X, thus causing a temporary hypercoagulable state.

To avoid this troublesome complication, when treating acute thrombosis, such as pulmonary embolism, overlap with heparin for at least 5 days is crucial, heparin should be stopped when the INR reached the therapeutic range for 2 consecutive days.

iii. **Warfarin Embryopathy:**

Warfarin is teratogenic if administered during organogenesis (weeks 6–12 of pregnancy). The typical syndrome consists of central nervous system defects, central facial hypoplasia, skeletal deformities, and microcephaly. Malformations are reported in 11–16% of exposed fetuses, miscarriage in up to 35% [34].

iv. **Other reported adverse effects of VKA**:

- Alopecia
- Osteoporosis [19]
- Purple toe syndrome: a rare complication, the ischemic changes resolve once VKA is stopped (Fig. 4).

Table 10 present advantages and shortcomings of VKAs for management of pulmonary embolism

3.3 Direct Oral Anticoagulants (DOACs)

The direct oral anticoagulants were introduced in the early 21st century as a solution for the shortcomings of the VKS and the parenteral LMWH. DOACs are small synthetic molecules with a molecular weight ranging from 430 to 670 Da. They are either direct thrombin inhibitors or factor Xa (FXa) inhibitors.

Dabigatran etexilate is the only approved oral direct thrombin inhibitor, and rivaroxaban, apixaban and edoxaban are oral FXa inhibitors. There are some pharmacokinetic differences between the drugs, especially regarding the way of elimination (Table 11).

The main advantages of DOACs over VKAs is their predictable pharmacokinetics and pharmacodynamics, rapid onset of action, a short half-life, a lower potential for food and drug interactions, and a wide therapeutic window. the stable pharmacological profile obviates the need for regular monitoring. These properties render the NOACs more user- friendly, thus improving compliance.

The efficacy and the safety of the DOACs was well established in a series of pivotal trials (Table 12) followed by real world experience based on world-wide registries such as the RIETE registry or the Dresden NOAC registry [4]. The

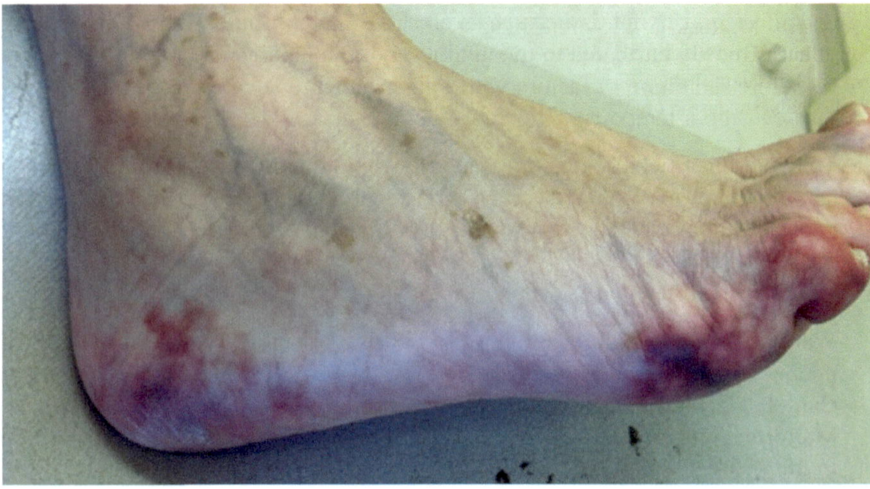

Fig. 4 Purple toe in a patient treated with warfarin for recurrent thrombotic events due to anti-phospholipid antibodies

Table.10 Advantages and shortcomings of VKAs for management of pulmonary embolism

Advantages	Shortcomings
Proven efficacy in a wide range of clinical settings	Narrow therapeutic range
Long half-life: less vulnerable to non-adherence	Long half-life: • $\geq$ 5d for effective anticoagulation, initial heparinization mandatory • several days of washout required (in case of bleeding, periprocedural)
Low cost	A wide range of drug and food interactions
	Constant monitoring needed
	Teratogenic

accumulating data support the initial finding in the pivotal studies, showing that the net clinical benefit is superior with the use of DOACS over VKAs, mostly due to reduction in the risk of major and clinically relevant non major bleeding in comparison to VKAs [4]. Given the higher bleeding risk in the elderly population, and the poorer control of INR observed in this population [35], DOACs seem to be a safer alternative. Another major advantage is a lower rate of intracranial bleeding and hemorrhagic stroke compared to VKAs, with an annual risk of 0.23–0.33 events per 100 patient-years for the different DOACs in the pivotal studies, compared to 0.7–0.85 events with warfarin in these studies [33].

These qualities make the DOACs an attractive "one stop shop" using the same medication for initial treatment, for the primary treatment and, if needed, also for

Table.11 Comparative pharmacokinetics of DOACs

	FII inhibitor	FXa inhibitors		
	Dabigatran	Rivaroxaban	Apixaban	Edoxaban
Route of administration	Oral	Oral	Oral	Oral
Molecular weight (Dalton)	627	435	459	548
Peak plasma level (h)	1–2	2–4	3–4	1–2
T1/2 (h)	12–17	5–13	9–14	10–14
Bioavailability (%)	3–10	>80 with food	50	62
Renal elimination (%)	80	33	27	50
CYP 3A4 metabolism (%)	non	66	25	<4
P-gp	yes	yes	yes	yes

Table.12 The efficacy and safety data for PE patients in the pivotal studies comparing DOACs to standard of care during the primary treatment period

	Dabigatran	Rivaroxaban	Apixaban	Edoxaban
Study name	RE-COVER and RE-COVER II pooled analysis	EINSTEIN-PE	AMPLIFY	HOKUSAI-VTE
Patients (N)	1602	4832	5395	8240
Symptomatic VTE recurrence vs. warfarin HR (95% CI); p value	0.93 (0.53–1.64); NR	1.12 (0.75–1.68); 0.003	0.84 (0.60–1.18); < 0.001	0.89 (0.70–1.13); < 0.001
Major or CRNM bleeding HR (95% CI); p value	0.65 (0.43–0.99); NR	0.90 (0.76–1.07); 0.23	0.44 (0.36–0.55); < 0.001	0.81 (0.71–0.94); 0.004
Patients with PE (%)	100	100	34	40.3

VTE Venous thromboembolism, *PE* pulmonary embolism, *CRNM* Clinically relevant non-major bleeding

extended long term prophylaxis. Table 13 present dosing schedules and considerations for special populations [4, 36, 37].

DOAC have potential drug–drug inter-actions. There are two primary known mechanisms by which other drugs may affect DOAC concentration: first by influence the absorption of DOACs by the intestinal P-glycoprotein (P-gp) transporter: DOAC are substrates of P-gp efflux, which pumps substrates back into the intestinal lumen. P-gp is also involved in the renal tubular excretion of medications. Thus, inhibition of P-gp may enhance absorption and reduce excretion of DOAC, leading to an increase in their bioavailability. The second mechanism is by changing the metabolism of DOACs in the hepatic cytochrome P450 (CYP) 3A4.

Table.13 Dosing schedules and considerations for special populations

	Dabigatran	Rivaroxaban	Apixaban*	Edoxaban
Lead-in with heparin	$\geq$ 5d	None	None	$\geq$ 5d
Initial dosing schedule	150 mg BID	15 mg BID for 21d	10 mg BID for 7d	
Dosing schedule	150 mg BID	20 mg/d	5 mg BID	60 mg/d
Extended dosing schedule	150 mg BID	10 mg/d	2.5 mg BID	60 mg/d
Dose adjustments				
Elderly	No dose adjustment. bleeding risk increases with age (consider dose reduction)	No dose adjustment. bleeding risk increases with age (consider dose reduction)	No dose adjustment	No dose adjustment
Low body weight	No dose adjustment	No dose adjustment	No dose adjustment	Reduce dose to 30 mg OD if weight < 60 kg
Kidney dysfunction	CrCl < 50 mL/min: avoid use if patient on P-gp inhibitor CrCl < 30 mL/min: avoid use	CrCl < 30 mL/min: avoid use	CrCl < 50 mL/min: avoid use if patient on P-gp inhibitor CrCl < 30 mL/min avoid use	CrCl 15–50 mL/min: reduce dose to 30 mg OD
Liver dysfunction	No dose adjustment with moderate impairment severe impairment: no dose recommendation	Avoid use in moderate or severe impairment or any hepatic injury with coagulopathy	No dose adjustment with mild impairment. no dose recommendation for moderate impairment	No dose adjustment with mild impairment not recommended in moderate or severe impairment
Pregnancy and breast-feeding	Safety unknown	Safety unknown	Safety unknown	Safety unknown
High risk APLA syndrome	Contra-indicated	Contra-indicated	Contra-indicated	Contra-indicated
Reversal agent	Idarucizumab	Andexanate	Andexanate	Andexanate

Dabigatran is a pro-drug with low bioavailability, and its plasma level highly depends on P-gp efflux transporter-mediated interactions but is not metabolized by nor induces any cytochrome P450 subtype. On the other hand, rivaroxaban, apixaban and edoxaban are all, at least to some extent, CYP450 and P-glycoprotein (P-gp) substrates, potentially leading to drug interaction [36]. Examples of drug interactions are listed in Table 14.

Table 14 Effect of drug-drug interactions and clinical factors on DOAC plasma levels and anticoagulant effects

		Dabigatran Etexilate	Rivaroxaban	Apixaban	Edoxaban
CYP3A4 inhibition; P-gp competition, elevate DOACs concentration, increase risk for bleeding	Ketoconazole/ Itraconazole/ Posconazole/ Voriconazole	Not advisable due to increased plasma levels	Not advisable due to increased plasma levels	Not advisable due to increased plasma levels	Dose reduction to 30 mg once daily for ketoconazole, no data for other Azoles
	Imatinib, Crizotinib, Vandetanib, Sunitinib	Not advisable due to increased plasma levels	Not advisable due to increased plasma levels	Not advisable due to increased plasma levels	Not advisable due to increased plasma levels
	Ritonavir/ Glecaprevir/ Pibrentasvir	Not advisable due to increased plasma levels	Not advisable due to increased plasma levels	not advisable due to increased plasma levels	No data yet
	Dronedarone	Not advisable due to increased plasma levels	Moderate effect especially in renal failure; should be avoided	With caution	Dose reduction to 30 mg once daily
	Verapramil	Dose reduction to 110 mg * 2 day	No dose reduction required	No dose reduction required	No dose reduction required
	Amiodarone	Consider monitoring level for patients with other risk factors	Consider monitoring level for patients with other risk factors	Consider monitoring level for patients with other risk factors	Consider monitoring level for patients with other risk factors
	Clarithromycin; Erythromycin	Consider monitoring level for patients	Consider monitoring level for patients with	Consider monitoring level for patients	Dose reduction to 30 mg once daily

(continued)

Table 14 (continued)

		Dabigatran Etexilate	Rivaroxaban	Apixaban	Edoxaban
		with other risk factors	other risk factors	with other risk factors	
	Abiraterone	Not advisable due to increased plasma levels	Not advisable due to increased plasma levels	Not advisable due to increased plasma levels	Not advisable due to increased plasma levels
	Venetoclax	Consider monitoring level	Consider monitoring level	Consider monitoring level	Consider monitoring level
	Ciclosporine/ Tacrolimus	Not advisable due to increased plasma levels	Consider monitoring level for patients with other risk factors	Consider monitoring level for patients with other risk factors	Dose reduction to 30 mg once daily
P-gp/BCRP and CYP3A4 induction, decrease DOACs concentration, increase risk for thrombosis	Rifampicin	Not advisable due to decreased plasma levels	Not advisable due to decreased plasma levels	Not advisable due to decreased plasma levels	Consider monitoring level
	Hypericum	Not advisable due to decreased plasma levels	Not advisable due to decreased plasma levels	Not advisable due to decreased plasma levels	Consider monitoring level
	Carbamazepine	Not advisable due to decreased plasma levels	Not advisable due to decreased plasma levels	Not advisable due to decreased plasma levels	Consider monitoring level
	Phenobarbital	Not advisable due to decreased plasma levels	Not advisable due to decreased plasma levels	Not advisable due to decreased plasma levels	Consider monitoring level
	Phenytoin	Not advisable due to decreased	Not advisable due to decreased	Not advisable due to decreased	Consider monitoring level

(continued)

Table 14 (continued)

		Dabigatran Etexilate	Rivaroxaban	Apixaban	Edoxaban
		plasma levels	plasma levels	plasma levels	
	Primidone	Not advisable due to decreased plasma levels	Not advisable due to decreased plasma levels	Not advisable due to decreased plasma levels	Consider monitoring level
	Enzalutamide	Consider monitoring level	Not advisable due to decreased plasma levels	Not advisable due to decreased plasma levels	Consider monitoring level

The latest ECS guidelines [3] and the 2020 ASH guidelines [2] recommend to prefer DOAC over VKA, when oral anticoagulation is started in a patient with PE who is eligible for a DOAC. (eligible patients are those with no contra indications such as pregnancy, high risk anti-phospholipid syndrome, prosthetic valve or moderate to severe liver dysfunction). Indirect comparison between the different DOACs showed similar efficacy for preventing recurrence of VTE with an advantage of apixaban versus rivaroxaban or edoxaban regarding the bleeding risk (RR 0.4795% CI 0.37–0.61 $p < 0.001$ for apixaban versus rivaroxaban, and RR 0.54 95% CI 0.42–0.70, $p < 0.001$ for apixaban versus edoxaban) [28].

Although regular monitoring of the anticoagulant effect of the DOACs is not necessary, there may be situations where such a laboratory test may be required or even crucial for management of a specific patient.

The relevant laboratory tests are measuring plasma level of dabigatran (e.g. Hemoclot) or calibrated chromogenic anti-FXa activity of the FXa inhibitors can be in order [38].

Examples for such cases include:

- Acute bleeding
- Periprocedural (urgent invasive procedure, high risk elective procedure, high risk patient)
- Elderly frail patient
- Overweight or underweight
- Impaired renal failure
- Concomitant use of strong inducer/inhibitor of CYP450 and/or P-gp efflux transmitter
- Use of concomitant anti-aggregating agent

- Coagulopathy/thrombocytopenia
- Patients after (sub)total gastrectomy or bariatric surgery
- Thrombotic event under treatment?

4 Chronic Long-Term Anticoagulation

4.1 Extended Duration Treatment

After the completion of the primary treatment period, lasting 3–6 months, a re-assessment of the risk for VTE recurrence or predisposing condition for chronic thromboembolic pulmonary hypertension, [3] should be weighed against the bleeding risk.

For patients with first PE/VTE secondary to a major transient/reversible risk factor, discontinuation of therapeutic oral anticoagulation is recommended after 3 months.

Long term treatment, preferably with a DOAC, should be considered, especially in men with unprovoked pulmonary embolus, or those with an ongoing risk factor [2, 3] since the risk for recurrence is as high about 40% in 10 years, with 4% of recurrent events resulting in death [39].

Another major consideration for long term anticoagulation is the presence of risk factors for thromboembolic pulmonary hypertension (CTEPH). These risk factors can be related to the extent and severity of the acute PE (e.g. large thrombus with echocardiographic evidence of RV dysfunction), previous PE or other venous thrombosis or other comorbidities predisposing to CTEPH such as major thrombophilias, history ofcancer or myeloproliferative neoplasms, history of splenectomy or chronic inflammation (e.g. inflammatory bowel disease) [3].

Extended duration treatment with reduced dose apixaban proved to reduce the recurrence rate by 80% (RR 0.19, 95% CI 0.11–0.33, compared to placebo, whereas the corresponding bleeding risk was 1.20 95% CI 0.69–2.10. Rivaroxaban in a reduced dose was compared to aspirin, the recurrence rate of VTE was significantly lower in the 10mg/d group (reduced dose) compared to aspirin with a hazard ratio of 0.26 (95% CI, 0.14–0.47; $P < 0.001$), aspirin alone reduced the recurrence rate in 32% with a similar rate of bleeding [40, 41].

As for warfarin and the other VKs, the annual risk for an major bleeding is estimated as 3%, with an annual case fatality rate of 0.6%, whereas the annual case fatality rate of recurrent pulmonary embolism exceeds 7% [42].

How to choose the right agent for my patient?

After the diagnosis of acute pulmonary embolism, once the patient is hemodynamically stable, the choice of the best suited anticoagulant is based on pharmacokinetic and pharmacodynamic properties of the different anticoagulants, co-morbidities or other patient related conditions and patient preferences [4, 36].

For example, if a PE occurred during pregnancy, the only option will be LMWH (or in rare, high-risk situation, unfractionated heparin), since all other option are contraindicated, or their safety is unknown during pregnancy.

With high risk antiphospholipid syndrome, the current recommendation are to prefer VKA since the efficacy and safety of DOAC in this setting are inferior to VKA [2, 3, 37].

On the other hand, in most patients without a contraindication, treatment with a DOAC is preferred over VKAs or long-term parenteral treatment with a LMWH [2–4, 39]. A "one stop shop" using the same agent throughout the whole therapy is a safe option with significant advantages regarding the patient's compliance and satisfaction.

In a patient with a high gastro-intestinal bleeding risk, dyspepsia or impaired absorption, apixaban or LMWH are preferred over rivaroxaban or dabigatran. With kidney impairment apixaban is the preferred choice. If ease of use is the main issue, once a day medication such as rivaroxaban or edoxaban can be offered. These considerations are illustrated in Fig. 5.

In case VKA is chosen as the preferred long-term anticoagulation (for example in patients with high-risk antiphospholipid syndrome), the INR should be frequently monitored in order to maintain the INR in the therapeutic range. A scheme for long term monitoring and dose adjustments is presented in Fig. 3.

An overview on the different treatment options is presented in Fig. 6.

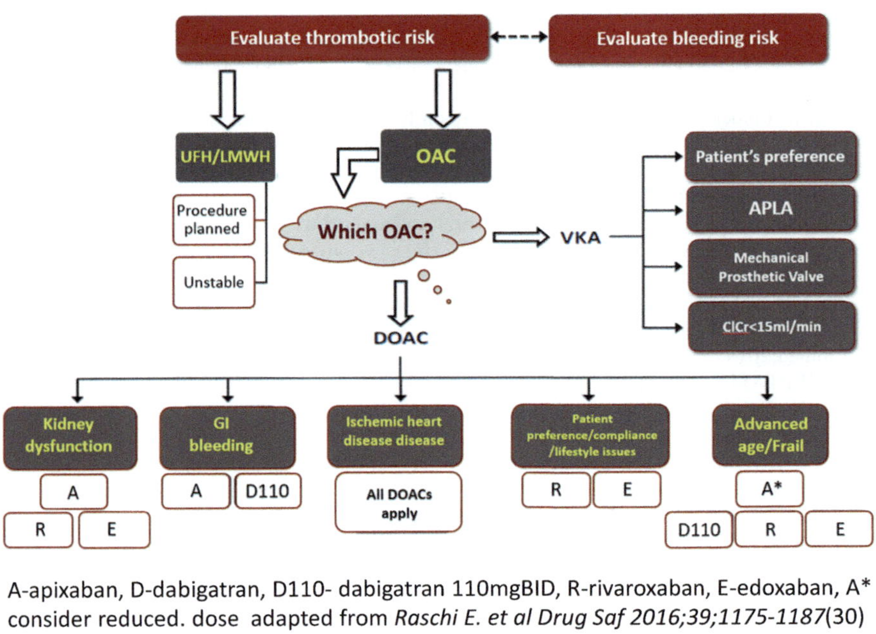

Fig. 5 A flowchart demonstrating the main is issues to be considered when choosing an anticoagulant

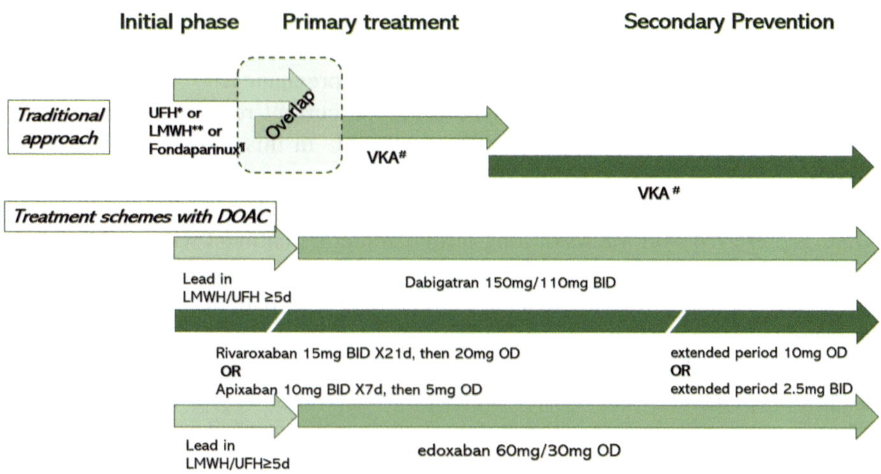

Fig. 6 Summary of treatment options: "one stop shop" versus traditional approach

References

1. Flinterman LE, van Hylckama Vlieg A, Cannegieter SC, Rosendaal FR. Long-term survival in a large cohort of patients with venous thrombosis: incidence and predictors. PLoS Med. 9 (1).
2. Ortel TL, Neumann I, Ageno W, Beyth R, Clark NP, Cuker A, et al. American society of hematology 2020 guidelines for management of venous thromboembolism: treatment of deep vein thrombosis and pulmonary embolism. Blood Adv. 2020;4(19):4693–738.
3. Konstantinides SV, Meyer G, Galié N, Simon R Gibbs J, Aboyans V, Ageno W, et al. ESC Guidelines for the diagnosis and management of acute pulmonary embolism developed in collaboration with the European Respiratory Society (ERS). Eur Respir J [Internet]. 54(3). https://doi.org/10.1183/13993003.01647-2019
4. Eldredge JB, Spyropoulos AC. Direct oral anticoagulants in the treatment of pulmonary embolism. Curr Med Res Opin [Internet]. 34(1):131–40. https://doi.org/10.1080/03007995.2017.1364227
5. Ali MR, Salim Hossain M, Islam MA, Saiful Islam Arman M, Sarwar Raju G, Dasgupta P, et al. Aspect of thrombolytic therapy: a review, vol. 2014. Scientific World Journal. Hindawi Limited;2014.
6. STREPTASE® [Internet]. 2007. https://pdf.hres.ca/dpd_pm/00003639.PDF.
7. fda. Kinlytic™ (urokinase for injection).
8. FDA. ACTIVASE (alteplase) Prescribing information. 2015.
9. Marti C, John G, Konstantinides S, Combescur C, Sanchez O, Lankeit M, et al. Systemic thrombolytic therapy for acute pulmonary embolism: a systematic review and meta-analysis, vol. 36. European Heart Journal. Oxford University Press;2015. p. 605–14.
10. Kucher N, Boekstegers P, Müller OJ, Kupatt C, Beyer-Westendorf J, Heitzer T, et al. Randomized, controlled trial of ultrasound-assisted catheter-directed thrombolysis for acute intermediate-risk pulmonary embolism. Circulation. 2014;129(4):479–86.
11. Schissler AJ, Gylnn RJ, Sobieszczyk PS, Waxman AB. Ultrasound-assisted catheter-directed thrombolysis compared with anticoagulation alone for treatment of intermediate-risk pulmonary embolism. Pulm Circ. 2018;8(4).

12. Piazza G, Hohlfelder B, Jaff MR, Ouriel K, Engelhardt TC, Sterling KM, et al. A prospective, single-arm, multicenter trial of ultrasound-facilitated, catheter-directed, low-dose fibrinolysis for acute massive and submassive pulmonary embolism: The SEATTLE II study. JACC Cardiovasc Interv. 2015;8(10):1382–92.
13. Jimenez D, Martin-Saborido C, Muriel A, Zamora J, Morillo R, Barrios D, et al. Efficacy and safety outcomes of recanalisation procedures in patients with acute symptomatic pulmonary embolism: systematic review and network meta-analysis. Thorax. 2018;73(5):464–71.
14. Bick RL, Frenkel EP, Walenga J, Fareed J, Hoppensteadt DA. Unfractionated heparin, low molecular weight heparins, and pentasaccharide: Basic mechanism of actions, pharmacology, and clinical use, vol. 19. Hematology/Oncology Clinics of North America. W.B. Saunders;2005. p. 1–51.
15. Kaatz S, Ahmad D, Spyropoulos AC, Schulman S. Definition of clinically relevant non-major bleeding in studies of anticoagulants in atrial fibrillation and venous thromboembolic disease in non-surgical patients: communication from the SSC of the ISTH. J Thromb Haemost. 2015;13(11):2119–26.
16. van Rein N, Biedermann JS, van der Meer FJM, Cannegieter SC, Wiersma N, Vermaas HW, et al. Major bleeding risks of different low-molecular-weight heparin agents: a cohort study in 12 934 patients treated for acute venous thrombosis. J Thromb Haemost. 2017;15(7):1386–91.
17. Lee GM, Arepally GM. Heparin-induced thrombocytopenia. http://ashpublications.org/hematology/article-pdf/2013/1/668/1249307/bep00113000668.pdf.
18. Warkentin TE, Pai M, Linkins L-A. Direct oral anticoagulants for treatment of HIT: update of Hamilton experience and literature review. Blood [Internet]. 2017;130(9):1104–13. http://ashpublications.org/blood/article-pdf/130/9/1104/1405076/blood778993.pdf.
19. Signorelli SS, Scuto S, Marino E, Giusti M, Xourafa A, Gaudio A. Anticoagulants and osteoporosis [Internet], vol. 20. International Journal of Molecular Sciences. MDPI AG;2019. www.mdpi.com/journal/ijms.
20. Trautmann A, Seitz CS. The complex clinical picture of side effects to anticoagulation. Med Clin North Am [Internet]. 2010;94(4):821–34. https://doi.org/10.1016/j.mcna.2010.03.003.
21. Hahn KJ, Morales SJ, Lewis JH, Net KJH. Enoxaparin-induced liver injury: case report and review of the literature and FDA Adverse Event Reporting System (FAERS). Drug Saf Case Reports. 2015;2.
22. Zirlik A, Bode C. Vitamin K antagonists: relative strengths and weaknesses vs. direct oral anticoagulants for stroke prevention in patients with atrial fibrillation. J Thromb Thrombolysis. 2017;43:365–79.
23. Beinema M. the effects of CYP2C9 polymorphisms on the pharmacokinetics and anticoagulant response are also least pronounced in the case of phenprocoumon. Thromb Haemost. 2008;100(6):1052–7.
24. Holbrook A, Schulman S, Witt DM, Vandvik PO, Fish J, Kovacs MJ, et al. Evidence-based management of anticoagulant therapy. Antithrombotic therapy and prevention of thrombosis, 9th ed: American College of Chest Physicians evidence-based clinical practice guidelines. Chest [Internet]. 2012;141(2 SUPPL.):e152S–e184S. https://doi.org/10.1378/chest.11-2295.
25. Di Minno A. Old and new oral anticoagulants: Food, herbal medicines and drug interactions. Blood Rev. 2017;31:193–203.
26. Mearns ES, Kohn CG, Song JS, Hawthorne J, Meng J, White CM, et al. Meta-analysis to assess the quality of international normalized ratio control and associated outcomes in venous thromboembolism patients. Thromb Res [Internet]. 2014;134(2):310–9. https://doi.org/10.1016/j.thromres.2014.05.035.
27. Kooistra HAM, Veeger NJGM, Khorsand N, Kluin-Nelemans HC, Meijer K, Piersma-Wichers M. Long-term quality of VKA treatment and clinical outcome after extreme overanticoagulation in 14,777 AF and VTE patients. Thromb Haemost. 2015;113(4):881–90.
28. Mantha S, Ansell J. Indirect comparison of dabigatran, rivaroxaban, apixaban and edoxaban for the treatment of acute venous thromboembolism. J Thromb Thromb. 2015;39(2):155–65.

29. Middeldorp S, Prins MH, Hutten BA. Duration of treatment with vitamin K antagonists in symptomatic venous thromboembolism [Internet], vol. 8, Cochrane Database of Systematic Reviews. 2014. www.cochranelibrary.com.
30. Budnitz DS, Lovegrove MC, Shehab N, Richards CL. Emergency hospitalization for adverse drug events in older Americans. N Eng J Med. 2011;365:2002–12.
31. Rydberg DM, Linder M, Malmström RE, Andersen M. Risk factors for severe bleeding events during warfarin treatment: the influence of sex, age, comorbidity and co-medication. Eur J Clin Pharmacol. 2020;76(6).
32. Lip GYH, Frison L, Halperin JL, Lane DA. Comparative validation of a novel risk score for predicting bleeding risk in anticoagulated patients with atrial fibrillation. J Am Coll Cardiol. 2011;57(2).
33. Verdecchia P, Angeli F, Aita A, Bartolini C, Reboldi G. Why switch from warfarin to NOACs? Intern Emerg Med. 2016;11(3).
34. Starling LD, Sinha A, Boyd D, Furck A. Fetal warfarin syndrome. BMJ Case Rep [Internet]. 2012. https://www.ncbi.nlm.nih.gov/pmc/articles/PMC3624665/.
35. Budnitz DS, Lovegrove MC, Shehab N, Richards CL. Emergency hospitalizations for adverse drug events in older Americans A BS T R AC T, vol. 365, N Engl J Med. 2011.
36. Leentjens J, Peters M, Esselink AC, Smulders Y, Kramers C. Initial anticoagulation in patients with pulmonary embolism: thrombolysis, unfractionated heparin, LMWH, fondaparinux, or DOACs? Br J Clin Pharmacol. 2017;83(11):2356–66.
37. Tektonidou MG, Andreoli L, Limper M, Amoura Z, Cervera R, Costedoat-Chalumeau N, et al. EULAR recommendations for the management of antiphospholipid syndrome in adults. Ann Rheum Dis. 2019;78(10):1296–304.
38. Douxfils J, Ageno W, Samama CM, Lessire S, ten Cate H, Verhamme P, et al. Laboratory testing in patients treated with direct oral anticoagulants: a practical guide for clinicians. J Thromb Haemost. 2018;16(2):209–19.
39. Khan F, Rahman A, Carrier M, Kearon C, Weitz JI, Schulman S, et al. Long term risk of symptomatic recurrent venous thromboembolism after discontinuation of anticoagulant treatment for first unprovoked venous thromboembolism event: systematic review and meta-analysis. BMJ. 2019;366.
40. Connors JM. Extended treatment of venous thromboembolism. N engl j med. 2013;8:368.
41. Weitz JI, Lensing AWA, Prins MH, Bauersachs R, Beyer-Westendorf J, Bounameaux H, et al. Rivaroxaban or aspirin for extended treatment of venous thromboembolism. N Engl J Med. 2017;376(13):1211–22.
42. Hirsh J, Fuster V, Ansell J, Halperin JL. American Heart Association/American College of Cardiology Foundation Guide to Warfarin Therapy. Circulation. 2003;107(12).

Catheter Directed Thrombolytic Therapy in Pulmonary Embolism

Gabby Elbaz-Greener, Ronny Alcalai, Eyal Herzog, Allan I. Bloom, and David Planer

1 Introduction

Pulmonary embolism (PE) is considered to be the third most common cause of cardiovascular death worldwide, with up to 100,000 deaths per year in the US [1].

Management of patients with PE is complex and depends on the severity of the event in addition to the resources and expertise of the health care system managing the patient.

Current clinical guidelines categorize PE severity into four main risk categories: low risk, intermediate-low risk, intermediate-high risk and high-risk PE [1–3]. This classification is based on the hemodynamic status of the patient, clinical parameters, severity of PE as assessed by the pulmonary embolism scoring index (PESI), right ventricle (RV) function and by the level of cardiac biomarkers [1–3].

A consensus document was recently issued by the Pulmonary Embolism Response Team (PERT) Consortium, which endorses a PERT approach to intermediate-high risk patients by a multidisciplinary team. This team includes cardiologists, interventional cardiologists, radiologists, interventional radiologists, cardiac surgeons, hematologists and critical care specialists who discuss the PE cases and expedite treatment decisions. The PERT team intends to influence PE outcomes by early diagnosis, management, treatment and follow-up [4]. PERT team decisions include three major components [4, 5]:

*Co-senior authors Allan I. Bloom and David Planer, equally contributed to the chapter.

G. Elbaz-Greener (✉) · R. Alcalai · E. Herzog · D. Planer
Department of Cardiology, Faculty of Medicine, Hadassah University Medical Center, Hebrew University of Jerusalem, Jerusalem, Israel
e-mail: Gabby@hadassah.org.il

A. I. Bloom
Department of Medical Imaging, Interventional and Vascular Radiology, Hadassah University Medical Center, Jerusalem, Israel

E. Herzog (ed.), *Pulmonary Embolism*,
https://doi.org/10.1007/978-3-030-87090-4_12

1. The anticoagulation treatment on admission and discharge (i.e. Heparin, Low Molecular Weight Heparin (LMWH), Vitamin K Antagonist (VKA), Direct Oral Anticoagulant (DOAC)).
2. The need for cardiopulmonary/hemodynamic support.
3. The reperfusion strategy: I. pharmacological alone (systemic anticoagulation); II. thrombolysis (i.e. systemic, CDT, USCDT or mechanical); III. embolectomy (i.e. surgical, catheter direct modalities).

2 The Rationale for CDT and Its Indications

Anticoagulation should be initiated as soon as the diagnosis of PE is suspected [1–3]. Unfractionated heparin may be preferred in patients who are candidates for further advanced therapies such as systemic thrombolysis, CDT, catheter directed or surgical embolectomy because it provides more flexibility for the procedures due to it is short half-life [1–3].

CDT is one of the newest, novel treatment options for intermediate-high risk PE and a small selected group of patients with high risk PE.

In general, there is consensus that patients with low-risk PE should be treated with anticoagulation alone, and that in patients with high-risk PE, systemic thrombolysis is recommended as first-line therapy unless contraindicated [1–3]. CDT or surgical embolectomy are reserved for patients who are not candidates for systemic thrombolysis [3] or for patients who have a higher risk of bleeding with systemic thrombolytic therapy and who have access to the expertise and resources required to perform CDT. Similarly, if the expert PERT team is likely to choose CDT over systemic thrombolytic therapy [6].

In contrast to patients with low-risk and high-risk PE, the optimal treatment for intermediate-risk pulmonary embolism remains controversial [7–9]. Because of the perception of a reduced risk of major hemorrhage, including intra-cranial, when compared to systemic thrombolysis, CDT is increasingly used for patients with intermediate-risk PE, based largely on the assumptions that it is more efficacious than anticoagulation alone and safer than systemic thrombolysis. The goal of therapy is to rapidly decrease the clot burden, to increase pulmonary arterial perfusion, to reduce the pulmonary artery (PA) and right heart pressures, thereby hastening resolution of RV strain. This strategy may improve short term survival, while preventing progression to chronic thromboembolic pulmonary hypertension (CTEPH) and thus improving long term outcome [7–9].

3 Contraindications

Absolute contraindications for CDT are similar to the contraindications for systemic thrombolysis. They include: patients with recent intracranial hemorrhage, structural cerebral vascular lesions, intracranial neoplasm, ischemic stroke within the past three months, possible aortic dissection, active bleeding or bleeding diathesis (excluding menses), significant head injury or facial trauma within the past three months, recent intracranial or spinal surgery, severe uncontrolled hypertension and for streptokinase, previous treatment within six months [10].

Relative contraindications include: severe, poorly controlled hypertension, severe hypertension at presentation (systolic blood pressure > 180 mmHg or diastolic blood pressure > 110 mmHg), prolonged (>10 min) cardiopulmonary resuscitation (CPR) or major surgery within three weeks, history of ischemic stroke, dementia, internal bleeding within 2–4 weeks, non-compressible vascular puncture, pregnancy, active peptic ulcer, current therapy of anticoagulant associated with an elevated international normalized ratio (INR) higher than 1.7 or a prothrombin time (PT) longer than 15 s [10].

3.1 The Procedure

The access to the pulmonary arteries is typically achieved via the femoral veins, however jugular vein access can also be used. Ultrasound guided venous puncture is recommended to reduce vascular and bleeding complications. A 4–6 French shaped diagnostic catheter (Multipurpose, Judkins Right or pigtail catheter) with the guide-wire is inserted via a 6-french introducer sheath and placed within the pulmonary artery (main, right and left) using fluoroscopic guidance. PA pressure is measured using a multi side hole catheter to assess the degree of pulmonary hypertension. Integrated information obtained by a pulmonary CT scan (Fig. 1a) and/or by pulmonary angiogram (Fig. 1b) may be used to choose the best target for the catheter thrombolysis procedure (Fig. 1c) using 5–6-french pigtail catheter. Figures 2a–d demonstrate the equipment for CDT that is used in our health care center. One or two therapeutic guiding catheters (i.e. Multipurpose or Judkins Right 6Fr) are inserted to the target arteries (Fig. 3a) and an infusion catheter (i.e. Cragg-McNamara™; Boston Scientific Infusion Catheter 4-5 Fr), is inserted through the guiding catheter and placed within the embolus (Fig. 3b, c). Typically, a dose of 3 mg tPA is given as a bolus in each catheter and this is followed by a continuous infusion of 1 mg/h of tPA for 12–18 h. This is done with combination of systemic heparin infusion to achieve a target PTT of 60–80. Alternatively, an ultrasound-assisted thrombolysis catheter (USCDT) (EKOS Corp) can be used, usually for a shorter duration of treatment.

The patient is monitored in the cardiac intensive care unit by staff who are familiar with the procedure, anticipated outcome and potential complications [11].

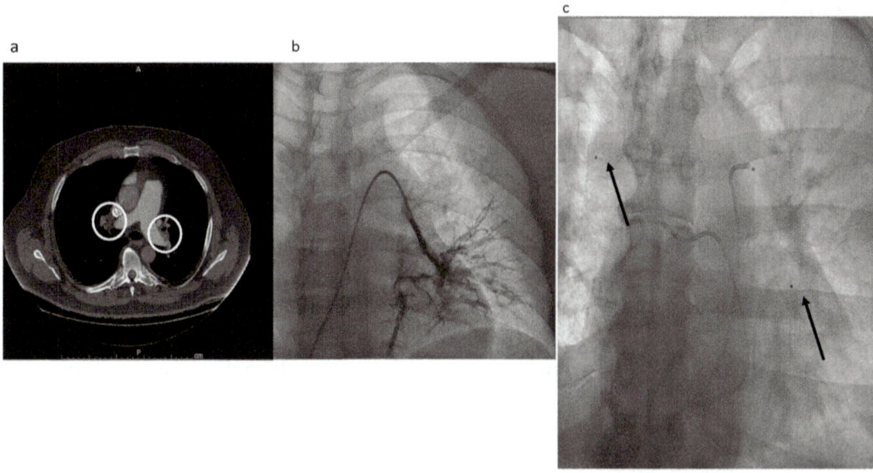

Fig. 1 Integrated information obtained by a pulmonary CT scan (**a**), white circles indicate right and left PA emboli) and by pulmonary angiogram (**b**), is used to select the best target for the catheter thrombolysis; black arrow (**c**)

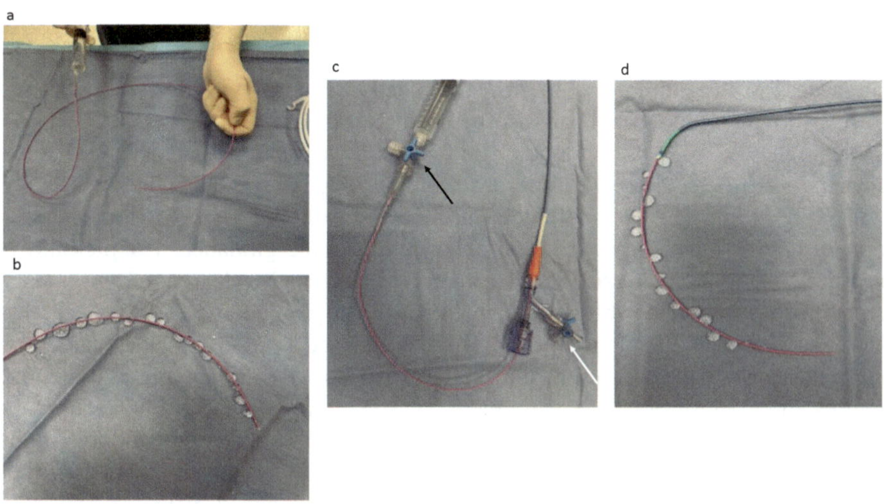

Fig. 2 Cragg-McNamara™; (Boston Scientific), Infusion-catheter is flushed with saline (**a**), Saline exiting the side holes (**b**), Infusion-catheter inserted into the guide-catheter, the distal port (black arrow) for tPA infusion and the side port (white arrow) for saline flushing (**c**, **d**)

Clinical evaluation of the patient after the completion of the infusion of the low dose thrombolytic therapy includes: transthoracic echocardiogram, CT angiography or in selected patients a repeated pulmonary angiogram (Fig. 4a, b) to evaluate the improvement in arterial perfusion, the reduction of clot burden, the change in the

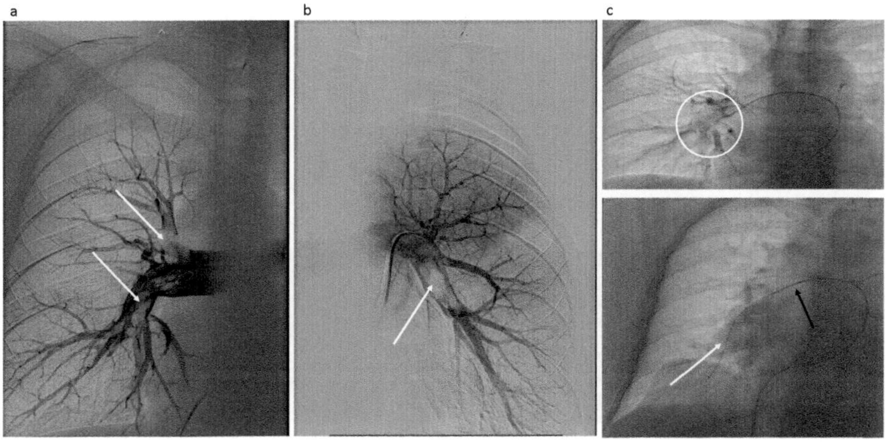

Fig. 3 Selective pulmonary angiogram demonstrates right and left PA with lobar emboli and reduced peripheral perfusion; white arrow (**a**, **b**), selective injection; white circle (**c** top), and catheter thrombolysis catheter; white arrow (**c** bottom) insertion via the guide catheter in the selected artery; black arrow (**c** bottom)

PA pressure (Fig. 5a, b) and to evaluate the RV size and function. Depending on these results, the decision is made to pursue additional thrombolytic therapy or to withdraw the CDT catheter with continuation of systemic anticoagulation.

Additional examples of CDT procedures from our health care center are shown in Figs. 6, 7, 8 and 9.

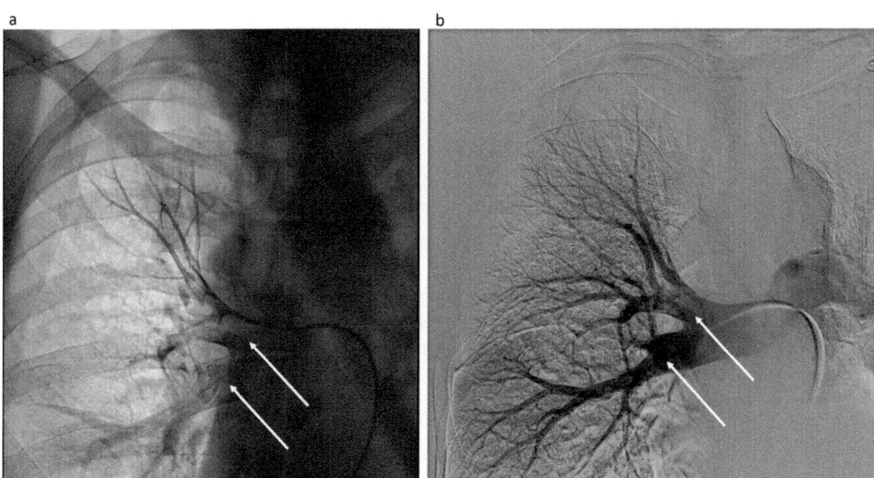

Fig. 4 Patient with Acute PE. Pulmonary angiogram before (**a**) and after CDT therapy (**b**) with decreased clot burden (white arrows)

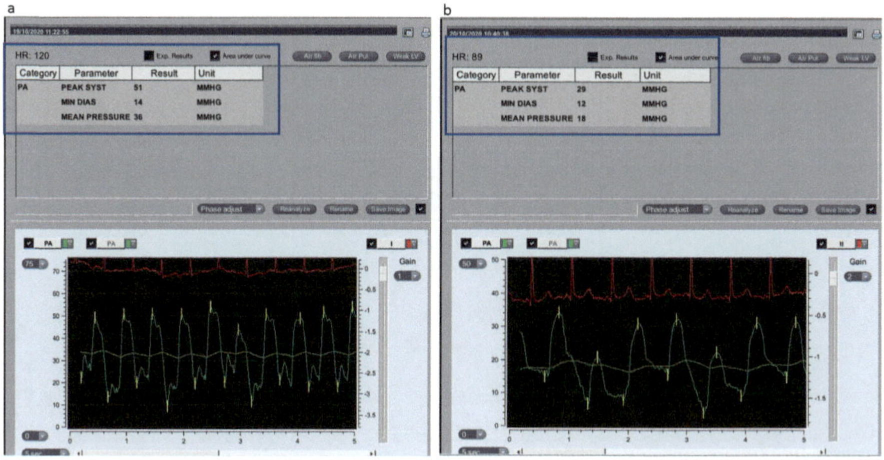

Fig. 5 Patient with Acute PE. Direct pressure measurements during Pulmonary angiography showed Peak systolic and mean pressure of 51 and 36 mmHg respectively before tPA CDT therapy (**a**) and decreased PA Peak systolic and mean pressures of 29 and 18 mmHg respectively after 14 h of CDT therapy (**b**)

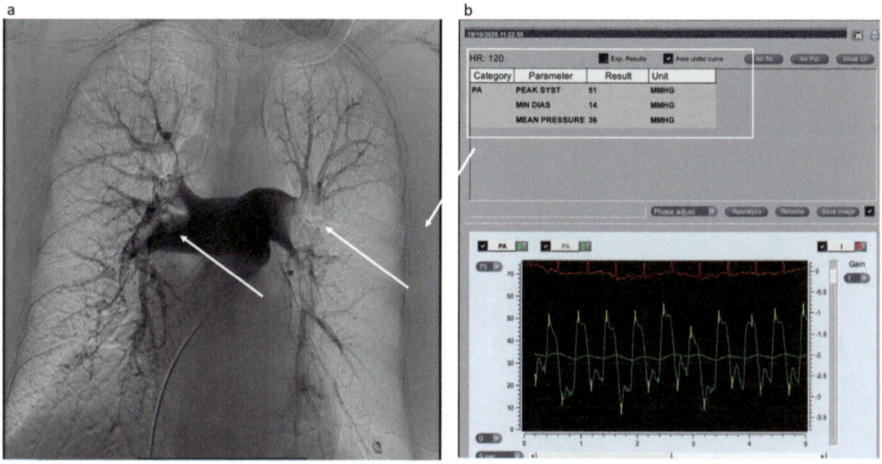

Fig. 6 Acute PE. Pulmonary angiogram from the main PA with large central emboli in both the left and right PA; white arrows (**a**). Note marked reduction of perfusion especially on the left side. Peak systolic and mean arterial pressure of 51 and 36 mmHg before CDT therapy (**b**)

a b

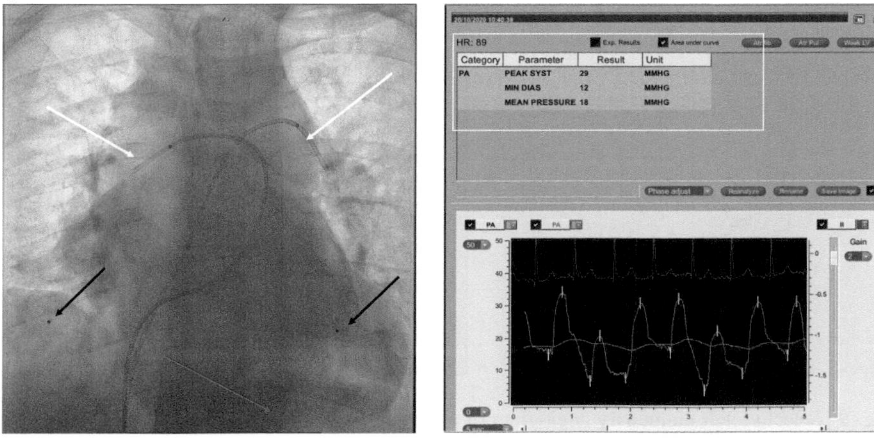

Fig. 7 Same patient that was described in Fig. 6: pulmonary angiogram with two guiding catheters; white arrows (**a**) and two infusion catheters; black arrows (**a**). There is a marked reduction in PA pressure after 11 h of CDT (**b**)

a b

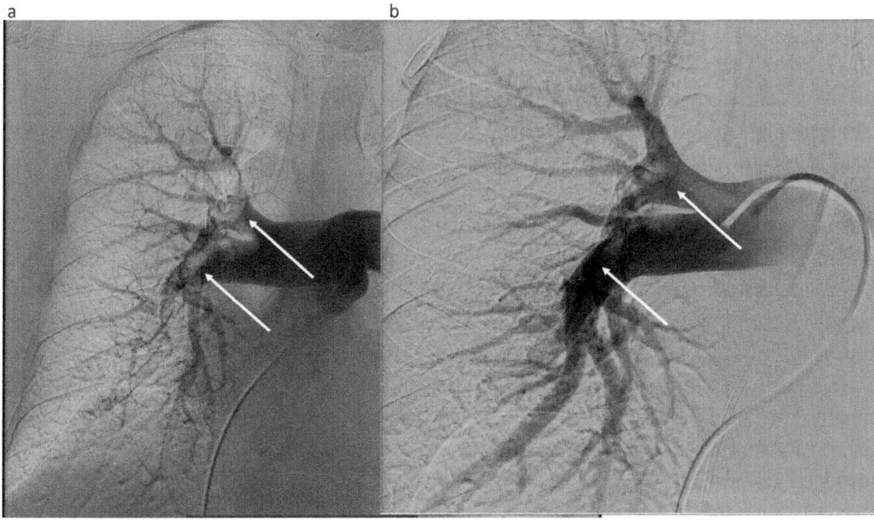

Fig. 8 Acute PE: Pulmonary angiogram before CDT shows central and lobar emboli in the right lung; white arrows (**a**). Post CDT therapy (**b**); white arrows demonstrate a marked reduction of clot burden and improved perfusion

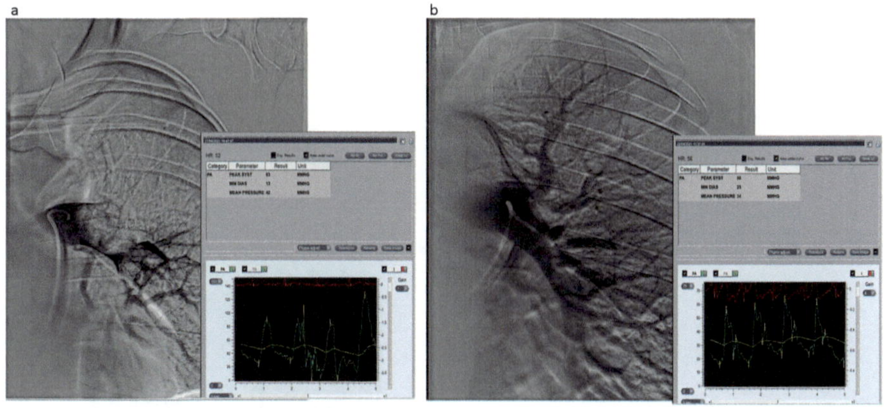

Fig. 9 Selective left pulmonary angiogram of a patient with acute PE before CDT with systolic PA pressure of 83 mmHg (**a**) and after CDT therapy with decreased clot burden, improved perfusion and a significant reduction in systolic PA pressure to 50 mmHg (**b**)

3.2 *Post Procedure Follow-Up*

At the time of this publication there is no clinical evidence to recommend a specific follow up regime post procedure, with the consensus being that the follow up of patients is similar to patients who received systemic thrombolysis.

Patients should undergo neurologic and cardiovascular evaluation with blood pressure monitoring every 15 min during and after the tPA infusion at least for 2 h, then every half an hour for the next 6 h and hourly for the next 16 h. Fibrinolytic therapy should be stopped immediately with any signs of neurologic deterioration, and the patient should receive an emergency full neurological assessment including computed tomography (CT) of the head. Furthermore, fibrinolytic agents must be stopped immediately with any evidence of a significant bleeding complication. Hemodynamic assessment should be performed, transfusion of blood products and volume support should be initiated. If the patient also has been on concomitant heparin, protamine sulfate can reverse the heparin effect [12]. If systemic anticoagulation cannot be continued at this time, the insertion of an optional IVC filter should be considered [13].

3.3 *Potential Complications of CTD*

Thrombolytic agents, also known as fibrinolytic or thrombolysis agents, aim to dissolve intravascular clots and to prevent ischemic damage by improving blood flow. Adverse effects of these agents include: systemic and local effects such as minor or major bleeding, allergic reactions, angioedema and hypotension [10–12].

Bleeding is the most frequent complication of thrombolytic therapy and can occur at the puncture site or spontaneously anywhere in the body, including pulmonary or retroperitoneal hemorrhage. Intracranial hemorrhage or hemorrhagic stroke is the greatest concern of this therapy with a potentially devastating outcome. To prevent this complication, the dose of the therapy must be adjusted to the body-weight of the patient. Other complications include: perforation or dissection of the pulmonary artery, cardiac arrhythmias, right-sided valvular regurgitation, pericardial tamponade, and contrast-induced nephropathy [10–12].

4 The Evidence to Support the Use of CDT

Table 1 summarizes current evidence for the use of CDT in PE [14–27].

Several clinical trials have investigated the use and the safety of CDT for the treatment of acute PE [28–30]. Kuo et al. [14] reported in the Pulmonary Embolism Response to Fragmentation, Embolectomy, and Catheter Thrombolysis (PERFECT) registry, that CDT has a lower risk of major bleeding compared to conventional systemic therapy. They concluded that CDT is a safe and effective treatment of both acute massive and sub-massive PE [14]. The Ultrasound-Assisted, Catheter-Directed Thrombolysis for Acute Intermediate-Risk Pulmonary Embolism (ULTIMA) [15] and the SEATLE II [16] studies compared USCDT to anticoagulation and thrombolytic therapy respectively. They concluded that CDT was superior to the other treatment options in reversing RV dilatation without increasing the risk of bleeding or mortality. The SEATLE II study also showed evidence of reduction in pulmonary hypertension, clot burden and a decreased intracranial bleeding rate compared to systemic thrombolysis.

Few studies however have reported conflicting results but had many limitations due to lack of data [14–27]. Accordingly, current European Society of Cardiology (ESC) and American College of Chest Physicians (ACCP) guidelines [1–3] recommend limiting the use of CDT for patients with:

1. Hemodynamic instability in whom systemic thrombolysis is contraindicated or has failed.
2. Patients with a high bleeding risk.
3. Patients in shock who are likely to die before systemic thrombolysis can take effect.

It is highly recommended that CDT be used only if appropriate expertise and resources are available [6].

Interestingly, since the establishment of a PERT team at our institution the use of systemic thrombolysis has decreased by whereas the use of CDT has increased.

Table 1 Current evidence for the use of CDT in PE

Publication	N	Intervention	Control	Outcomes
Kuo et al. 2015 [14]	101	CDT		Improvement in right-sided heart strain There were no major procedure-related complications, major hemorrhages, or hemorrhagic strokes
Kucher et al. 2014 [15]	59	USCDT		USCDT found to be superior regarding improving RV function. USCDT appears safe from bleeding complications
Piazza et al. 2015 [16]	150	USCDT		USCDT decreased RV dilation, reduced pulmonary hypertension, decreased anatomic thrombus burden, and minimized intracranial bleeding
Yoo et al. 2016 [17]	72	CDT	Thrombolysis	Similar outcomes regarding; 7-day mortality, in-hospital mortality and bleeding
Avgerinos et al. 2016 [18]	128	CDT/ USCDT	Anticoagulation	Similar outcomes in PE related mortality or major bleeding In the CDT group faster restoration of RV function, shorter ICCU stay, higher rate of minor bleeding were found
Liang et al. 2017 [19]	2860	CDT	Thrombolysis	Systemic thrombolysis for acute pulmonary embolism may not improve in-hospital mortality compared to CDT but increases the overall risk of hemorrhagic stroke compared to catheter-directed intervention
Arora et al. 2017 [20]	4426	CDT	Thrombolysis	Lower rate of in-hospital mortality as well as bleeding in the CDT group. Similar readmission rates between groups
Avgerinos et al. 2018 [21]	317	CDT/ USCDT	Thrombolysis	CDT provides similar recovery of right ventricular function compared with ST. Major bleeding and stroke complications may be lower
Sista et al. 2018 [22]	87	CDT	Anticoagulation	Rates of mortality and bleeding did not correlate with treatment arm
Schissler et al. 2018 [23]	104	USCDT	Anticoagulation	USCDT treatment was not associated with mortality benefit or increased resolution of RV dysfunction
Sharifi et al. 2019 [24]	97	USCDT	Thrombolysis	The results indicate that both USCDT and CDT lead to rapid reduction of PASP and RV/LV pressures. The individual components of death, bleeding, and transfusion at 30 days were not different between the groups

(continued)

Table 1 (continued)

Publication	N	Intervention	Control	Outcomes
Stein et al. 2020 [25]	1,500	CDT	Anticoagulation	Mortality was lower with CDT than with anticoagulants in unmatched patients There were no fatal or nonfatal adverse events associated with CDT
D'Auria et al. 2020 [26]	198	CDT	Anticoagulation	CDT reduced mortality at 30-days and 1-year when compared without increase in bleeding
Beyer et al. 2020 [27]	5,436	CDT/ USCDT	Thrombolysis	Rates of bleeding events, vasopressor use, and mechanical ventilation were similar between therapeutic strategies. Following adjustment, in-hospital mortality and 30-day readmission rates were not significantly different between USCDT and CDT alone

CDT Catheter Direct Thrombolysis; *USCDT* Ultrasound Assist Catheter Direct Thrombolysis)

5 Conclusions

CDT is one of the newest, novel treatment options for patients with acute PE who are risk stratified to the "intermediate-high risk" PE group, in addition to selected patients with "high risk" PE. There is increasing evidence in the current literature to support extending it's use in many health care systems worldwide.

References

1. Benjamin EJ, Muntner P, Alonso A, Bittencourt MS, Callaway CW, Carson AP, Chamberlain AM, Chang AR, Cheng S, Das SR, Delling FN, Djousse L, Elkind MSV, Ferguson JF, Fornage M, Jordan LC, Khan SS, Kissela BM, Knutson KL, Kwan TW, Lackland DT, Lewis TT, Lichtman JH, Longenecker CT, Loop MS, Lutsey PL, Martin SS, Matsushita K, Moran AE, Mussolino ME, O'Flaherty M, Pandey A, Perak AM, Rosamond WD, Roth GA, Sampson UKA, Satou GM, Schroeder EB, Shah SH, Spartano NL, Stokes A, Tirschwell DL, Tsao CW, Turakhia MP, VanWagner LB, Wilkins JT, Wong SS, Virani SS, American Heart Association Council on E, Prevention Statistics C and Stroke Statistics S. Heart disease and stroke statistics-2019 update: a report from the American Heart Association. Circulation. 2019;139:e56–e528.
2. Konstantinides SV, Meyer G, Becattini C, Bueno H, Geersing GJ, Harjola VP, Huisman MV, Humbert M, Jennings CS, Jimenez D, Kucher N, Lang IM, Lankeit M, Lorusso R, Mazzolai L, Meneveau N, Ni Ainle F, Prandoni P, Pruszczyk P, Righini M, Torbicki A, Van Belle E, Zamorano JL and Group ESCSD. 2019 ESC Guidelines for the diagnosis and management of acute pulmonary embolism developed in collaboration with the European Respiratory Society (ERS). Eur Heart J. 2020;41:543–603.

3. Jaff MR, McMurtry MS, Archer SL, Cushman M, Goldenberg N, Goldhaber SZ, Jenkins JS, Kline JA, Michaels AD, Thistlethwaite P, Vedantham S, White RJ, Zierler BK, American Heart Association Council on Cardiopulmonary CCP, Resuscitation, American Heart Association Council on Peripheral Vascular D, American Heart Association Council on Arteriosclerosis T and Vascular B. Management of massive and submassive pulmonary embolism, iliofemoral deep vein thrombosis, and chronic thromboembolic pulmonary hypertension: a scientific statement from the American Heart Association. Circulation. 2011;123:1788–830.
4. https://pertconsortium.org/about/. Accessed July 2021.
5. Herzog E, Elbaz-Greener G, Planer D, Koren T, Amir O, Shapiro J and Kalish Y. Pathway for the diagnosis and management of pulmonary embolism. Crit Pathw Cardiol. 2021;20:57–62.
6. Kearon C, Akl EA, Ornelas J, Blaivas A, Jimenez D, Bounameaux H, Huisman M, King CS, Morris TA, Sood N, Stevens SM, Vintch JRE, Wells P, Woller SC, Moores L. Antithrombotic therapy for VTE disease: CHEST guideline and expert panel report. Chest. 2016;149:315–52.
7. Busse LW, Vourlekis JS. Submassive pulmonary embolism. Crit Care Clin. 2014;30:447–73.
8. Piazza G. Submassive pulmonary embolism. JAMA. 2013;309:171–80.
9. Kabrhel C, Rosovsky R, Channick R, Jaff MR, Weinberg I, Sundt T, Dudzinski DM, Rodriguez-Lopez J, Parry BA, Harshbarger S, Chang Y, Rosenfield K. A multidisciplinary pulmonary embolism response team: initial 30-month experience with a novel approach to delivery of care to patients with submassive and massive pulmonary embolism. Chest. 2016;150:384–93.
10. Baig MU, Bodle J. Thrombolytic therapy. In: StatPearls [Internet]. Treasure Island (FL): StatPearls Publishing; 2021. https://www.ncbi.nlm.nih.gov/books/NBK557411. Accessed July 2021.
11. Brown KN, Devarapally SR, Lee LS, et al. Catheter directed thrombolysis of pulmonary embolism. In: StatPearls [Internet]. Treasure Island (FL): StatPearls Publishing; 2021 Jan–. https://www.ncbi.nlm.nih.gov/books/NBK536918. Accessed July 2021.
12. Kaufman C, Kinney T, Quencer K. Practice trends of fibrinogen monitoring in thrombolysis. J Clin Med. 2018;7:111–21.
13. DeYoung E, Minocha J. Inferior vena cava filters: guidelines, best practice, and expanding indications. Semin Intervent Radiol. 2016;33:65–70.
14. Kuo WT, Banerjee A, Kim PS, DeMarco FJ Jr, Levy JR, Facchini FR, Unver K, Bertini MJ, Sista AK, Hall MJ, Rosenberg JK, De Gregorio MA. Pulmonary Embolism Response to Fragmentation, Embolectomy, and Catheter Thrombolysis (PERFECT): initial results from a prospective multicenter registry. Chest. 2015;148:667–73.
15. Kucher N, Boekstegers P, Müller OJ, Kupatt C,Beyer-Westendorf J, Heitzer T, ,Tebbe U, Horstkotte J, Müller R, Blessing E, Greif M, Lange P, Thorsten Hoffmann R, Werth S, Barmeyer A, Härtel D, Grünwald H, Empen K, Baumgartner I. Randomized, controlled trial of ultrasound-assisted catheter-directed thrombolysis for acute intermediate-risk pulmonary embolism. Circulation. 2014;129:479–86.
16. Piazza G, Hohlfelder B, Jaff MR, Ouriel K, Engelhardt TC, Sterling KM, Jones NJ, Gurley JC, Bhatheja R, Kennedy RJ, Goswami N, Natarajan K, Rundback J, Sadiq IR, Liu SK, Bhalla N, Raja ML, Weinstock BS, Cynamon J, Elmasri FF, Garcia MJ, Kumar M, Ayerdi J, Soukas P, Kuo W, Liu PY, Goldhaber SZ; SEATTLE II Investigators. A prospective, single-arm, multicenter trial of ultrasound-facilitated, catheter-directed, low-dose fibrinolysis for acute massive and submassive pulmonary embolism: the SEATTLE II study. JACC Cardiovasc Interv. 2015;10:1382–92.
17. Yoo Jw, Choi HC, Lee SJ, Cho YJ, Lee JD, Kim HC. American Journal of Emergency Medicine comparison between systemic and catheter thrombolysis in patients with pulmonary embolism. Am. J. Emerg. Med. 2016;34:985–8.
18. Avgerinos ED, Liang NL, El-Shazly OM, Toma C, Singh MJ, Makaroun MS, Chaer RA. Improved early right ventricular function recovery but increased complications with catheter-directed interventions compared with anticoagulation alone for submassive

pulmonary embolism presented in the plenary session at the 2015 vascular annual meeting. J Vasc Surg Venous Lymphat Disord. 2016;4:268–75.
19. Liang NL, Avgerinos ED, Singh MJ, Makaroun MS. Systemic thrombolysis increases hemorrhagic stroke risk without survival bene fi t compared with catheter-directed intervention for the treatment of acute pulmonary embolism. J. Vasc. Surg. 2017; 5:171–176.e1
20. Arora S, Panaich SS, Ainani N, Kumar V, Patel NJ, Tripathi B, Shah P, Patel N, Lahewala S, Deshmukh A, Badheka A, Grines C. Comparison of in-hospital outcomes and readmission rates in acute pulmonary embolism between systemic and catheter-directed thrombolysis (from the national Readmission Database). Am J Cardiol. 2017;120:1653–61.
21. Avgerinos ED, Abou Ali AN, Liang NL, Lebron BR, Toma C, Maholic R, Makaroun MS, Chaer R. Catheter-directed interventions compared with systemic thrombolysis achieve improved ventricular function recovery at a potentially lower complication rate for acute pulmonary embolism. J Vasc Surg Venous Lymphat Disord. 2018;6:425–32.
22. Sista AK, Friedman OA, Dou E, Denvir B, Askin G, Stern J, Estes J, Salemi A, Winokur RS, Horowitz JM. A pulmonary embolism response team's initial 20 month experience treating 87 patients with submassive and massive pulmonary embolism. Vasc Med. 2018;23:65–71.
23. Schissler AJ, Gylnn RJ, Sobieszczyk PS, Waxman AB. Ultrasound-assisted catheter-directed thrombolysis compared with anticoagulation alone for treatment of intermediate-risk pulmonary embolism. Pulm. Circ. 2018;8. https://doi.org/10.1177/2045894018800265.
24. Sharifi M, Awdisho A, Schroeder B, Jimenez J, Lyer P, Bay C. Retrospective comparison of ultrasound facilitated catheter-directed thrombolysis and systemically administered half-dose thrombolysis in treatment of pulmonary embolism. Vasc Med. 2019;24:103–9.
25. Stein PD, Matta F, Hughes MJ. Catheter-directed thrombolysis in submassive pulmonary embolism and acute cor pulmonale. Am J Cardiol. 2020;131:109–14.
26. D'Auria S, Sezer A, Thoma F, Sharbaugh M, McKibben J, Maholic R, Avgerinos ED, Rivera Lebron BL, Toma C. Outcomes of catheter-directed thrombolysis vs. standard medical therapy in patients with acute submassive pulmonary embolism. Pulm. Circ. 2020;10. https://doi.org/10.1177/2045894019898368.
27. Beyer SE, Shanafelt C, Pinto DS, Weinstein JL, Aronow HD, Weinberg I, Yeh RW, Secemsky EA, Carroll BJ. Utilization and outcomes of thrombolytic therapy for acute pulmonary embolism: a nationwide cohort study. Chest. 2020;157:645–53.
28. Jimenez D, Martin-Saborido C, Muriel A, Zamora J, Morillo R, Barrios D, Klok FA, Huisman MV, Tapson V, Yusen RD. Efficacy and safety outcomes of recanalisation procedures in patients with acute symptomatic pulmonary embolism: systematic review and network meta-analysis. Thorax. 2018;73:464–71.
29. Lou BH, Wang LH, Chen Y. A meta-analysis of efficacy and safety of catheter-directed interventions in submassive pulmonary embolism. Eur Rev Med Pharmacol Sci. 2017;21:184–98.
30. Konstantinides S. 2019 ESC guidelines on pulmonary embolism: novelties and unanswered questions. Eur J Intern Med. 2020;74:1–4.

Surgical Treatment of Acute Pulmonary Embolism

Sandhya K. Balaram and Minh Quan Vu

1 Introduction

The history of surgical pulmonary embolectomy (SPE) is closely linked to the history of cardiac surgery itself. Friedrich Trendelenburg, a German surgeon, was credited as the first to study and describe surgical removal of pulmonary embolism (PE) in 1908 [1]. Working initially on animal models, he developed a technique later termed the Trendelenberg Procedure, that allowed access to the pulmonary artery through a left parasternal thoracotomy [1]. Unfortunately, neither of his two patients who underwent the procedure survived the early postoperative period. Years later, his pupil Martin Kirschner reported the first successful pulmonary embolectomy at the German Surgical Conference in Berlin in 1924 [2].

Critical developments followed that affected the treatment of pulmonary embolism. For instance, the discovery of heparin as a systemic anticoagulant in 1916 became the cornerstone of pulmonary embolism management [3]. Futhermore, it was a patient who died of pulmonary embolism after a cholecystectomy that inspired John Gibbon to develop the cardiopulmonary bypass (CPB) circuit which was completed in 1953 [4]. This invention has helped millions of patients with cardiac and pulmonary disease since its inception.

The modern treatment of acute pulmonary embolism has evolved with the creation of a multidisciplinary team-based program termed PERT: pulmonary embolism response teams. This approach to care occurs in real time upon patient presentation and provides expert opinions from multiple specialties for the care of each individual patient [5]. These patients are often ill, regardless of the size of their PE. Large prospective databases and registries demonstrate a marked difference between overall outcomes of massive versus submassive PE. Submassive PE without hemodynamic instability is associated with a mortality between 3 and 15%

S. K. Balaram (✉) · M. Q. Vu
Department of Cardiovascular Surgery, Mount Sinai Morningside, New York City, NY, USA
e-mail: sandhya.balaram@mountsinai.org

E. Herzog (ed.), *Pulmonary Embolism*,
https://doi.org/10.1007/978-3-030-87090-4_13

while massive PE with CPR-requiring cardiogenic shock carries a mortality of 50–80% [6–8].

Given this range of mortality, there remains some discussion and controversy about optimal treatment for acute PE. There is little debate about small emboli with no hemodynamic compromise benefitting from anticoagulation alone. Yet right ventricular (RV) dysfunction with an elevated troponin or lactate, a saddle embolus with large clot burden, or the presence of even transient hypotension, can increase the mortality rate dramatically. Patients may appear stable with minimal oxygen requirements. It can be difficult to predict which patients may rapidly decompensate, even as high risk features are noted. For this subset of patients, it is important to recognize those that can significantly benefit from operative intervention versus those that may be treated with catheter-directed thrombolysis, lytic therapy, or anticoagulation alone.

Published formal indications for surgery are based on European guidelines most recently updated in 2019 [9]. Systemic thrombolysis is considered a class I recommendation for patients with hemodynamic deterioration and catheter directed thrombolysis and surgical embolectomy are considered alternative Class IIa recommendations. Other recommendations for surgical intervention involve the presence of right sided PE, or clots in transit, or the presence of an interatrial defect that would make a left sided ischemic stroke a possibility [9] (Table 1).

Recent studies suggest that patients with evidence of marked RV strain despite hemodynamic stability should be considered for early surgery [10]. Very early reports of mortality of over 60% have markedly improved, first dropping to 20–30% [11–13]. Current studies report 3–6% postoperative mortality for SPE [10, 14–16]. This large drop in mortality occurred due to technical improvements of cardiopulmonary bypass, better management of right ventricular dysfunction in the intensive care unit, and improved options for anticoagulation. The overall numbers of patients taken to the operating room for embolectomy after cardiac arrest have fallen as alternative treatments have become available. In today's era, improved surgical outcomes are a reflection of a careful selection of patients, comprehensive management in centers of expertise, and vigilant perioperative care.

Table 1 Indications for Surgical Pulmonary Embolectomy

Massive or Submassive PE with Hemodynamic instability
Contraindication to Lytic Therapy
Clot in Transit
Large PFO or ASD
Moderate to Severe Right Ventricular Dysfunction
Failed Catheter Directed or Systemic Thrombolysis

2 Preoperative Evaluation

Obtaining a detailed history from the patient requires specific questions regarding the presence or absence of syncope, duration of symptoms, trigging event, prior pulmonary emboli or DVT, and family history of PE or clotting disorders. Any comorbidities or neurological deficits should be noted. Exact hemodynamic status, oxygenation requirements, and tachycardia should be recorded. A formal physical exam should be performed. Preoperative studies, including the diagnostic CT angiogram (CTA), should be obtained in a timely manner and a TTE and electrocardiogram (EKG) should be available for immediate interpretation, preferably by the entire PERT team. Ultrasound examination of bilateral legs should be performed to rule out or document the presence of thrombus. Laboratory studies including troponin, D-dimer, beta natriuretic peptide (BNP), complete blood count (CBC), chemistries, lactate, coagulation studies, liver enzymes, fibrinogen, and arterial blood gas, should be obtained.

This preoperative evaluation of a patient with a massive or submissive PE is a critical component of the decision making process. Current guidelines reserve the use of surgical embolectomy for patients with massive PE in whom thrombolysis is contraindicated and who have documented hypoxemia, shock, or hypotension that is refractory to medical management [9]. The diagnostic CTA and TTE should be carefully evaluated and reviewed so that the patient may be risk-stratified. A clot in transit or a patent foramen oval with or without impending paradoxical embolism are immediate indications for surgical intervention (Table 1). Accurate assessment of the degree of right ventricular (RV) dysfunction by TTE is a vital part of this evaluation, as the possibility of impending instability may be identified based on severe RV dilation and hypokinesis as well as the occurrence of syncope; early surgery may be indicated. Given the marked improvement in recent surgical results, it is important that patients not wait for failed medical management to the point of hemodynamic collapse before the surgical team is involved. Thus the introduction of PERT groups has been a revolutionary advance in patient care by making these decisions in real time.

Formal contraindications should also be identified (Table 2). Some of these contraindications are relative, but would include patients with acute on chronic PE who are at high risk of right ventricular failure. In the setting of chronic endothelial changes in the pulmonary vasculature, these patients are at risk for pulmonary hemorrhage at the time of endarterectomy. Active bleeding is also a contraindication given the need for high dose heparin anticoagulation for cardiopulmonary bypass. The presence of a cerebrovascular accident (CVA), without evidence of hemorrhage, may change therapy depending on the clinical status of the patient and the findings on transthoracic echocardiography (TTE). Risk–benefit ratios with the requirement of heparinization for CPB clearly play a role in this setting. Pulmonary embolectomy may be justified in patients who have suffered a small ischemic stroke, if the patients are critically ill as a result of a large centrally located PE, and if there is no alternative rescue procedure available [10].

Table 2 Contraindications to Surgical Pulmonary Embolectomy

Use of Fibrinolytic Therapy
Hemorrhagic Stroke
Recent Major Trauma or Surgery
Active GI or other Bleed
Acute on Chronic Pulmonary Embolism (relative)
Recent TIA or Ischemic Stroke (relative)
Failed Thrombolysis (relative)

The timing of a recent surgical intervention that may act as a precursor to acute PE may also prevent the use of systemic lytic therapy. In fact, surgical embolectomy with controlled anticoagulation may be the patients best option if high risk features are present. While immediate preceding thrombolysis is not an absolute contraindication to SPE, the patient will be at significant risk for bleeding post-operatively [17]. This group of patients may benefit more from immediate extra corporeal membrane oxygenation (ECMO) to stabilize their hemodynamic status, followed by delayed SPE if needed [18–20] (Fig. 1). SPE in the setting of acute on chronic PE is generally contraindicated because of complications that may include persistent pulmonary hypertension, right heart failure, and intractable pulmonary hemorrhage [9]. Active bleeding from the gastrointestinal tract or post-surgical site is also a contraindication for SPE.

3 Operative Procedure

3.1 Preparation

In the operating room, the surgeon should expect hemodynamic instability at anesthetic induction in up to 19% of cases [7]. It is mandatory to have a surgical team available who are ready for an expeditious sternotomy and institution of cardiopulmonary bypass once the patient arrives. Many surgeons favor placement of monitoring lines while the patient is awake, and have the patient prepped for surgery prior to anesthesia induction. Transesophageal echocardiography (TEE) is standard in cardiac surgery, and provides immediate assessment of ventricular function and the presence of valvular disease or wall motion abnormalities and can confirm the presence of intra-atrial or right ventricular thrombus. The location of an atrial septal defect (ASD) or a patent foramen ovale (PFO) should also be reviewed at this time. Supine standard positioning is indicatd with the chest and legs prepped in a sterile fashion. A fluoroscopy table is indicated if a postoperative inferior vena cave (IVC) filter placement is planned.

3.2 *Surgical Technique*

Embolectomy alone can be performed under full cardiopulmonary support and a beating heart. Standard cardiopulmonary bypass is required including an aortic cannula and either bi-caval or double lumen right atrial cannulation for venous drainage. Bi-caval venous cannulation is required if the right atrium needs to be opened for closure of a PFO or ASD, or in the presence of right atrial clot in-transit. A single venous cannula can be used if SPE through the pulmonary arteries is the only procedure planned. An aortic root vent is placed for de-airing at the end of the procedure. We suggest a mild degree of hypothermia (32–34 °C). A left superior pulmonary vein vent can be placed to drain the left ventricle if needed.

Once high dose heparin is delivered and the activated clotting time is adequate, cardiopulmonary bypass is initiated. If there is an intra-cardiac thrombus, the right atrium is opened first through a vertical incision. Thrombus is removed carefully from the right atrium and right ventricle. An ASD or PFO should be closed at this

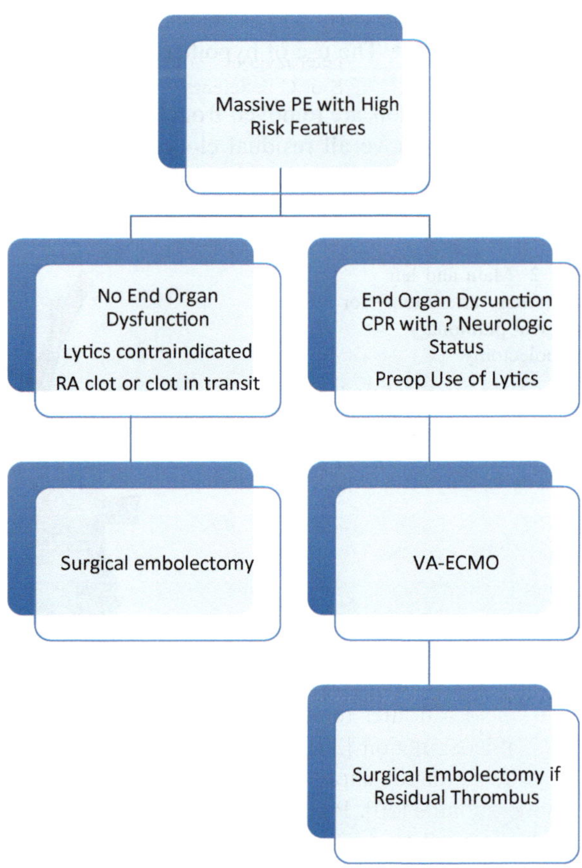

Fig. 1 Decision tree for surgical embolectomy and veno-arterial ECMO

time. A bovine pericardial patch may be needed if the defect is large. The right atrium is then closed and the main pulmonary artery (PA) is opened longitudinally 1.5 cm above the pulmonary valve. This incision can be extended to about 2–3 cm into the left main PA (Fig. 2). Optimal exposure is assured by using gentle traction with a nerve root or vein retractor. One should be careful with the use of pledgeted retraction sutures as the pulmonary artery wall is vulnerable to excessive traction. Continuous suctioning of any blood return aids visualization. Straight and angled ring forceps are used to gently remove all visible thrombus, preferably in a single specimen if possible. Large saddle emboli can usually be removed completely just with this incision.

Care should be taken not to injure the intima, particularly in the setting of acute on chronic pulmonary embolism. Each arterial branch should be inspected carefully and cleared. A Fogarty catheter can be used to retrieve distal thrombi but this does come with some risk of distal arterial injury not amenable to repair. Intermittent reduction in bypass flow facilitates clot removal by reducing pulmonary blood return, thus improving exposure. It is advisable to further cool the patient if frequent flow reduction periods are required. This decreases the metabolic rate and flow requirements. In the case of refractory high blood return, one can consider cross-clamping the aorta and ischemic arrest with delivery of cold blood cardioplegia to the heart. The use of hypothermic circulatory arrest is rarely needed in the current era.

Once all the clots are removed from the left side, copious irrigation with saline is suggested to remove all residual clots or debris in the PA. The right PA in then exposed and incised longitudinally (Fig. 3). The surgeon typically moves to the

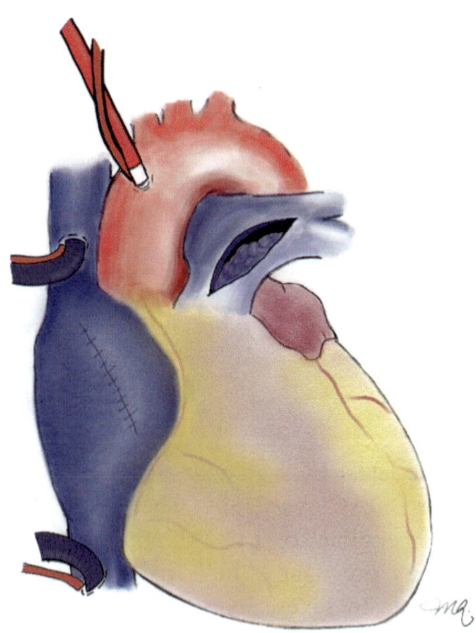

Fig. 2 Main and left pulmonary arteriotomy for surgical pulmonary embolectomy

patient's left side for better visualization of the right segmental branches. Again, continuous suction of blood return and adequate retraction are key for optimal exposure. Clots are removed in the same systematic way as on the left side. A Fogarty balloon catheter can be used at the discretion of the surgeon to remove distal clots if needed. The right PA is then closed with 4–0 prolene suture, followed by the main PA incision. In this way, large clots may be removed in total, a benefit of acute SPE (Fig. 4).

During PA closure, the heart is allowed to fill for routine de-airing maneuvers and the aortic root vent is opened. Valsalva maneuvers are performed by the anesthesia team in order to evacuate any remaining left-sided air. The patient is carefully weaned off the bypass machine, with care taken to monitor right and left ventricular function. Use of inotropes, epoprostenol, or nitric oxide may be required to lower PA pressure and aid postoperative recovery.

3.3 *Retrograde Pulmonary Embolectomy*

The technique of retrograde pulmonary embolectomy has been described and is used in some centers. It is a complementary technique to the standard embolectomy procedure, usually completed after antegrade removal of clots from the PA [21]. A cannula is inserted in the left superior pulmonary vein and a vascular clamp is applied to both left pulmonary veins, proximal to the cannula. One liter of cold

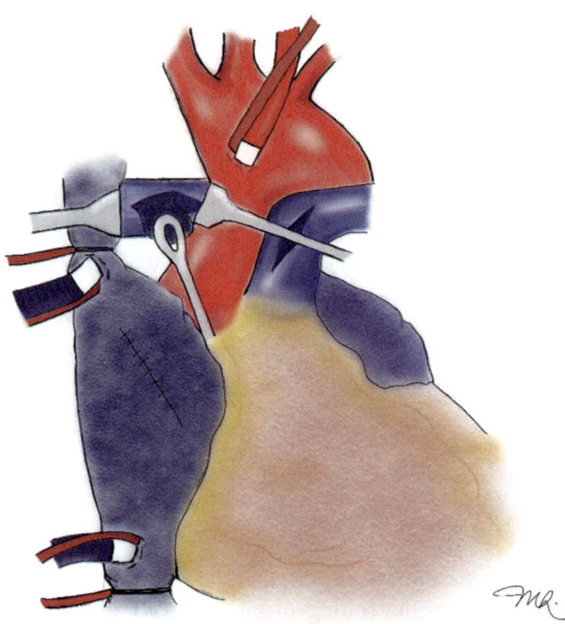

Fig. 3 Exposure and right pulmonary arteriotomy for surgical embolectomy

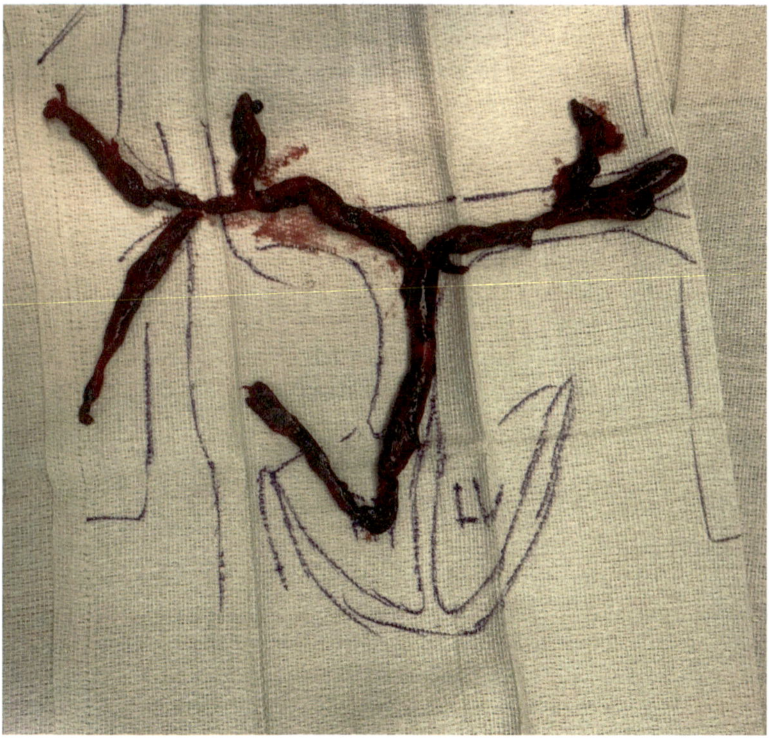

Fig. 4 Complete surgical specimen of large pulmonary clot-in-transit

blood at a flow of 200 mL/minute is flushed. Blood return with residual clots should be expected from the main PA incision [21]. An adequate perfusion pressure must be obtained to flush backward but not increase pulmonary edema. Opening the pleura will allow massage of the lung in order to facilitate dislodgement of the clots [21]. This technique is somewhat controversial, as manual compression may further injure an already fragile and infarcted lung [22]. Although retrograde flushing seems effective to remove distal and smaller clots, one should weigh the risk of a longer procedure, pulmonary edema, pulmonary vein trauma and possible pulmonary vein stenosis against the actual clinical benefits of removing residual clots. Smaller distal clots will likely resolve with anticoagulation and cause little hemodynamic compromise [10].

3.4 *IVC Filter*

Once the sternum is closed, an IVC filter may be inserted through the femoral vein, particularly in the setting of known DVT diagnosed preoperatively by ultrasound.

Adequate placement is guided by fluoroscopy. According to the current guidelines (the American Heart Association, the American College of Chest Physicians and the European Society of Cardiology), IVC filters are used when anticoagulation or thrombolysis are contraindicated or have failed [9]. Relative indications for IVC placement include large floating DVT, non-compliance to anticoagulation, recurrent PE, chronic PE treated with thromboendarterectomy, and massive PE treated with thrombolysis/thrombectomy [23]. Although the routine use of IVC filter is not recommended in all cases of PE, hemodynamically significant PE presents a higher risk that may warrant an IVC filter. In fact, data from the International Cooperative Pulmonary Embolism Registry (ICOPER) reported that among patients presenting with massive PE, those who received an IVC filter had higher survival rates and lower recurrence of PE [24]. These numbers should be interpreted with caution because of the low rates of IVC insertion ($\leq 10\%$), different patient characteristics between both groups,, and the retrospective nature of the study [24].

4 ECMO

Peripheral veno-arterial extracorporeal membrane oxygenation (ECMO) support can be considered in patients with massive pulmonary embolism with marked hemodynamic instability who are not immediate surgical candidates due to contraindications such as prior lytic therapy [18, 19]. This technique can offer early and reliable organ perfusion. It can also provide support in case of a suspected imminent circulatory collapse during anesthetic induction. VA-ECMO should also be considered for PE with cardiac arrest or refractory shock in combination with systemic thrombolysis as the initial management. This can be followed by delayed surgical pulmonary embolectomy if required.

ECMO is typically performed using a Seldinger technique with cannulas placed after sequential dilations of the target vessel over guidewires. A 16F or 18F cannula is used in the femoral artery and a 23F or 25F venous cannula is placed in the femoral vein, advanced up into the IVC for drainage. This can be done percutaneously or by using an open technique, with pursestrings placed around the cannula for hemostasis. The importance of the cannula placement, particularly the venous cannula, is critical and should be confirmed by x-ray fluoroscopy or by TEE.

4.1 *Postoperative Care and Follow-Up*

In addition to careful postoperative care in the surgical intensive care unit, patients require a formal Hematology consult and laboratory studies to rule out primary coagulation disorders such as Protein C and S deficiency, lupus anticoagulant, or Factor V Leiden deficiency. Patients are started on heparin initially and once no operative/surgical site bleeding is confirmed, direct oral anticoagulants (DOACs) are initiated. If DOACs are contraindicated, warfarin is begun. Patients are seen at one week and one month postoperatively and echocardiograms are done at one month, three months, six months, and then yearly to assess right ventricular function. Functional status can be objectively measured with six-minute walks.

5 Outcomes

In the current era, surgical embolectomy has become a viable option for patients who present with large PE and high-risk features. Published outcomes come from large volume tertiary medical centers with well-established systems in place. But in fact, in a query of isolated SPE performed between 2011 and 2015, only 310 centers out of 1144 eligible hospitals enrolled in the STS database performed at least one SPE, while only 7 centers reported an average of more than 5 per year [25]. Despite these low numbers, improvements in perioperative management, right ventricular support, and the use of ECMO in salvage situations, may all be contributing to overall improved outcomes.

As interest in SPE increases, more data is being collected. In the most recent STS database review, operative mortality was 16%, but only 8% in those patients who underwent surgery without the presence of shock [25]. Of those patients that required preoperative CPR, there was an overall mortality rate of 44%. In determining patient selection, it is important to look at predictors of mortality, which include age > 55, obesity BMI > 30, cardiogenic shock, preoperative CPR, neurologic coma, and moderate to severe chronic lung disease [25]. Also statistically significant were evidence of end organ injury: previous recent MI, low EF, RV dysfunction, renal failure, or elevated bilirubin [25]. Preoperative intraaortic balloon pump (IABP), inotropes, or need for ECMO are all obviously significant risk factors. Reoperation and prolonged ventilation are the most common morbidities in terms of postoperative outcomes and can occur in 50% of all patients [25].

A retrospective database study of over 58,000 acute PE patients who underwent surgical embolectomy, systemic thrombolysis, or catheter-directed therapy from 2010 to 2014, was recently published [26]. 3085 of these patients were treated with SPE with an overall mortality of 19.8%. Lower rates of major bleeding and intracranial hemorrhage were observed when compared to systemic thrombolysis [26]. Although overall in-hospital mortality was higher than less invasive treatments, this group was also at higher risk of death than the other two groups. Predictors of mortality from surgery in this study included age > 60, atrial fibrillation, congestive heart failure, and non-saddle embolus [26]. Once CPR is required, the increase in mortality rose from 16% to 44% [26].

The importance of preoperative cardiac arrest is significant for in-hospital mortality in all studies. SPE should be considered before this occurs, and perhaps also before escalating cardiogenic shock. Careful evaluation of the patient's history, physical exam, laboratory studies, and TTE, will help predict in which patients this decompensation may occur.

As experience increases and careful patient selection is used, outcomes will continue to improve. Depending on the center, early referral for SPE may be indicated. In fact, the surgical team is a critical element of most PERT systems. Benefits of early surgical intervention include marked improvement in RV function that has been shown to persist over midterm followup and supports early intervention [27, 28]. Surgical bail-out of failed lytic therapy presents a more complicated problem to manage due to the excessive risk of perioperative bleeding. Some evidence shows that surgery has similar early mortality rates and less bleeding complications when compared to systemic thrombolysis as the first line management of massive PE [29]. Surgery can be more efficient than thrombolysis to relieve strain on the RV and decrease pulmonary artery pressure [30]. In addition, outcomes in surgical embolectomy following failed thrombolysis were found to be superior to repeat thrombolysis, with lower mortality and recurrence of PE [30].

6 Conclusion

Recent reports have shown excellent outcomes achieved by early surgical intervention that occurs before deterioration of the hemodynamic state. Cardiogenic shock and poor neurologic status are strong risk factors for mortality after SPE and suggest that intervention prior to these secondary effects of a large PE will result in even better survival for these group.

The use of venoarterial ECMO may also play an important role going forward for those patients with marked hemodynamic instability, cardiopulmonary arrest, and questionable neurologic status. This device gives the surgeon time to stabilize the hemodynamic status of the patient, rest the right ventricle, and assess neurologic status, prior to proceeding with a more definitive operation.

References

1. Trendelenburg F. Uber die operative Behandlung der Embolie der Lungenarterie. Arch Klin Chir. 1908;86:686–700.
2. Kirschner M. Ein durch die Trendelenburgsche Operation geheilten Fall von Embolie der Art Pulmonalis. Arch Klin Chir. 1924;133:312–59.
3. Galanaud JP, Laroche JP, Righini M. The history and historical treatments of deep vein thrombosis. J Thromb Haemost. 2013;11(3):402–11.
4. Gibbon JH Jr. The development of the heart–lung apparatus. Am J Surg. 1978;135:608–19.
5. Chaudhury P, Gadre SK, Schneider E, Renapurkar RD, Gomes M, Haddadin I, Heresi GA, Tong MZ, Bartholomew JR. Impact of multidisciplinary pulmonary embolism response team availability on management and outcomes. Am J Cardiol. 2019;124(9):1465–9.

6. Bova C, Pesavento R, Marchiori A, et al. Risk stratification and outcomes in hemodynamically stable patients with acute pulmonary embolism: a prospective, multicentre, cohort study with three months of follow-up. J Thromb Haemost. 2009;7:938–44.
7. Kasper W, Konstantinides S, Geibel A, et al. Management strategies and determinants of outcome in acute major pulmonary embolism: results of a multicenter registry. J Am Coll Cardiol. 1997;30:1165–71.
8. Righini M, Roy PM, Meyer G, Verschuren F, Aujesky D, Le Gal G. The Simplified Pulmonary Embolism Severity Index (PESI): validation of a clinical prognostic model for pulmo- nary embolism. J Thromb Haemost. 2011;9:2115.
9. Konstantinides SV, Meyer G, Becattini C, Bueno H, Geersing GJ, Harjola VP, Huisman MV, Humbert M, Jennings CS, Jiménez D, Kucher N, Lang IM, Lankeit M, Lorusso R, Mazzolai L, Meneveau N, Ní Áinle F, Prandoni P, Pruszczyk P, Righini M, Torbicki A, Van Belle E, Zamorano JL; ESC Scientific Document Group. 2019 ESC Guidelines for the diagnosis and management of acute pulmonary embolism developed in collaboration with the European Respiratory Society (ERS). Eur Heart J. 2020;41(4):543–603.
10. Fukuda I, Daitoku K. Surgical Embolectomy for Acute Pulmonary Thromboembolism. Ann Vasc Dis. 2017;10(2):107–14.
11. Kalra R, Bajaj NS, Arora P, Arora G, Crosland WA, McGiffin DC, Ahmed MI. Surgical Embolectomy for acute pulmonary embolism: systematic review and comprehensive meta-analyses. Ann Thorac Surg. 2017;103(3):982–90.
12. Stein PD, Alnas M, Beemath A, Patel NR. Outcome of pulmonary embolectomy. Am J Cardiol. 2007;99:421–3.
13. Yavuz S, et al. Surgical embolectomy for acute massive pulmonary embolism. Int J Clin Exp Med. 2014;7(12):5362–75.
14. Leacche M, et al. Modern surgical treatment of massive pulmonary embolism: results in 47 consecutive patients after rapid diagnosis and aggressive surgical approach. J Thorac Cardiovasc Surg. 2005;129(5):1018–23.
15. Neely, R.C., et al., Surgical embolectomy for acute massive and submassive pulmonary embolism in a series of 115 patients. Ann Thorac Surg. 2015;100(4):1245–51; discussion 1251–2.
16. Pasrija, C., et al., Outcomes after surgical pulmonary embolectomy for acute submassive and massive pulmonary embolism: a single-center experience. J Thorac Cardiovasc Surg. 2018;155(3): 1095–1106 e2.
17. Meneveau N. Therapy for acute high-risk pulmonary embolism: thrombolytic therapy and embolectomy. Curr Opin Cardiol. 2010;25(6):560–7.
18. Weinberg A, Tapson VF, Ramzy D. Massive pulmonary embolism: extracorporeal membrane oxygenation and surgical pulmonary embolectomy. Semin Respir Crit Care Med. 2017;38 (1):66–72.
19. Tahir UA, Carroll B, Pinto DS. Massive pulmonary embolism: embolectomy or extracorporeal membrane oxygenation? Curr Opin Crit Care. 2019;25(6):630–7.
20. Meneveau N, Guillon B, Planquette B, Piton G, Kimmoun A, Gaide-Chevronnay L, Aissaoui N, Neuschwander A, Zogheib E, Dupont H, Pili-Floury S, Ecarnot F, Schiele F, Deye N, de Prost N, Favory R, Girard P, Cristinar M, Ferré A, Meyer G, Capellier G, Sanchez O. Outcomes after extracorporeal membrane oxygenation for the treatment of high-risk pulmonary embolism: a multicenter series of 52 cases. Eur Heart J. 2018 Dec 14;39 (47):4196–204.
21. Hussain ST, Bartholomew JR, Leacche M, Zhen-Yu TM. Retrograde pulmonary embolectomy for acute pulmonary embolism: a simplified technique. Ann Thorac Surg. 2017;103(5): e473–4. https://doi.org/10.1016/j.athoracsur.2016.11.082 PMID: 28431732.
22. Yavuz S, Toktas F, Goncu T, Eris C, Gucu A, Ay D, Erdolu B, Tenekecioglu E, Karaagac K, Vural H, Ozyazicioglu A. Surgical embolectomy for acute massive pulmonary embolism. Int J Clin Exp Med. 2014;7(12):5362–75. PMID: 25664045; PMCID: PMC4307492.
23. DeYoung E, Minocha J. Inferior Vena cava filters: guidelines, best practice, and expanding indications. Semin Intervent Radiol. 2016;33(2):65–70.

24. Kucher N, Rossi E, De Rosa M, Goldhaber SZ. Massive pulmonary embolism. Circulation. 2006;113(4):577–82.
25. Kon ZN, Pasrija C, Bittle GJ, Vemulapalli S, Grau-Sepulveda MV, Matsouaka R, Deatrick KB, Taylor BS, Gammie JS, Griffith BP. The incidence and outcomes of surgical pulmonary embolectomy in North America. Ann Thorac Surg. 2019;107(5):1401–8.
26. Percy ED, Shah R, Hirji S, Tartarini RJ, Yazdchi F, Harloff M, Kaneko T, Pelletier MP. National outcomes of surgical embolectomy for acute pulmonary embolism. Ann Thorac Surg. 2020;110(2):441–7.
27. Keeling WB, Leshnower BG, Lasajanak Y, Binongo J, Guyton RA, Halkos ME, Thourani VH, Lattouf OM. Midterm benefits of surgical pulmonary embolectomy for acute pulmonary embolus on right ventricular function. J Thorac Cardiovasc Surg. 2016;152 (3):872–8.
28. Keeling WB, Sundt T, Leacche M, Okita Y, Binongo J, Lasajanak Y, Aklog L, Lattouf OM; SPEAR Working Group. Outcomes after surgical pulmonary embolectomy for acute pulmonary embolus: a multi-institutional study. Ann Thorac Surg. 2016;102(5):1498–502.
29. Aymard, T., et al., Massive pulmonary embolism: surgical embolectomy versus thrombolytic therapy—should surgical indications be revisited? Eur J Cardiothorac Surg. 2013;43(1): 90–4; discussion 94.
30. Azari A, et al. Surgical embolectomy versus thrombolytic therapy in the management of acute massive pulmonary embolism: short and long-term prognosis. Heart Lung. 2015;44(4):335–9.

Pulmonary Embolism Response Team: A Multidisciplinary Approach to Improve Pulmonary Embolism Management

James S. Salonia, David Steiger, and Janet M. Shapiro

1 Introduction

Pulmonary embolism (PE) is a potentially life-threatening condition, accounting for an estimated 150,000–250,000 hospitalizations and up to 100,000 deaths every year in the United States [4, 15]. Diagnosis of PE has significantly improved with advances in CT angiography imaging. At the time that PE is diagnosed, risk stratification is mandatory to determine appropriate management.

Various classification systems have been created to identify patients presenting with PE who have a higher risk of death. The European Society of Cardiology stratifies patients presenting with PE into high, intermediate, and low risk groups to predict in-hospital or 30 day mortality. This risk classification is based on the presence of hemodynamic instability (cardiac arrest, shock, and vasopressor requirement), right ventricular dysfunction, elevated cardiac troponin levels, and pulmonary embolism severity scores [12]. The intermediate risk group is further divided into intermediate high and intermediate low (Table 1) [12]. Mortality rates vary significantly depending on pulmonary embolism severity, with low risk PE mortality rate of 1%, intermediate risk PE of 5–25%, and high risk PE of 18–65% [3].

Available treatments for PE comprise systemic anticoagulation, reduced or full-dose dose systemic thrombolysis, catheter-directed thrombolysis (CDT), catheter embolectomy, and surgical embolectomy. Additionally, circulatory support may be provided with the use of extracorporeal membrane oxygenation (ECMO). The decision as to which therapeutic option to select is complex and can vary greatly based on institutional expertise and practice. A paucity of randomized

J. S. Salonia (✉) · D. Steiger · J. M. Shapiro
Division of Pulmonary, Critical Care, and Sleep Medicine, Mount Sinai Morningside-Mount Sinai West, Icahn School of Medicine at Mount Sinai, New York, NY, USA
e-mail: James.salonia@mountsinai.org

E. Herzog (ed.), *Pulmonary Embolism*,
https://doi.org/10.1007/978-3-030-87090-4_14

Table 1 European Society of Cardiology classification of pulmonary embolism severity and risk for in-hospital or 30 day mortality

Mortality risk	Hemodynamic instability	Right ventricular dysfunction	Elevated cardiac troponin level	PESI class III-V or sPESI > 1
High	+	+	+	+
Intermediate—high	−	+	+	+
Intermediate—low	−	+	±	±
Low	−	−	−	−

clinical trials make already complex treatment decisions even more challenging, so that even professional societies cannot give definitive evidence-based recommendations.

Thus, we advocate for the formation of a multidisciplinary group of specialists, a Pulmonary Embolism Response Team (PERT), to select the right treatment for the individual patient at the bedside.

2 Pulmonary Embolism Response Team (PERT) Structure and Organization

A multidisciplinary team approach with collaboration among specialty services has been successfully implemented to diagnose and rapidly manage complex life-threatening medical conditions such as acute myocardial infarction, acute stroke, and a difficult airway [10, 13, 14]. Given the increasing patient complexity and multitude of therapeutic interventions for the management of patients presenting with PE, the multidisciplinary Pulmonary Embolism Response Team is created to collaborate in the diagnosis, management, and follow-up of these acutely ill patients. This PERT approach for the comprehensive care of patients with PE is a class IIa recommendation (should be considered) by the European Society of Cardiology [12].

Pulmonary embolism response team composition and process is based on the institutional resources. The PERT may include representation from pulmonary and critical care medicine, interventional radiology, cardiac surgery, cardiology, hematology, emergency medicine, and clinical pharmacy. The vast array of specialty services included in PERT provides an expedited and comprehensive approach to the management of patients presenting with PE.

There is no standard approach to a PERT activation or a singular platform for multidisciplinary communication. Additionally, since patients with acute PE may present in various clinical locations such as the emergency department, the general medical or surgical wards, intensive care units, or specialty service wards, the site and nature of the initial physician–patient contact is highly variable. Each institution must consider their resources and limitations when developing a customized policy describing the PERT activation. It is imperative that this PERT policy be communicated to front-line providers.

In general, we recommend that PERT be activated for patients presenting with acute PE who are classified as intermediate or high risk according to the European Society of Cardiology risk classification system (Table 1) [12]. The rationale behind this recommendation is based on data demonstrating a higher risk of in-hospital or 30 day mortality compared to low risk group patients [3].

We recommend that a critical care physician or cardiologist evaluate the patient and make the determination to activate the PERT. Patients presenting with acute PE who are being considered for advanced therapeutic interventions may be clinically unstable, with significant cardiopulmonary abnormalities and medical comorbidities, making the clinical course of these patients extremely unpredictable. The physician activating the PERT must be comfortable with performing a rapid evaluation of the unstable patient, interpreting and communicating laboratory and radiographic information, and managing patients who have the potential to rapidly deteriorate. Furthermore, skill in point of care ultrasound (POCUS) is highly desirable as it allows for rapid bedside assessment of the cardiac, pulmonary, and vascular systems, providing real-time information that is essential for the PERT decision making process [8].

One of the most critical components of the PERT is the effective and secure communication of important patient information. There is no preferred platform to activate and communicate patient information with the multidisciplinary PERT, however, several factors should be considered when deciding on the means of communication. The platform should have the capacity for team members to engage in a virtual online forum and allow for the rapid transmission of data, including videos of scans and echocardiograms to all members of the PERT. Ideally, the communication platform should be encrypted and PERT member access limited to ensure patient security. Finally, the format of communication should be standardized to allow for effective transmission of crucial time sensitive information.

Effective communication to the members of the PERT should include the patient's clinical presentation, relevant comorbidities, vital signs and physical exam, relevant laboratory and radiographic information, and all treatments provided prior to the PERT activation. Clinical presentation and a thorough evaluation of the patient’s relevant medical and surgical history may identify risk factors for the development of venous thromboembolism (VTE). Particular attention should be paid to the patient's mental status, respiratory status and oxygen requirements, and cardiovascular status including heart rate, blood pressure and the need for vasopressors, and peripheral perfusion. Asymmetric edema of an extremity may indicate the presence of a deep venous thrombosis (DVT). Laboratory information should include a complete blood count, basic metabolic panel, troponin, brain natriuretic peptide (BNP), and lactate. Computed tomography angiography performed to diagnose acute PE will provide valuable information such as location and extent of thrombosis in the pulmonary arteries and may provide evidence of right heart strain. Cardiac POCUS or an official transthoracic echocardiography (TTE) examination allows for a more comprehensive evaluation of the cardiac chambers and can provide direct evidence of right heart strain through assessment of the right ventricular size and function. Furthermore, cardiac ultrasonography can detect the presence of a clot-in-transit, a particularly worrisome finding associated with increased mortality [2]. Vascular ultrasonography can be utilized to diagnose the presence of a DVT. Video and image media should be uploaded to the PERT communication platform for review by the various specialty services.

The clinical, laboratory, and radiographic information should be integrated into one of the validated scoring systems to predict 30-day mortality in patients with acute PE. The scoring systems most frequently utilized include the pulmonary embolism severity index (PESI), simplified PESI (sPESI), and BOVA score (Tables 2 and 3) [1, 5, 7, 11]. A combination of clinical data, cardiac biomarkers, presence of right ventricular dysfunction on echocardiography, and calculated score from one of the scoring systems allows the PERT to classify patients according to the European Society of Cardiology guidelines [12]. Finally, it is critical to identify all relevant treatments and interventions that were performed prior to the PERT activation. All of this information must be effectively communicated to the PERT to facilitate a multidisciplinary discussion and expedite management decisions and potentially life-saving interventions.

Table 2 Pulmonary embolism severity index (PESI) and simplified pulmonary embolism severity index (sPESI)

Patient characteristics	PESI	sPESI
Age	Score in years	Age $\geq$ 80 = 1
Male sex	10	
Cancer present	30	1
History of heart failure	10	1
History of chronic lung disease	10	1
Heart rate $\geq$ 110	20	1
Systolic blood pressure < 100 mmHg	30	1
Respiratory rate $\geq$ 30	20	
Temperature < 36 °C	20	
Altered mental status	60	
Oxygen saturation < 90%	20	1
PESI Score	30 day mortality (%)	sPESI risk of death
<65	0–1.6	0 points = 1.1%
66–85	1.7–3.5	$\geq$ 1 points = 8.9%
86–105	3.2–7.1	
106–125	4.0–11.4	
>125	10.0–24.5	

Table 3 Bova score to predict pulmonary embolism related 30-day mortality and 30-day complications

Patient characteristics	Score
Systolic blood pressure < 100	2
Elevated cardiac troponin	2
Right ventricular dysfunction	2
Heat rate $\geq$ 110	1

Bova score	Stage	PE-related 30 day complications (%)	PE-related 30 day mortality (%)
0–2	I (low risk)	4.2	1.7
3–4	II (intermediate risk)	10.8	5.0
>4	III (high risk)	29.2	15.5

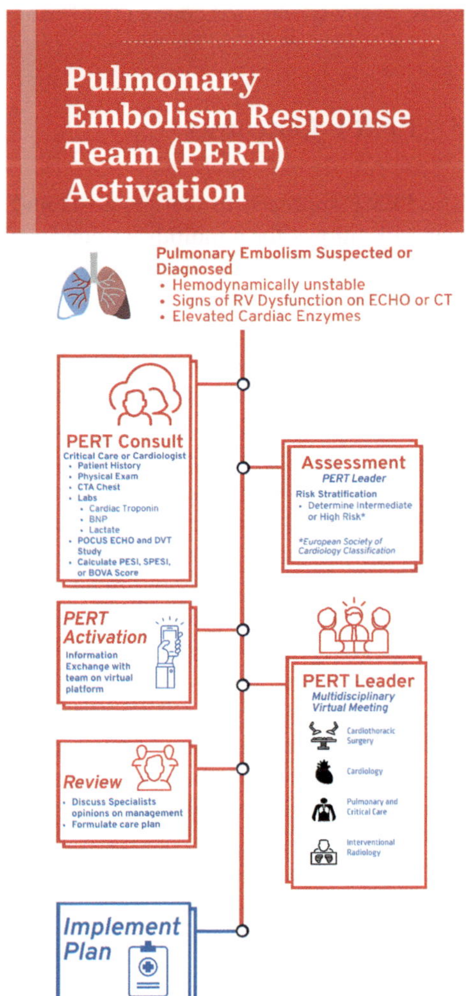

Fig. 1 Algorithm for the activation of the Pulmonary Embolism Response Team

The paucity of randomized control trials evaluating outcomes among the various advanced therapeutic modalities and consequent lack of uniform recommendations create a challenge in the management of these critically ill patients. It is essential that all information be communicated and thoroughly discussed among the multidisciplinary PERT, so that expert consensus can be achieved. All specialty services provide their expert recommendation and articulate the rationale, risks, and benefits behind that recommendation. Differences in opinion in proposed treatment recommendations are to be expected and should be encouraged, so that all appropriate therapeutic interventions are explored. While discussing complex management, careful consideration is given to the unique values and preferences of each patient. The potential risks and benefits of all proposed interventions should be thoroughly discussed with the patient and/or family representative. A consensus plan incorporating expert medical opinion and patient values is then implemented. Finally, the PERT should determine the appropriate level of patient monitoring and coordinate for the safe transfer of care. We recommend utilizing an algorithm to assist with diagnosis, management, and continuity of care for patients with acute PE (Fig. 1) [9, 15].

3 PERT Outcomes

The PERT approach to the diagnosis and management of patients presenting with acute PE allows for a multidisciplinary collaboration to provide expert guidance in the absence of comprehensive evidence-based guidelines. While this multidisciplinary approach may potentially improve patient access to advanced therapeutic interventions and expedite care, the ultimate goal of the PERT is to improve clinical outcomes. Presently, there is a paucity of published data evaluating the impact of PERT on patient centered clinical outcomes. A recent analysis showed that PERT was associated with a shorter time to therapeutic anticoagulation, decreased bleeding complications and decreased all-cause 30 day mortality [6]. An increase in the proportion of patients undergoing advanced therapeutic interventions, mainly catheter directed therapy, has been reported; there was no increased risk of major bleeding or mortality benefit in this study [16]. Ambiguity in the published literature regarding a definitive mortality benefit with the PERT can be attributed to the lack of prospective randomized controlled trials comparing interventional with surgical therapies in the management of patients with acute PE. Additional research is needed in the form of high quality randomized controlled trials evaluating catheter-directed thrombolysis, interventional embolectomy, and surgical embolectomy and their respective impact on mortality. Other important factors which need to be explored are the impact of PERT on hospital and intensive care unit length of stay, hospital re-admission rates, healthcare costs, patient follow-up, and quality of life.

Patients with acute PE who required PERT activation should have close outpatient follow-up upon discharge. This is especially important for any patient that received advanced therapeutic interventions. Outpatient specialty follow-up should be tailored to the clinical needs of the patient and address specific areas such as evaluation of the cause of PE, duration of systemic anticoagulation, removal of IVC filter, bleeding complications, repeat echocardiography, evaluation for chronic thromboembolic pulmonary hypertension (CTEPH), and quality of life. In general, all patients should have follow-up with their primary care provider and a pulmonologist. If the patient had evidence of right ventricular dysfunction, follow-up with a cardiologist is also recommended. Any patient who underwent a surgical intervention should have close follow-up with cardiothoracic surgery. Concern for malignancy or hematological abnormalities require close hematology and oncology follow-up. A multidisciplinary PERT outpatient clinic with ability to assess cardiac, pulmonary, hematologic, and vascular systems may provide an efficient and comprehensive follow up.

4 PERT Quality Improvement and Continuing Education

There has been an expansion of the published literature describing the institutional development, implementation, and outcomes of this multidisciplinary PERT approach [6, 15, 16]. However, it is important to understand that the PERT model is still in its infancy and therefore requires constant assessment for areas of improvement. The literature surrounding the diagnosis, severity classification, and management of acute PE extends across a vast array of medical and surgical specialties. Consequently, it is not possible for a single specialist to remain informed on all the published literature. Thus, a successful PERT requires a commitment of all specialty services to quality improvement, patient safety, and continuing education.

This quality improvement and continuing education process should be customized to meet the specific needs of the PERT group and individual members. Involvement in national and international PERT societies, such as the PERT Consortium, promotes education and allows for the free exchange of information. Periodic multidisciplinary meetings of the hospital PERT should be organized to review cases and outcomes such as: review of complex and challenging medical or surgical cases, patient morbidity and mortality, concerns from the various specialty services, and analysis of PERT data with a focus on patient-centered clinical outcomes. Potential opportunities for improvement in patient care and the PERT process should be explored and discussed in a collegial manner. Finally, applicable literature and guidelines from the various specialty services should be presented and discussed so they may be incorporated into the PERT model to provide optimal patient care.

5 Conclusion

In conclusion, a pulmonary embolism response team brings expert opinions and appropriate care to the bedside of patients with acute pulmonary embolism who are at increased risk of mortality. The complexity and acuity of these patients demand an integrated, multidisciplinary evaluation to explore all therapeutic options. As the interventional, surgical, and medical therapies in the treatment of pulmonary embolism continue to rapidly evolve, so must the PERT approach to the management and follow-up of these acutely ill patients.

References

1. Blood Clots: A Serious but Preventable Medical Condition. http://www.cdc.gov/ncbddd/dvt/documents/blood-clots-fact-sheet.pdf. Updated May 4, 2016. Accessed 6 May 2016.
2. Rivera-Lebron B, McDaniel M, Ahrar K, Alrifai A, Dudzinski DM, Fanola C, Blais D, Janicke D, Melamed R, Mohrien K, Rozycki E, Ross CB, Klein AJ, Rali P, Teman NR, Yarboro L, Ichinose E, Sharma AM, Bartos JA, Elder M, Keeling B, Palevsky H, Naydenov S, Sen P, Amoroso N, Rodriguez-Lopez JM, Davis GA, Rosovsky R, Rosenfield K, Kabrhel C, Horowitz J, Giri JS, Tapson V, Channick R, PERT Consortium. Diagnosis, treatment and follow up of acute pulmonary embolism: consensus practice from the PERT Consortium. Clin Appl Thromb Hemost. 2019;25. https://doi.org/10.1177/1076029619853037.
3. Konstantinides SV, Meyer G. 2019 ESC Guidelines for the diagnosis and management of acute pulmonary embolism developed in collaboration with the European Respiratory Society: The Task Force for the diagnosis and management of acute pulmonary of the European Society of Cardiology (ESC). Eur Respir J. 2019;54(3):1901647.
4. Bělohlávek J, Dytrych V, Linhart A. Pulmonary embolism, part I: Epidemiology, risk factors and risk stratification, pathophysiology, clinical presentation, diagnosis and nonthrombotic pulmonary embolism. Exp Clin Cardiol. 2013 Spring;18(2):129–38.
5. Holmes DR Jr, Rich JB, Zoghbi WA, Mack MJ. The heart team of cardiovascular care. J Am Coll Cardiol. 2013;61(9):903–7.
6. Nazir FS, Petre I, Dewey HM. Introduction of an acute stroke team: an effective approach to hasten assessment and management of stroke in the emergency department. J Clin Neurosci. 2009;16(1):21–5.
7. Mark LJ, Herzer KR, Cover R, Pandian V, Bhatti NI, Berkow LC, Haut ER, Hillel AT, Miller CR, Feller-Kopman DJ, Schiavi AJ, Xie YJ, Lim C, Holzmueller C, Ahmad M, Thomas P, Flint PW, Mirski MA. Difficult airway response team: a novel quality improvement program for managing hospital-wide airway emergencies. Anesth Analg. 2015;121(1):127-39
8. Filopei J, Acquah SO, Bondarsky EE, Steiger DJ, Ramesh N, Ehrlich M, Patrawalla P. Diagnostic Accuracy of Point-of-Care Ultrasound Performed by Pulmonary Critical Care Physicians for Right Ventricle Assessment in Patients With Acute Pulmonary. Crit Care Med. 2017;45(12):2040–5.
9. Barrios D, Rosa-Salazar V, Jiménez D, Morillo R, Muriel A, Del Toro J, López-Jiménez L, Farge-Bancel D, Yusen R, Monreal M; RIETE investigators. Right heart thrombi in pulmonary embolism. Eur Respir J. 2016 Nov;48(5):1377–85.

10. Aujesky D, Obrosky DS, Stone RA, Auble TE, Perrier A, Cornuz J, Roy PM, Fine MJ. Derivation and validation of a prognostic model for pulmonary embolism. Am J Respir Crit Care Med. 2005;172(8):1041–6.
11. Donzé J, Le Gal G, Fine MJ, Roy PM, Sanchez O, Verschuren F, Cornuz J, Meyer G, Perrier A, Righini M, Aujesky D. Prospective validation of the Pulmonary Embolism Severity Index. A clinical prognostic model for pulmonary embolism. Thromb Haemost. 2008 Nov;100(5):943–8.
12. Jiménez D, Aujesky D, Moores L, Gómez V, Lobo JL, Uresandi F, Otero R, Monreal M, Muriel A, Yusen RD; RIETE Investigators. Simplification of the pulmonary embolism severity index for prognostication in patients with acute symptomatic pulmonary embolism. Arch Intern Med. 2010;170(15):1383–9.
13. Bova C, Sanchez O, Prandoni P, Lankeit M, Konstantinides S, Vanni S, Jiménez D. Identification of intermediate-risk patients with acute symptomatic pulmonary embolism. Eur Respir J. 2014;44(3):694–703.
14. Herzog E; Elbaz-Greener G; planner D; Koren T; Amir O, Shapiro J, Kalish, Y. Pathway for the diagnosis and management of pulmonary embolism. Crit Pathw Cardiol. January 11, 2021 —Volume Publish Ahead of Print.
15. Chaudhury P, Gadre SK, Schneider E, Renapurkar RD, Gomes M, Haddadin I, Heresi GA, Tong MZ, Bartholomew JR. Impact of Multidisciplinary Pulmonary Embolism Response Team Availability on Management and Outcomes. Am J Cardiol. 2019;124(9):1465–69.
16. Rosovsky R, Chang Y, Rosenfield K, Channick R, Jaff MR, Weinberg I, Sundt T, Witkin A, Rodriguez-Lopez J, Parry BA, Harshbarger S, Hariharan P, Kabrhel C. Changes in treatment and outcomes after creation of a pulmonary embolism response team (PERT), a 10-year analysis. J Thromb Thrombolysis. 2019;47(1):31–40.

Pulmonary Embolism in Pregnancy and the Postpartum Period

Joshua I. Rosenbloom, Eyal Herzog, and Donna R. Zwas

1 Background

Venous thromboembolism (VTE) is the fifth leading cause of maternal death in the United States, accounting for 9.6% of maternal deaths (https://www.cdc.gov/reproductivehealth/maternal-mortality/pregnancy-mortality-surveillance-system.htm#causes). Pregnancy increases the risk of VTE approximately fivefold, and the risk is 60 times higher in the postpartum period [1, 2]. In pregnancy, there is physiologic hypercoagulability, as seen in increased levels of pro-thrombotic factors including Factors VII, VIII, X, fibrinogen, and von Willebrand factor, and decreased function of free protein S [2]. These changes, combined with venous stasis and often immobility, lead to the increased risk of VTE in pregnant women. At the same time, many of the presenting signs and symptoms of pulmonary embolism (PE), such as tachycardia and dyspnea, are also seen in healthy pregnant women. Therefore, a very high index of suspicion is required to make the timely diagnosis of PE in pregnancy.

J. I. Rosenbloom (✉)
Department of Obstetrics and Gynecology, Hadassah Hebrew University Medical Center, Jerusalem, Israel
e-mail: joshuar@hadassah.org.il

Department of Obstetrics and Gynecology, Washington University in St Louis School of Medicine, St. Louis, MO, USA

E. Herzog · D. R. Zwas
Department of Cardiology, Heart Institute, Hadassah Hebrew University Medical Center, Jerusalem, Israel

E. Herzog (ed.), *Pulmonary Embolism*,
https://doi.org/10.1007/978-3-030-87090-4_15

2 Pathophysiology of Thromboembolism in Pregnancy

Pregnancy, both pre and post-delivery, is associated with all three components that pre-dispose to thrombus formation described in Virchow's triad: venous stasis, hypercoagulability and endothelial damage. Venous studies demonstrate greater blood volume and an increase in the diameter of the venous system of the lower limbs in pregnant women [3], and greater distensibility of veins associated with decreased flow velocity [4]. The gravid uterus compresses the pelvic veins, and the preponderance of DVT on the left side and in the more proximal veins in pregnant women suggests that compression of the left iliac vein by the right common iliac artery as it crosses over to the inferior vena cava engenders left sided stasis [5].

Hypercoagulability begins in the first trimester of pregnancy, increases during the second and third and peaks during the first week post-partum. The pro-coagulant Factors VII, VIII, X, XII and von Willebrand factor rise significantly during the course of pregnancy, and there is a marked increase in the concentration of plasma fibrinogen [6]. Free and total protein S levels decrease starting during the first trimester and remain decreased, and more than half of pregnant women may develop 'activated protein C resistance' on peripheral testing, whereby plasma fails to be anticoagulated by the addition of activated protein C in vitro. The increase in pro-coagulant activity leads to an increase in fibrin turnover, which leads to the increase in measured D-Dimers [7]. At the same time, there is a reduction in plasma fibrinolytic activity during pregnancy, and it remains low until after delivery of the placenta [6]. This may be mediated by increased levels of plasminogen activator inhibitors, some of which derive from the placenta, which inhibit tissue plasminogen activator activity. At the same time there are increases in platelet adhesion and aggregation, despite the lower platelet counts found in pregnancy [8]. During the course of pregnancy, the placenta also sheds and secretes microparticles of different sizes and contents into the maternal circulation. These microparticles and exosomes have immune-modulatory effects in the local and more distant circulation, but may also be pro-inflammatory and pro-coagulant [9]. The relative pro-coagulant state may confer a survival advantage in the setting of hemorrhage, at the cost of increased VTE.

Normal pregnancy is associated with reduced endothelial sensitivity to vasoconstrictors and adaptive increases in endothelial cell vasodilator production. In pre-eclampsia, there are pathologically elevated levels of cytokines and growth factors that may promote endothelial dysfunction by acutely inhibiting key Ca^{2+} signaling events that lead to vasodilatation and promoting the breakdown of endothelial cell–cell contacts [10]. The breakdown of the endothelial monolayer and loss of vascular integrity are associated with the clinical manifestations of pre-eclampsia including hypertension, proteinuria, renal dysfunction, as well as liver dysfunction and pulmonary, visual and cerebral dysfunction. In more severe pre-eclampsia, endothelial dysfunction in the setting of damaged endothelial cells may lead to the release of thrombotic factors.

3 Risk Assessment

The vast majority of women who present with PE during pregnancy have identifiable risk factors (RFs) for VTE, and the risk may be considerable even in the first trimester. Every woman should undergo a risk assessment for PE as part of pre-conception or early pregnancy evaluation. If the women is admitted to the hospital during pregnancy or develops new medical issues, her risk should be re-assessed. The risk evaluation should be repeated before delivery or immediately post-partum [11]. Risk factors for VTE can be divided into pre-existing risk factors, obstetric risk factors and transient, potentially reversible risk factors. Risk factors differ for ante-natal versus post-natal VTE (Table 1). The women at risk should be informed as to the signs and symptoms of VTE, and how to seek help in these situations.

Of the pre-existing risk factors, thrombophilia and history of VTE are associated with the highest risk of pregnancy-associated VTE [12], in particular if the prior event was not associated with surgery. Patients at the highest risk include those who developed recurrent VTE or VTE in the setting of estrogen-containing medications, patients with anti-phospholipid antibody syndromes, and anti-thrombin deficiency. Those who are on chronic anti-coagulation should be transitioned to non-teratogenic anticoagulants prior to pregnancy, or initiate anticoagulation as early as possible in pregnancy, and should be managed in conjunction with a hematologist with expertise in pregnancy-related thrombosis. Other thrombophilic

Table 1 Risk factors for postpartum VTE

Maternal risk factors	Age >35
	Obesity (BMI ≥ 30 kg/m^2)
	Parity ≥ 3
	Varicose veins
	Thrombophilia
	Smoking
	History of VTE
	Current systemic disease (malignancy, auto-immune, inflammatory, cardiac)
	Immobility
Obstetric risk factors	Preeclampsia
	Fetal growth restriction
	Multiple pregnancy
	Current stillbirth
	Prolonged labor
	Caesarean section
	Postpartum hemorrhage
	Prolonged hospitalization

diagnoses associated with pregnancy-related VTE include Factor V Leiden mutation, which is reported to be the most common hematologic abnormality [13], protein C or S deficiency, compound heterozygosity for Factor V Leiden and prothrombin gene mutation (G20210A). Women with previous history of VTE or with a family history of VTE in a first-degree relative under age 50 should undergo an evaluation for thrombophilia. A history of superficial venous thrombosis is also associated with significantly increased risk [14].

Other maternal characteristics that increase the risk for VTE include obesity, which is associated with five times the risk of VTE compared with non-obese pregnant women. Of note, obese women also have a higher incidence of PE in the setting of VTE and a higher risk of mortality in the setting of VTE [15]. Active smoking may increase the risk of VTE during pregnancy by two to five times [15]. Intravenous drug users are also at increased risk. Multiparity after the third pregnancy is also associated with increased risk [15]. Black women may also be at increased likelihood of developing VTE [12].

Multiple medical co-morbidities are associated with increased risk of VTE during pregnancy and should be considered as part of the risk assessment. The presence of malignancy, heart failure or cardiovascular disease requiring hospital admission, as well as nephrotic syndrome, or type 1 diabetes with nephropathy are recognized risk factors for VTE while pregnant [11]. Systemic lupus erythematosus is a risk factor even if the patient has no evidence of APLA [16], as are inflammatory bowel disease and inflammatory arthritis. Anemia and in particular, sickle cell anemia, are associated with increased risk. Medical conditions that lead to immobility such as paraplegia are also risk conditions. If the patient undergoes any surgical procedure during pregnancy, or there is evidence of systemic infection or dehydration, the patient should be considered at increased risk for the duration of the event. Long-distance travel can also be considered a short-term risk for VTE.

There are also noteworthy obstetric risk factors for VTE. In-vitro fertilization is associated with an increased risk of VTE, particularly in the first trimester [17]. Hyperemesis, similar to dehydration, is associated with increased risk. Twin and multiple-pregnancies also increase the risk during pregnancy. Later in pregnancy, intra-uterine growth restriction and pre-eclampsia are associated with increased VTE after delivery [18]. The combination of pre-eclampsia and fetal growth restriction further increases the risk [19]. Bedrest is not recommended in pregnancy, as this is also a risk factor for VTE. Peripartum risk factors for VTE include cesarean birth, with planned cesarean birth conveying a smaller increase in risk but unplanned surgery associated with a higher risk. Ante- and post-partum hemorrhage, in particular loss of more than 1000 ml of blood or transfusion requirement, and infection are associated with high risk for postpartum VTE [12], and the combination of these events with cesarean birth further increases the risk [19].

4 VTE Prevention in Pregnancy

Unfortunately, data assessing VTE prevention largely consist of case–control studies and expert opinions with limited evidence from randomized controlled trials or meta-analyses. Furthermore, there are limited data to enable the clinician to quantify the risk of VTE in a given patient, and while it is assumed that the co-existence of multiple risk factors conveys additive risk, this has been documented only in select cases. Although there is overlap in the recommendations of the differing guidelines for high and low risk women, there remain differences in recommendations as to women with combinations of risk factors. Given the lack of data and consensus, different choices may be appropriate for individual patients, and discussion and decision-aids may help each patient arrive at a management decision consistent with her values and preferences (Table 2).

When indicated, low molecular weight heparin is the prophylactic agent of choice, with dose adjustments based on whether the risk assessment suggests low, intermediate or high risk. The present guidelines suggest that there is no need to monitor Factor Xa levels.

Table 2 Approach to VTE prevention in pregnancy and the puerperium

Condition	Notes	Antepartum management	Postpartum management
High risk conditions			
Previous history of VTE-unprovoked or during previous pregnancy or estrogen exposure	Other than related to major surgery, trauma or immobility	LMWH throughout pregnancy	6 weeks post-partum treatment with LMWH
VTE during current pregnancy		LMWH throughout pregnancy (treatment dose)	At least 6 weeks post-partum treatment with LMWH. Can consider NOAC if not breastfeeding or warfarin if breastfeeding
High risk thrombophilia without prior VTE	Anti-thrombin deficiency, homozygosity for Factor V Leiden or prothrombin gene 20210a, or heterozygosity for both Factor V Leiden and prothrombin gene 20210a	LMWH throughout pregnancy (prophylactic or intermediate dose)[b]	6 weeks post-partum treatment with LMWH

(continued)

Table 2 (continued)

Condition	Notes	Antepartum management	Postpartum management
High risk thrombophilia with prior VTE	Anti-thrombin deficiency, homozygosity for Factor V Leiden or prothrombin gene 20210a, or heterozygosity for both Factor V Leiden and prothrombin gene 20210a	LMWH throughout pregnancy	6 weeks post-partum treatment with LMWH
Receiving long-term anticoagulation therapy		Treatment with LMWH throughout pregnancy	At least 6 weeks post-partum treatment with LMWH. Can consider NOAC if not breastfeeding or warfarin if breastfeeding. Consultation with hematologist for long-term management
Low-risk thrombophilia with previous VTE	Factor V Leiden heterozygote, prothrombin gene mutation heterozygote, protein S or C deficiency	LMWH throughout pregnancy (prophylactic or intermediate dose)	6 weeks post-partum LMWH
Intermediate risk conditions			
Previous h/o VTE-provoked	Related to major surgery, trauma or immobility	Observation	Consider anti-coagulation in the setting of cesarean delivery, obesity, immobility, or other risk factors
Low-risk thrombophilia without previous VTE	Factor V Leiden heterozygote, prothrombin gene mutation heterozygote, protein S or C deficiency	Observation	Consider anti-coagulation in the setting of cesarean delivery, obesity, immobility, or other risk factors
Low-risk thrombophilia with a family history of VTE	Factor V Leiden heterozygote, prothrombin gene mutation heterozygote, protein S or C deficiency	Observation or prophylactic dose LMWH	6 weeks post-partum LMWH

(continued)

Table 2 (continued)

Condition	Notes	Antepartum management	Postpartum management
Short term indications for anticoagulation	Surgery Immobilization Hospitalization	LMWH during acute event	LMWH during acute event

[a]There is no clear recommendation for prophylactic, intermediate dose, or adjusted-dose (treatment) LMWH
[b]There is a difference of opinion regarding necessity for prophylaxis in patients with homozygous prothrombin gene mutations or anti-thrombin deficiency without a history of prior VTE
VTE venous thromboembolism, including deep venous thrombosis
LMWH low molecular weight heparin

5 Diagnosis

A pregnant patient presenting with concerning signs or symptoms for PE, including tachycardia, tachypnea, dyspnea, pleural chest pain, hemoptysis, or hypoxemia, should be immediately evaluated for PE [2] (Fig. 1). Additionally, the presence of risk factors such as obesity or thrombophilia should be sought.

There are no validated risk prediction scores (such as the Wells criteria) for use during pregnancy. The use of D-dimer in pregnancy is controversial. D-dimer levels increase throughout pregnancy and decline postpartum. However, there are no validated reference ranges. A negative (low) D-dimer level has a reasonably high negative predictive value, but an elevated D-dimer level is not useful in predicting PE. Currently, use of D-dimer testing in pregnancy as a screening test for PE is not recommended [20].

Although not necessary for the diagnosis, an electrocardiogram (ECG) is often performed during the workup of a patient with a suspected PE. The most common finding on ECG in patients with PE is sinus tachycardia, and other findings may include S1Q3T3, right ventricular strain, right axis deviation, or P pulmonale [21]. A finding of right ventricular dysfunction on echocardiography also supports the diagnosis and is associated with a worse prognosis [22].

The mainstay of PE diagnosis in pregnancy, as in non-pregnant patients, is imaging. If the patient has signs or symptoms suggestive of a deep venous embolism (DVT), compression ultrasonography is recommended. If this is positive, and the patient is hemodynamically stable, no further imaging is required [23]. However, if this is negative, or if the patient has no symptoms of DVT, chest imaging is necessary.

Controversy exists over the best imaging mode. Spiral CT angiography (CTA) is readily available and provides a very low radiation dose to the fetus [2]. Specifically, the fetal radiation dose is estimated to be between 0.03 and 0.66 mGy [23]. In general, cumulative fetal radiation doses <50 mGy in pregnancy are not thought to be teratogenic or otherwise harmful [24]. Therefore, withholding CTA in a patient with a possible PE, due to fears of radiation, is not justified.

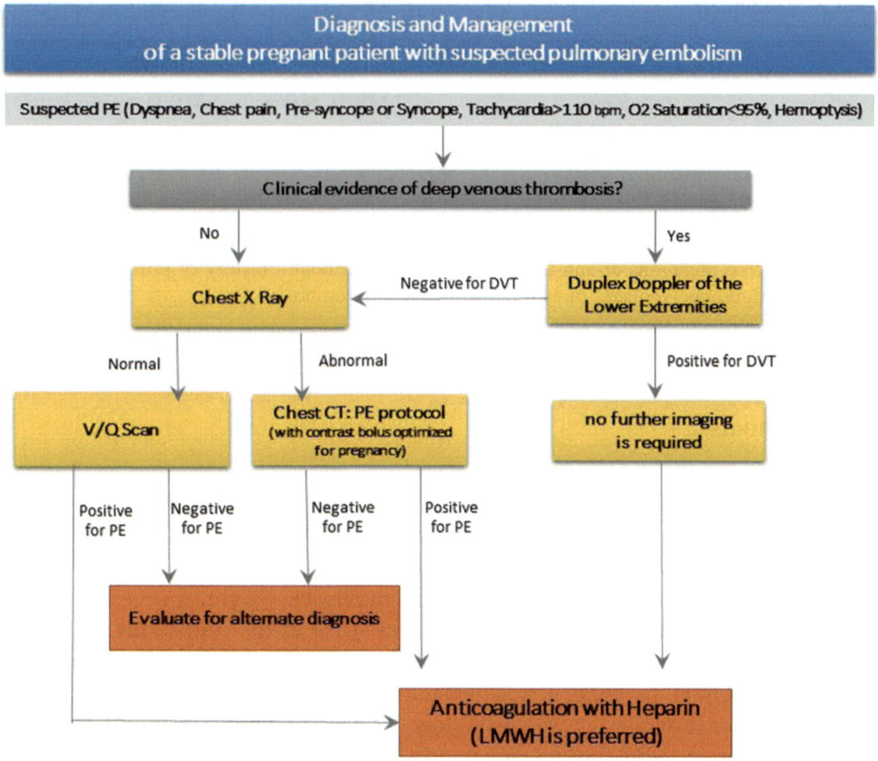

Fig. 1 Evaluation and management of the stable pregnant or postpartum patient with signs and symptoms of venous thromboembolic disease

However, compared to the non-pregnant population, there is a higher incidence of non-diagnostic CTA in pregnancy, generally related to suboptimal contrast bolus timing resulting in reduced opacification of the pulmonary arterial tree [23, 25]. Therefore, it is important to inform the radiology technician that the patient is pregnant, both so that appropriate shielding can be provided and so that the contrast bolus can be timed correctly.

Due to the issues outlined above, ventilation/perfusion scintigraphy (V/Q scanning) is preferred over CTA for PE diagnosis in pregnancy and the immediate postpartum period [23]. V/Q scanning provides a similar radiation dose to the fetus as CTA but a lower dose to the mother [23]. Exposure to ionizing radiation in pregnancy and the postpartum period is associated with an increased risk of breast cancer, due to the proliferative changes that take place in breast tissue during pregnancy and lactation. Therefore, reducing the maternal radiation dose as much as possible is of key importance [26]. Furthermore, V/Q scanning may have a higher diagnostic yield than CTA, although results are inconclusive [25, 27]. Prior to performing V/Q scanning, a chest X-ray should be obtained. If the patient has a normal chest X-ray, proceed to V/Q scanning. However, patients with an abnormal chest X-ray require CTA instead of V/Q scanning [2].

Although the main priority is establishing the diagnosis and treating PE as required, attention should be paid also to fetal wellbeing during the period of evaluation, particularly in unstable patients. Patients at a viable gestational age should have fetal monitoring performed where feasible. A neonatologist should be consulted in cases of preterm delivery.

6 Treatment

Patients with PE should be treated by a multidisciplinary team including a maternal–fetal medicine specialist or high risk obstetrician and an expert in thromboembolism. An obstetric anesthesiologist should be consulted if delivery is required, and a neonatologist should be consulted if preterm delivery is being contemplated. Additional members of the team may include a critical care specialist, cardiologist and a pharmacist.

The first question in treating a pregnant patient with suspected PE is if she is stable or unstable. Stable patients can be treated in labor and delivery, the antepartum ward, or an internal medicine floor according to hospital protocol (Fig. 1. Hemodynamically unstable patients (Fig. 2) should be moved to the intensive care unit, and fetal monitoring should be performed if the fetus is viable. If a pulmonary embolism response team is available, they should be immediately called [28]. If the patient requires continuous cardiopulmonary resuscitation, current guidelines should be followed, including emergency cesarean delivery after four minutes of unsuccessful CPR in pregnancies of at least 20 weeks gestation [29]. If she has restoration of spontaneous circulation, obstructive shock or persistent hypotension, hemodynamic resuscitation with intravenous fluids and vasopressors should be instituted, and anticoagulation should be initiated as discussed below. Fluids should be used judiciously in patients with right ventricular dysfunction to avoid exacerbating right heart failure. Oxygen should be provided to maintain oxygen saturation above 95%. If the patient does not stabilize and continues with obstructive shock or persistent hypotension, further intervention such as catheter-directed thrombolysis or embolectomy should be considered.

Data regarding thrombolysis and thrombectomy in pregnancy are limited [30, 31]. Although thrombolytics are not thought to be teratogenic and do not cross the placenta, they greatly increase the risk of maternal hemorrhage, particularly if delivery is indicated [30]. Delivery within 8 h of thrombolysis significantly increases the risk of serious hemorrhage. Therefore thrombolytics are generally used only in patients with life-threatening PE. Catheter-based thrombolysis is the option of choice in patients who do not have a contraindication to thrombolysis, due to reduced risk of hemorrhage (consensus opinion). If catheter-based thrombolysis is not an option and the patient can tolerate transfer, the patient should be transferred to a center that provides that option. For those patients who are not a

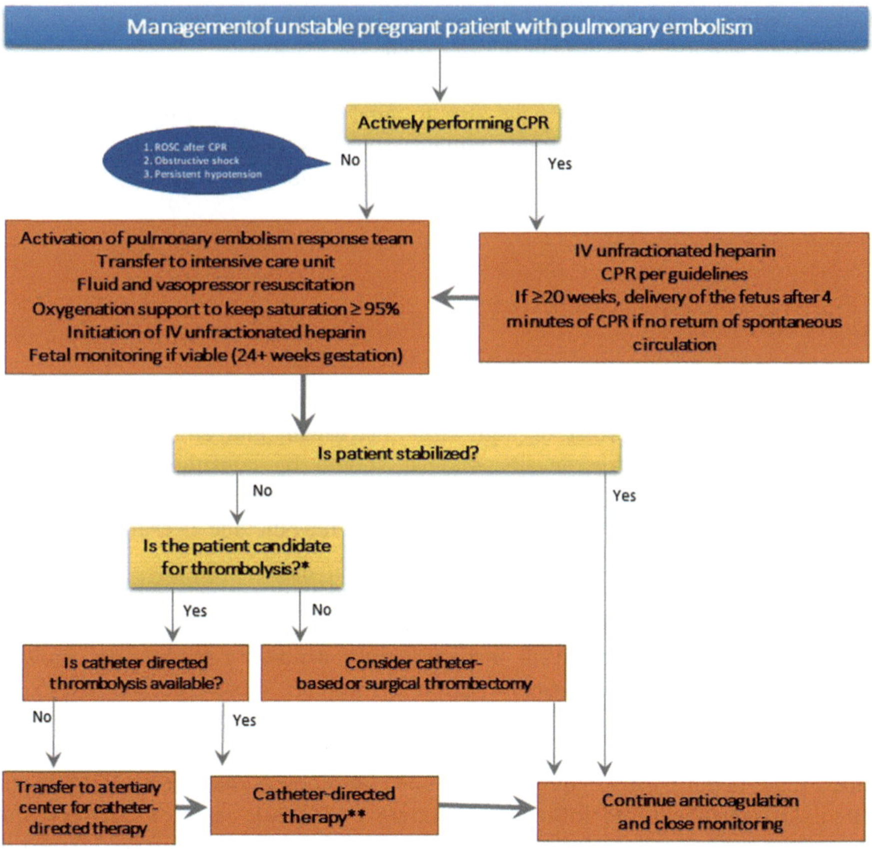

* Absolute contraindications to thrombolysis include recent surgery including delivery, prior intracranial hemorrhage, known intracranial malformation, suspected dissection, recent head trauma, ischemic stroke within prior 3 months, bleeding diathesis. Relative contraindications include use of anticoagulants, pregnancy, CPR >10 minutes, uncontrolled hypertension, major surgery in prior 3 weeks, history of ischemic stroke, or recent internal bleeding

** Expert opinion suggests catheter-directed treatment over systemic thrombolysis or thrombectomy.

ROSC Restoration of spontaneous circulation

Fig. 2 Evaluation and management of the unstable pregnant or postpartum patient with signs and symptoms of venous thromboembolic disease

candidate for catheter-directed thrombolysis, thombectomy may also be considered as a last resort. Extracorporeal membrane oxygenation has been used successfully in pregnant patients with pulmonary embolism [32].

Treatment for PE in pregnancy consists of anticoagulation. Low-molecular weight heparin (LMWH) and unfractionated heparin (UFH) are the only anticoagulants that can be safely used in pregnancy [2, 30]. Warfarin is a known teratogen. In early pregnancy it is associated with warfarin embryopathy, while later in pregnancy it can cause fetal hemorrhage. Data on the safety of novel oral anticoagulants are still emerging but they are not considered safe in pregnancy at this time [33].

LMWH and UFH do not cross the placenta and are not associated with adverse fetal effects [34]. In choosing between LMWH and UFH, in general LMWH is preferred because, at least in non-pregnant patients, it is more effective. Furthermore, its dosing is more predictable, and there are fewer maternal adverse effects such as osteoporosis [30]. However, in patients who may need imminent intervention (such as delivery) or who are unstable, IV UFH may be preferable because it is reversible with protamine and has a shorter half-life [30].

LMWH is usually dosed at 1 mg/kg enoxaparin twice daily or 2 mg/kg daily. The anti-Xa level is checked four hours after the fourth dose and should be between 0.6 and 1.0 IU/mL. In patients with a very high suspicion for PE, the first dose of LMWH should be given prior to confirmation of the diagnosis.

It is unknown if the dose should be adjusted in as pregnancy progresses. Some clinicians advocate checking monthly anti-Xa levels or adjusting the dose based on the increasing maternal weight throughout the pregnancy; but there is no firm evidence underlying this practice [2, 35].

If IV UFH is used, the normal dose is 80 units/kg bolus and then a constant infusion of 18 units/kg/hour, titrated to achieve a therapeutic aPTT [30]. The patient may be transitioned to LMWH after stabilization. The use of IVC filters may be considered in patients with a contraindication to anticoagulation or who fail anti-coagulation, although their use in pregnancy is associated with an increased rate of complications [2, 36].

7 Delivery

The management of anticoagulation around the time of delivery is dependent on the clinical scenario. If the PE is remote, therapeutic dose anticoagulation can be stopped 24 h prior to scheduled delivery (induction of labor or scheduled cesarean delivery) [2]. Delivery timing is not altered by the presence of PE, and delivery timing should be based on standard obstetric indications.

Patients who are anticoagulated at the time of delivery cannot receive neuraxial anesthesia, due to the risk of spinal hematoma [37]. Therefore, anesthesiology consultation prior to delivery is essential in all patients receiving anticoagulation [37].

In patients in whom stopping the anticoagulation prior to delivery is considered ill-advised, patients can be transitioned to an IV UFH infusion which is stopped only 4–6 h prior to delivery (i.e. the drip can be continued also during the beginning of the induction of labor). IVC filter placement can also be considered in rare circumstances if even a short period without anticoagulation is thought to be problematic.

After delivery, anticoagulation should be restarted: 6 h after vaginal delivery and 12 h after cesarean delivery. However, the timing of anticoagulation should be discussed with the anesthesiologist if the patient received neuraxial anesthesia [37]. In particular, current guidelines recommend waiting 24 h after any neuraxial procedure and 4 h after removal of the epidural catheter before resuming therapeutic dose anticoagulation [37].

Anticoagulation should be given until six weeks postpartum and for a minimum of three months [30]. Patients who will be receiving long-term anticoagulation may be transitioned to warfarin, which is compatible with breastfeeding. On the other hand, NOACs are not compatible with breastfeeding.

8 Conclusion

PE is one of the most common medical complications in pregnancy and is a leading cause of maternal mortality. Every woman should undergo a risk assessment for PE as part of pre-conception or early pregnancy evaluation and reassessment peri-delivery. Prompt diagnosis and treatment is essential for both maternal and fetal health. A multidisciplinary team should be used to manage these patients.

References

1. Pomp ER, Lenselink AM, Rosendaal FR, Doggen CJ. Pregnancy, the postpartum period and prothrombotic defects: risk of venous thrombosis in the MEGA study. J Thromb Haemost. 2008;6(4):632–7.
2. American College of Obstetricians, Gynecologists' Committee on Practice B-O. ACOG Practice Bulletin No. 196: thromboembolism in pregnancy. Obstet Gynecol. 2018;132(1):e1–7.
3. Goulart VB, Cabral AC, Reis ZS, Navarro TP, Alves SL, de Miranda PR, Sarquis AL, de Lima Rezende CA. Anatomical and physiological changes in the venous system of lower limbs in pregnant women and findings associated with the symptomatology. Arch Gynecol Obstet. 2013;288(1):73–8.
4. Wood JE 3rd, Goodrich SM. Dilation of the veins with pregnancy or with oral contraceptive therapy. Trans Am Clin Climatol Assoc. 1964;76:174–80.
5. DeStephano CC, Werner EF, Holly BP, Lessne ML. Diagnosis and management of iliac vein thrombosis in pregnancy resulting from May-Thurner Syndrome. J Perinatol. 2014;34(7):566–8.
6. Bremme KA. Haemostatic changes in pregnancy. Best Pract Res Clin Haematol. 2003;16(2):153–68.
7. Siennicka A, Kłysz M, Chełstowski K, Tabaczniuk A, Marcinowska Z, Tarnowska P, Kulesza J, Torbe A, Jastrzębska M. Reference values of D-Dimers and fibrinogen in the course of physiological pregnancy: the potential impact of selected risk factors—a pilot study. Biomed Res Int. 2020;2020:3192350.
8. Holthe MR, Staff AC, Berge LN, Lyberg T. Different levels of platelet activation in preeclamptic, normotensive pregnant, and nonpregnant women. Am J Obstet Gynecol. 2004;190(4):1128–34.

9. Mincheva-Nilsson L, Baranov V. Placenta-derived exosomes and syncytiotrophoblast microparticles and their role in human reproduction: immune modulation for pregnancy success. Am J Reprod Immunol. 2014;72(5):440–57.
10. Boeldt DS, Bird IM. Vascular adaptation in pregnancy and endothelial dysfunction in preeclampsia. J Endocrinol. 2017;232(1):R27–44.
11. Royal College of Obstetricians and Gynaecologists. Reducing the risk of venous thromboembolism during pregnancy and the puerperium. Green Top Guideline No. 37a. London (UK): RCOG; 2015.
12. James AH, Jamison MG, Brancazio LR, Myers ER. Venous thromboembolism during pregnancy and the postpartum period: incidence, risk factors, and mortality. Am J Obstet Gynecol. 2006;194(5):1311–5.
13. Thornton P, Douglas J. Coagulation in pregnancy. Best Pract Res Clin Obstet Gynaecol. 2010;24(3):339–52.
14. Danilenko-Dixon DR, Heit JA, Silverstein MD, Yawn BP, Petterson TM, Lohse CM, Melton LJ 3rd. Risk factors for deep vein thrombosis and pulmonary embolism during pregnancy or post partum: a population-based, case-control study. Am J Obstet Gynecol. 2001;184(2):104–10.
15. Larsen TB, Sørensen HT, Gislum M, Johnsen SP. Maternal smoking, obesity, and risk of venous thromboembolism during pregnancy and the puerperium: a population-based nested case-control study. Thromb Res. 2007;120(4):505–9.
16. Clowse ME, Jamison M, Myers E, James AH. A national study of the complications of lupus in pregnancy. Am J Obstet Gynecol. 2008;199(2):127.e1-6.
17. Henriksson P, Westerlund E, Wallén H, Brandt L, Hovatta O, Ekbom A. Incidence of pulmonary and venous thromboembolism in pregnancies after in vitro fertilisation: cross sectional study. BMJ. 2013;346:e8632.
18. Lindqvist P, Dahlbäck B, Marŝál K. Thrombotic risk during pregnancy: a population study. Obstet Gynecol. 1999;94(4):595–9.
19. Jacobsen AF, Skjeldestad FE, Sandset PM. Ante- and postnatal risk factors of venous thrombosis: a hospital-based case-control study. J Thromb Haemost. 2008;6(6):905–12.
20. Van der Pol LM, Mairuhu AT, Tromeur C, Couturaud F, Huisman MV, Klok FA. Use of clinical prediction rules and D-dimer tests in the diagnostic management of pregnant patients with suspected acute pulmonary embolism. Blood Rev. 2017;31(2):31–6.
21. Thomson D, Kourounis G, Trenear R, Messow CM, Hrobar P, Mackay A, Isles C. ECG in suspected pulmonary embolism. Postgrad Med J. 2019;95(1119):12–7.
22. Cho JH, Kutti Sridharan G, Kim SH, Kaw R, Abburi T, Irfan A, Kocheril AG. Right ventricular dysfunction as an echocardiographic prognostic factor in hemodynamically stable patients with acute pulmonary embolism: a meta-analysis. BMC Cardiovasc Disord. 2014;14:64.
23. Leung AN, Bull TM, Jaeschke R, Lockwood CJ, Boiselle PM, Hurwitz LM, James AH, McCullough LB, Menda Y, Paidas MJ, Royal HD, Tapson VF, Winer-Muram HT, Chervenak FA, Cody DD, McNitt-Gray MF, Stave CD, Tuttle BD, Pregnancy ASCoPEi. An official American Thoracic Society/Society of Thoracic Radiology clinical practice guideline: evaluation of suspected pulmonary embolism in pregnancy. Am J Respir Crit Care Med. 2011;184(10):1200–8.
24. Committee Opinion No. 723. Guidelines for diagnostic imaging during pregnancy and lactation. Obstet Gynecol. 2017;130(4):e210–6.
25. Cahill AG, Stout MJ, Macones GA, Bhalla S. Diagnosing pulmonary embolism in pregnancy using computed-tomographic angiography or ventilation-perfusion. Obstet Gynecol. 2009;114(1):124–9.
26. Tirada N, Dreizin D, Khati NJ, Akin EA, Zeman RK. Imaging pregnant and lactating patients. Radiographics. 2015;35(6):1751–65.
27. van Mens TE, Scheres LJ, de Jong PG, Leeflang MM, Nijkeuter M, Middeldorp S. Imaging for the exclusion of pulmonary embolism in pregnancy. Cochrane Database Syst Rev. 2017;1:CD011053.

28. Parikh M, Chahine NM, Hammad TA, Tefera L, Li J, Carman T, Schilz R, Shishehbor MH. Predictors and potential advantages of PERT and advanced therapy use in acute pulmonary embolism. Catheter Cardiovasc Interv. 2021.
29. Jeejeebhoy FM, Zelop CM, Lipman S, Carvalho B, Joglar J, Mhyre JM, Katz VL, Lapinsky SE, Einav S, Warnes CA, Page RL, Griffin RE, Jain A, Dainty KN, Arafeh J, Windrim R, Koren G, Callaway CW. Cardiac arrest in pregnancy: a scientific statement from the American Heart Association. Circulation. 2015;132(18):1747–73.
30. Bates SM, Greer IA, Middeldorp S, Veenstra DL, Prabulos AM, Vandvik PO. VTE, thrombophilia, antithrombotic therapy, and pregnancy: antithrombotic therapy and prevention of thrombosis, 9th ed: American College of Chest Physicians evidence-based clinical practice guidelines. Chest. 2012;141(2 Suppl):e691S-e736S.
31. Rodriguez D, Jerjes-Sanchez C, Fonseca S, Garcia-Toto R, Martinez-Alvarado J, Panneflek J, Ortiz-Ledesma C, Nevarez F. Thrombolysis in massive and submassive pulmonary embolism during pregnancy and the puerperium: a systematic review. J Thromb Thrombolysis. 2020;50 (4):929–41.
32. Naoum EE, Chalupka A, Haft J, MacEachern M, Vandeven CJM, Easter SR, Maile M, Bateman BT, Bauer ME. Extracorporeal life support in pregnancy: a systematic review. J Am Heart Assoc. 2020;9(13):e016072.
33. Rosenbloom JI, Macones GA. Future research directions for prevention and treatment of obstetric venous thromboembolism. Semin Perinatol. 2019;43(4):213–7.
34. Greer IA, Nelson-Piercy C. Low-molecular-weight heparins for thromboprophylaxis and treatment of venous thromboembolism in pregnancy: a systematic review of safety and efficacy. Blood. 2005;106(2):401–7.
35. Boban A, Paulus S, Lambert C, Hermans C. The value and impact of anti-Xa activity monitoring for prophylactic dose adjustment of low-molecular-weight heparin during pregnancy: a retrospective study. Blood Coagul Fibrinolysis. 2017;28(3):199–204.
36. Rottenstreich A, Kalish Y, Elchalal U, Klimov A, Bloom AI. Retrievable inferior vena cava filter utilization in obstetric patients. J Matern Fetal Neonatal Med. 2019;32(18):3045–53.
37. Leffert L, Butwick A, Carvalho B, Arendt K, Bates SM, Friedman A, Horlocker T, Houle T, Landau R, Dubois H, Fernando R, Houle T, Kopp S, Montgomery D, Pellegrini J, Smiley R, Toledo P, Members of the SVTET. The Society for Obstetric Anesthesia and Perinatology consensus statement on the anesthetic management of pregnant and postpartum women receiving thromboprophylaxis or higher dose anticoagulants. Anesth Analg. 2018;126 (3):928–44.

Pulmonary Embolism in Cancer Patients

Ariela Arad, Aron Popovtzer, and Dan Gilon

1 Introduction

Cancer patients have an increased risk of venous thromboembolism (VTE). The pathogenesis of thrombosis in cancer is multifactorial and includes stasis due to prolonged bed rest, treatment side effects or extrinsic compression of blood vessels by the tumor. They include also vascular injury due to direct invasion by the tumor, central venous catheters, endothelial damage as result of chemotherapy, immunotherapy, radiation therapy or tumor cytokines release.

Hypercoagulable state—may be due to increased levels of leukocytes, platelets, and tissue factor—bearing microparticles and increase soluble P selectin.

For example, patients with lung or colorectal cancer often exhibit leukocytosis. Neutrophils could increase VTE in cancer patients by releasing neutrophil extra-cellular traps whereas monocytes may express Tissue Factor and release tissue factor- bearing microparticles to the blood stream. Thrombocytosis is often observed in gastrointestinal, lung, breast, and ovarian cancer. Increased level of soluble P-selectin is a biomarker of activation of platelets and endothelium in cancer patients.

A. Arad
Department of Hematology, Hadassah Medical Center, Faculty of Medicine, Hebrew University of Jerusalem, Jerusalem, Israel

A. Popovtzer
Department of Oncology, Hadassah Medical Center, Faculty of Medicine, Hebrew University of Jerusalem, Jerusalem, Israel

D. Gilon (✉)
Cardio-Oncology, Heart Institute, Hadassah Medical Center, Hebrew University of Jerusalem, Jerusalem, Israel
e-mail: dangi@ekmd.huji.ac.il; gilond@hadassah.org.il

E. Herzog (ed.), *Pulmonary Embolism*,
https://doi.org/10.1007/978-3-030-87090-4_16

Table 1 Risk factors for thrombosis in Cancer patients

Patient-related factors	Tumor-related factors	Treatment-related factors
Advance age	Site—hematological malignancies, lung, pancreas, stomach, brain, kidney	Chemotherapy
Prior VTE	Stage—advanced stage, tumor bulk leading to vascular compression or pathological fracture	Hormonal therapy
Prolonged immobilization	Mutational status: jak II mutation, acute promyelocytic leukemia	Anti-angiogenic therapy
Inherited or acquired thrombophilia		Need for surgical removal
Central venous catheter necessity		Erythropoiesis-stimulating agents
Hospitalization		

A better understanding of the pathogenesis of thrombosis in cancer patients and a better risk stratification will help us choose patients for primary VTE prevention [1].

The main risk factors for thrombosis are summarized in Table 1. In order to identify patients with cancer at elevated risk for VTE, the Khorana score (range, 0–6, with higher scores indicating a higher risk of venous thromboembolism) can be used (Table 2).

They have been validated to identify higher risk patients and improve selection of those who could benefit from thromboprophylaxis [2].

Newer trials of thromboprophylaxis have used score of ≥ 2 as eligibility criterion [3].

In a single tertiary referral medical center study of PE patients between 2014 and 2016 based on computed tomography scan 581 patients were diagnosed with PE of

Table 2 Khorana score

Patient characteristics	Risk score
Site of cancer	
Very high risk (stomach, pancreas)	2
High risk (lung, lymphoma, gynecologic, bladder, testicular)	1
Platelet count $\geq 350 \times 10^9$/L before chemotherapy	1
Hemoglobin level <10 mg/ml or use of Erythropoiesis-stimulating agents	1
Leukocyte count >11 $\times 10^9$/L before chemotherapy	1
BMI ≥ 35 kg/m^2	1

Abbreviations: BMI, body mass index, VTE, venous thromboembolism
Original risk cutoffs: High-risk score ≥ 3; intermediate-risk score 1–2; low risk score, 0
Adapted from Ref. [2]

which 187 (33%) had cancer. They tended to be older (64.8 vs. 58.5 years), had a lower body mass index and were less likely to be active smokers compared to non-cancer patients. There was no difference in hospital stay and hospital mortality [4].

2 Specific Groups and Clinical Considerations in Oncology Patients with PE

2.1 Asymptomatic (Incidental) Pulmonary Embolism

These are patients with cancer undergoing periodically computed tomography scans for staging purposes and for treatment response evaluation. The incidence of pulmonary Embolism (PE) ranges from 1 to 5% which probably represents an underestimation. Approximately one-half of these events are incidentally detected.

In most patients a retrospective anamnesis will reveal symptoms of PE that were obscured or mistakenly considered as related to other causes.

The prognosis of incidental VTE in this patient population appears to be similar to symptomatic events, with comparably high rates of recurrent VTEs. In the absence of major contraindications, anticoagulant treatment for 3–6 months is generally recommended for incidental pulmonary embolism that involves multiple subsegmental or more proximal pulmonary arteries.

Extension treatment should be considered for patients with active malignant disease [5, 6].

2.2 Subsegmental Pulmonary Embolism

The clinical relevance of a single incidental subsegmental pulmonary embolism without concomitant deep vein thrombosis is uncertain and either a watchful approach or a shorter course of anticoagulation to minimize the bleeding risk may also be considered. In the recent American Society of Hematology (ASH) guidelines, the panel suggested short-term anticoagulation treatment rather than observation (conditional recommendation, very low certainty of evidence.) [7].

2.3 Catheter-Related PE in Cancer Patients

One of the risk factors for thrombosis in cancer patients is insertion of central line catheters, commonly used in these patients. Thrombosis and embolism related to central line are one of the leading complications, along with infections and blood vessels trauma. Kang et al. showed in a cohort of 477 patients that included 50,841 catheter days of which 36 patients (7.5%) had their catheter removed. The most common reasons for removal of catheter were skin allergy (4.6%), occlusion (3.4%) and accidental withdrawal (2.3%). Nine patients (1.9%) developed symptomatic upper extremity deep vein thrombosis and six (1.3%) developed blood stream infection [8].

Central line catheters: vary in their type, size, route of insertion and intended placement of their tip. Accordingly, the rate of complications, including development of thrombosis and possible embolism varies significantly:

2.3.1 Totally Implantable Venous Access Ports (TIVAPs) for Chemotherapy

Thromboembolism (VTE) associated with totally implanted venous access ports (TIVPAs) for chemotherapy compared with peripherally inserted central catheters are associated with a decreased risk of VTE and a trend with lower VTE risk for Hickman catheters [9]. However, single centered based study by Akhthar et al. showed that the rate of VTE and Catheter related thrombosis (CRT) were similar for both CVAD types [10]. Peripherally inserted central catheter-related deep vein thrombosis rate appears to be low when evidence-based technical factors are taken into consideration during the insertion procedure [11].

2.3.2 Catheter Tip Placement: Right Atrium (RA) Versus Superior Vena Cava (SVC)

Hickman catheter insertion is associated with high incidence (12.5%) of early formation of right atrial (RA) thrombus. The formation of these thrombi is asymptomatic and highly associated ($p < 0.001$) with the catheter tip position in the RA, in contrast to their positioning in the superior vena cava or in its junction with the right atrium. On the basis of these findings, as reported in the study by Gilon et al., placing the (Hickman) catheter tip in the superior vena cava in preference to its placement in the RA should be considered with the intention to prevent catheter-associated thrombus formation [12].

2.3.3 Treatment

Central venous access device (CVAD)-related thrombosis (CRT) is a common complication among patients requiring central venous access as part of their medical care including cancer patients. Venous duplex is recommended for the diagnosis of CRT. Anticoagulation for at least 3 months or the duration of the indwelling CVAD is recommended for treatment of CRT. Thrombolysis should be considered for patients at low risk for bleeding who have limb-threatening thrombosis. CVAD removal should be considered for patients with bacteremia, persistent symptoms despite anticoagulation, and if the CVAD is no longer needed [13].

For patients with cancer and a central venous catheter (CVC), the ASH guidelines panel suggests not using parenteral or oral thromboprophylaxis [7].

3 Thrombolytic Therapy in Cancer Patients

The use of Thrombolytic therapy is indicated for high-risk Pulmonary Embolism.

There is relatively little data describing thrombolysis in cancer patients. A retrospective study using the US national inpatient sample (NIS) between the years 2013–2014 was performed to identify PE admission [14]. Out of 72,546 admissions for acute PE 14.7% (10,673) had comorbid cancer, 3.4% (2439) received thrombolysis. Comorbid cancer was associated with decreased odds of receiving thrombolysis. When restricting analysis to PE admission receiving thrombolysis, mortality occurred in 12.9% (315) of patients with no difference between those with cancer compared to those without cancer.

Rescue thrombolytic therapy is recommended for patients with hemodynamic deterioration on anticoagulation treatment [15]. The hemodynamic improvements are associated with reduction of RV dilatation on echocardiography. It may lead to more rapid improvement in pulmonary obstruction, pulmonary artery pressure and pulmonary vascular resistance in patients with PE compared to treatment with unfractionated heparin alone. The level of recommendation by the European Society of Cardiology (ESC) guidelines from 2019 is Ib (Class I level b).

A meta-analysis of patients with high-risk PE, with mainly cardiogenic shock, showed a significant reduction in the combined outcome of mortality and recurrent PE. This successful intervention was associated with 9.9% rate of severe bleeding and a 1.7% rate of intracranial bleeding [16].

Thrombolysis can be administered either systemically or by percutaneous catheter-based delivery intended to act locally within the pulmonary artery tree. The purpose of using this pharmacological tool is to accelerate resolution of acute pulmonary emboli, to lower pulmonary artery pressure and to improve arterial oxygenation.

The greatest benefit of this intervention is observed in the first 48 eight hours of symptoms onset, but can still be relevant in patient who have symptoms for up to 6–14 days [15, 17].

The American Society of Hematology (ASH) guidelines (2020) concur with the ESC recommendation for the use of thrombolysis followed by anticoagulation for "PE and hemodynamic compromise" considering it as strong recommendation [18]. The recommendation for the use of thrombolysis in this setting of PE is not specific for cancer patients, but needs to be personalized case by case also in this specific group. In cancer patients with metastatic brain tumor or central nervous system involvement, the risk of bleeding should be considered versus the risk of thrombosis. Brain (and spine if symptoms of cord compression exist) imaging (CT or MRI) should be done before considering thrombolysis [19, 20].

4 Treatment of Pulmonary Embolism in Thrombocytopenic Patients

Thrombocytopenia in cancer patients is very common and can be related to chemotherapy and non-chemotherapy drug reactions, radiotherapy, bone marrow involvement, sepsis and disseminated intravascular coagulation, immune thrombocytopenia, Vitamin B 12 deficiency, APLA syndrome and more rare causes such as thrombotic microangiopathy (TMA), Heparin induced thrombocytopenia and Hypersplenism.

Approach to the thrombocytopenic patient should include the following:

1. Peripheral blood smear- to rule out pseudo-thrombocytopenia, look for schistocytes, (Thrombotic Microangiopathy) large platelets (Immune Thrombocytopenia), tear drops and nucleated red blood cells (bone marrow involvement) hyper segmented neutrophils (Vitamin B12 deficiency) left shift and or toxic granulation (sepsis).
2. PT PTT Fibrinogen, Lupus anticoagulant Anticardiolipin IgM IgG AntiB2 glycoprotein 1 IgG IgM,
3. Evaluate spleen size (r/o splenomegaly)
4. Check every medication (prescribed and over the counter) that is given and stop if suspected as a cause of thrombocytopenia

There are limited data to guide treatment decision to administer therapeutic anticoagulation and appropriated dosing.

As the risk of recurrent VTE is highest in the acute period (i.e. within the first 30 days) [17, 18], during this time utilization of a full therapeutic dose of anticoagulation is recommended for patients with acute VTE and platelet counts of >50,000. If the thrombocytopenia is caused by a known factor and is temporary, therapeutic doses of anticoagulation with platelet transfusion support to maintain platelet counts above 40,000–50,000 may be considered.

For patients with platelet count between 25,000 and 50,000, a dose-modification strategy using 50% or prophylactic-dose low molecular weight heparin (LMWH) may be considered.

In patients with prolonged thrombocytopenia below 25,000 and acute pulmonary embolism or in patients with refractory thrombocytopenia we recommend to consider insertion of Inferior Vena Cava filter (IVC).

We recommend to restart anticoagulation once the platelet counts are rising and to consider removal of the IVC filter if no longer necessary.

Data on the use of Direct Oral Anticoagulants (DOAC's) in Cancer associated thrombosis and severe thrombocytopenia (<50 000) are lacking. Dose adjusted LMWH should be the treatment of choice [21, 22].

5 Preventive Treatment in Cancer Patients

Current clinical guidelines recommend against the use of routine primary thromboprophylaxis in unselected ambulatory cancer patients but the decision to treat the patient should be personalized.

To identify the patients with high risk for thrombotic complication, the assessment of the cancer patient should be in every clinic visit or at list every 3 month.

The Khorana score (Table 2) should be used as a risk assessment tool. Other factors that should be observed at every clinic visit include: mobility, COVID-19 status, treatment with anti-angiogenic drugs, hormonal therapy, recently performed orthopedic/surgical procedures recently, signs of hemolysis and post-partum period.

All patients at bed rest or with evidence of recent COVID-19 infection, recent surgery, post-partum period, active hemolysis and primary brain tumor should receive primary thromboprophylaxis unless contraindicated.

The use of apixaban and rivaroxaban for the prevention of cancer-associated thrombosis in ambulatory patients at intermediate to high risk of VTE (Khorana score ≥ 2) was assessed in two randomized controlled trials and found to reduce the risk of VTE in these patient population without a significant increase in major bleeding [23, 24].

Until the guidelines will adapt the use of primary thromboprophylaxis in ambulatory cancer patients at intermediate to high risk of VTE who do not have any apparent risk factors for bleeding, the decision of their use should be based on a case by case basis.

6 Direct Oral Anticoagulants for Treatment of VTE in Cancer Patients

The HOKUSAI-VTE CANCER trial was a large, international, open-label, non-inferiority randomized control trial comparing edoxaban with Low molecular weight heparin (LMWH) for the treatment of VTE in cancer patients (2018) [25].

Cancer Patients who had acute symptomatic or incidental venous thromboembolism were randomly to receive either low-molecular-weight heparin for at least 5 days followed by oral edoxaban at a dose of 60 mg once daily (edoxaban group) or subcutaneous dalteparin at a dose of 200 IU per kilogram of body weight once daily for 1 month followed by dalteparin at a dose of 150 IU per kilogram once daily (dalteparin group). Treatment was given for at least 6 months and up to

12 months. The primary outcome was a composite of recurrent venous thromboembolism or major bleeding during the 12 months after randomization, regardless of treatment duration. In the edoxaban group, 12.8% of patients developed a recurrent VTE or major bleeding compared with 13.5% in the LMWH group for an Hazard Ratio (HR) of 0.97 (95% CI, 0.70–1.36; *P* value for noninferiority of 0.006). There were fewer episodes of recurrent VTE in the edoxaban group (HR = 0.71; 95% CI, 0.48–1.06; *P* value = 0.09) but more episodes of major bleeding (HR = 1.77; 95% CI, 1.03–3.04; *P* value = 0.04).

Major bleeding events due to upper gastrointestinal bleeding complications, occurred mostly in gastrointestinal cancer patients.

The SELECT-D study was a multicenter, randomized, open-label, pilot trial in the United Kingdom.

Patients with active cancer who had symptomatic pulmonary embolism (PE), incidental PE, or symptomatic lower-extremity proximal deep vein thrombosis (DVT) were recruited. Allocation was to dalteparin (200 IU/kg daily during month 1, then 150 IU/kg daily for months 2–6) or rivaroxaban (15 mg twice daily for 3 weeks, then 20 mg once daily for a total of 6 months). The primary outcome was VTE recurrence over 6 months. Safety was assessed by major bleeding and clinically relevant nonmajor bleeding (CRNMB).

A total of 203 patients were randomly assigned to each group, 58% of whom had metastases. Twenty-six patients experienced recurrent VTE (dalteparin, n = 18; rivaroxaban, n = 8). The 6-month cumulative VTE recurrence rate was 11% (95% CI, 7–16%) with dalteparin and 4% (95% CI, 2–9%) with rivaroxaban (hazard ratio [HR], 0.43; 95% CI, 0.19–0.99). The 6-month cumulative rate of major bleeding was 4% (95% CI, 2–8%) for dalteparin and 6% (95% CI, 3–11%) for rivaroxaban (HR, 1.83; 95% CI, 0.68–4.96). There was also a disproportionate number of bleeding events in this trial, which were gastrointestinal or urological bleeding.

After an interim safety analysis, patients with esophageal and gastroesophageal cancer were excluded from the study (2018) [26].

The results of the ADAM-VTE trial, an open-label RCT, cancer patients diagnosed with VTE were randomized to apixaban or LMWH. The main aim of the ADAM-VTE trial is to test the hypothesis that apixaban is associated with a significantly lower rate of major bleeding compared to dalteparin in the treatment of cancer patients with acute VTE. The primary safety outcome was the rate of major bleeding. Secondary efficacy objective was to assess the rates of recurrent VTE or arterial thromboembolism. Cancer patients with acute VTE (n = 300) were randomized to receive apixaban (10 mg twice daily for 7 days followed by 5 mg twice daily thereafter) or dalteparin (200 IU/Kg daily for 30 days followed by 150 IU/kg daily thereafter) for 6 months. Stratification factors used for randomization included cancer stage and cancer specific risk of venous thromboembolism using the Khorana score.

No patient suffered a major bleeding event in the apixaban arm compared with 2 patients (1.4%) in the LMWH arm (*P* value = 0.14). In the apixaban group, 1 patient (0.7%) was diagnosed with recurrent VTE, whereas 9 patients (6.3%) in the LMWH group experienced this complication (*P* value = 0.03). Oral apixaban was associated with low major bleeding and VTE recurrence rates for the treatment of VTE in cancer patients (2017) [27].

In the recent ASH guidelines the panel suggests the use of Direct oral anticoagulants (apixaban, edoxaban, or rivaroxaban) over LMWH for the treatment of cancer-associated thrombosis (CAT) [7].

An increased bleeding risk in patients with gastrointestinal cancer was reported when using edoxaban and rivaroxaban. The Caravaggio study compared apixaban and dalteparin for the treatment of patients with CAT. Results from the Caravaggio study showed that Apixaban is a safe alternative to LMWH for the treatment in patients with CAT. No excess in gastrointestinal bleeding was observed in patients who received apixaban, including those with gastrointestinal cancer [28].

7 Duration of Treatment

After initial anticoagulant treatment for 6 months, all cancer patients should be evaluated for symptoms related to PE and or DVT, assessment of their bleeding risk, status of their malignant disease (remission, progressive, stable, risk of recurrence), residual thrombus (duplex of both legs), pulmonary hypertension (by Echo) and current treatment plan.

For cancer patients with pulmonary hypertension full dose anticoagulation should be considered. Right heart catheterization for more accurate diagnosis and to rule out other causes of pulmonary hypertension is needed. The use of DOAC'S in Chronic Thromboembolic Pulmonary Hypertension (CTPH) is controversial. We recommend considering treatment with LMWH for these patients.

For patients with active cancer and no signs of pulmonary hypertension consider secondary prophylaxis with low dose apixaban or rivaroxaban and repeat patient evaluation at least every 6 months.

In cancer patients with active treatment (chemotherapy, immunotherapy) or patients included in clinical trials where drug interaction is possible/suspected—consider drug level testing (apixaban, rivaroxaban) few days after initiating the new treatment protocol.

References

1. Hisada Y, Mackman N. Cancer-associated pathways and biomarkers of venous thrombosis. Blood. 2017;130:1499–506.
2. Khorana AA, Kuderer NM, Culakova E, Lyman GH, Francis CW. Development and validation of a predictive model for chemotherapy-associated thrombosis. Blood. 2008;111:4902–7.
3. Khorana AA, et al. Prediction and prevention of cancer-associated thromboembolism. Oncologist. 2021;26:e2–7.

4. Au C, et al. Clinical presentations and outcomes in pulmonary embolism patients with cancer. J Thromb Thrombolysis. 2021;51:430–6.
5. van Es N, Bleker SM, Di Nisio M. Cancer-associated unsuspected pulmonary embolism. Thromb Res. 2014;133(Suppl 2):S172–8.
6. Di Nisio M, et al. Diagnosis and treatment of incidental venous thromboembolism in cancer patients: guidance from the SSC of the ISTH. J Thromb Haemost JTH. 2015;13:880–3.
7. Lyman GH, et al. American Society of Hematology 2021 guidelines for management of venous thromboembolism: prevention and treatment in patients with cancer. Blood Adv. 2021;5:927–74.
8. Kang J, et al. Peripherally inserted central catheter-related complications in cancer patients: a prospective study of over 50,000 catheter days. J Vasc Access. 2017;18:153–7.
9. Jiang M, Li C-L, Pan C-Q, Cui X-W, Dietrich CF. Risk of venous thromboembolism associated with totally implantable venous access ports in cancer patients: a systematic review and meta-analysis. J Thromb Haemost JTH. 2020;18:2253–73.
10. Akhtar N, Lee L. Utilization and complications of central venous access devices in oncology patients. Curr Oncol Tor Ont. 2021;28:367–77.
11. Balsorano P, et al. Peripherally inserted central catheter-related thrombosis rate in modern vascular access era-when insertion technique matters: a systematic review and meta-analysis. J Vasc Access. 2020;21:45–54.
12. Gilon D, et al. Right atrial thrombi are related to indwelling central venous catheter position: insights into time course and possible mechanism of formation. Am Heart J. 1998;135:457–62.
13. Rajasekhar A, Streiff MB. How I treat central venous access device-related upper extremity deep vein thrombosis. Blood. 2017;129:2727–36.
14. Weeda ER, Hakamiun KM, Leschorn HX, Tran E. Comorbid cancer and use of thrombolysis in acute pulmonary embolism. J Thromb Thrombolysis. 2019;47:324–7.
15. Konstantinides SV, et al. 2019 ESC Guidelines for the diagnosis and management of acute pulmonary embolism developed in collaboration with the European Respiratory Society (ERS): The Task Force for the diagnosis and management of acute pulmonary embolism of the European Society of Cardiology (ESC). Eur Respir J. 2019;54.
16. Barrios D, et al. Prognostic significance of right heart thrombi in patients with acute symptomatic pulmonary embolism: systematic review and meta-analysis. Chest. 2017;151:409–16.
17. Konstantinides SV, et al. Impact of thrombolytic therapy on the long-term outcome of intermediate-risk pulmonary embolism. J Am Coll Cardiol. 2017;69:1536–44.
18. Ortel TL, et al. American Society of Hematology 2020 guidelines for management of venous thromboembolism: treatment of deep vein thrombosis and pulmonary embolism. Blood Adv. 2020;4:4693–738.
19. Meyer G, et al. Fibrinolysis for patients with intermediate-risk pulmonary embolism. N Engl J Med. 2014;370:1402–11.
20. Jimenez D, et al. Efficacy and safety outcomes of recanalisation procedures in patients with acute symptomatic pulmonary embolism: systematic review and network meta-analysis. Thorax. 2018;73:464–71.
21. Samuelson Bannow BT, et al. Management of cancer-associated thrombosis in patients with thrombocytopenia: guidance from the SSC of the ISTH. J Thromb Haemost JTH. 2018;16:1246–9.
22. Napolitano M, et al. Platelet cut-off for anticoagulant therapy in thrombocytopenic patients with blood cancer and venous thromboembolism: an expert consensus. Blood Transfus. 2019;17:171–80.
23. Carrier M, et al. Apixaban to prevent venous thromboembolism in patients with cancer. N Engl J Med. 2019;380:711–9.
24. Khorana AA, et al. Rivaroxaban for thromboprophylaxis in high-risk ambulatory patients with cancer. N Engl J Med. 2019;380:720–8.

25. Raskob GE, et al. Edoxaban for the treatment of cancer-associated venous thromboembolism. N Engl J Med. 2018;378:615–24.
26. Young AM, et al. Comparison of an oral factor Xa inhibitor with low molecular weight heparin in patients with cancer with venous thromboembolism: results of a randomized trial (SELECT-D). J Clin Oncol Off J Am Soc Clin Oncol. 2018;36:2017–23.
27. McBane Ii R, et al. Apixaban and dalteparin in active malignancy associated venous thromboembolism. The ADAM VTE trial. Thromb Haemost. 2017;117:1952–61.
28. Ageno W, et al. Bleeding with apixaban and dalteparin in patients with cancer-associated venous thromboembolism: results from the Caravaggio study. Thromb Haemost. 2020. https://doi.org/10.1055/s-0040-1720975.

Chronic Thromboembolic Pulmonary Hypertension (CTEPH)

Rabea Asleh, Offer Amir, and Neville Berkman

1 Introduction

Chronic thromboembolic pulmonary hypertension (CTEPH) refers to pulmonary hypertension attributable to the presence of post-thrombotic deposits in the pulmonary vascular tree [1]. CTEPH is classified as group IV PH. The definition of pulmonary hypertension in general was modified in 2018 and is now defined by the presence of mean pulmonary artery pressure (PAP) >20 mmHg (rather than 25 mmHg). and pulmonary vascular resistance $\geq$3WU, precapillary PH also requires PAWP $\leq$15 mmHg) [2]. Persistent symptoms due to chronic thromboembolic disease in the absence of pulmonary hypertension is referred to as "chronic thromboembolic pulmonary disease" or CTEPD. A time element of at least three months on adequate anticoagulant therapy is required to differentiate acute from chronic thromboembolic disease.

2 Pathogenesis

CTEPH is considered most likely a consequence of acute pulmonary embolism. In most cases, acute pulmonary emboli (PE) is followed by complete or partial resolution, leaving minimal or no residual vascular abnormalities. Aberrant clot

R. Asleh · O. Amir
Department of Cardiology, Hadassah-Hebrew University Medical Center, Jerusalem, Israel

N. Berkman (✉)
Institute of Pulmonary Medicine, Hadassah-Hebrew University Medical Center, Jerusalem, Israel
e-mail: neville@hadassah.org.il

E. Herzog (ed.), *Pulmonary Embolism*,
https://doi.org/10.1007/978-3-030-87090-4_17

resolution results in either partial or complete obstruction of the pulmonary vessels by organized scar tissue and subsequent development of a secondary micro-vasculopathy [2].

The basis for this abnormal resolution remains unclear and has been ascribed to several factors, including impaired fibrinolysis, presence of fibrinogen mutations, endothelial dysfunction and impaired neo-angiogenesis. Plasmin-mediated lysis was found to be impaired in patients with CTEPH compared with healthy controls [3].

Involvement of large proximal vessels accounts for the radiological lesions typically observed in CTEPH. The microvascular lesions are analogous to those seen in idiopathic PAH, including medial hypertrophy, intimal proliferation and microvascular thrombosis [4].

Pulmonary vascular bed occlusion leads to increased pulmonary vascular resistance and pulmonary hypertension, with an increase in right ventricular (RV) afterload and RV failure. In untreated patients, CTEPH has an estimated 5-year survival of 30% in patients with mean pulmonary artery pressure (mPAP) >40 mmHg and 10% with mPAP >50 mmHg [5].

3 Epidemiology and Risk Factors

The true incidence of acute PE remains unknown, it is estimated that there are approximately 300,000 incident PE events per year in the United States. Despite the high prevalence of acute pulmonary embolism, CTEPH appears to be relatively rare. This may be attributable in part to under diagnosis. Data from several PH registries has been published and an estimate of 40–50 cases per million seems consistent between studies [6]. Approximately half of the patients diagnosed with CTEPH have a prior history of acute PE.

CTEPD is likely to be far more prevalent but this entity has only recently been acknowledged and there is little data as to its prevalence. In addition, as opposed to CTEPH, which is fairly straightforward to define and simple to diagnose with echocardiography (in patients with previous documented PE), CTEPD is a more amorphous entity [7].

An important question relates to the frequency of CTEPH following acute PE [2]. In studies that used active surveillance after PE to estimate CTEPH incidence, estimates ranged between 0.1 and 8.8% within 2 years of PE diagnosis [8, 9]. In a large meta-analysis of 16 studies that included 4,047 patients followed after an episode of PE, the overall weighted pooled incidence of CTEPH across all 16 studies was 2.3%. A more recent study found the incidence of CTEPH in patients following acute PE to be 0.79% at 2 years [10]. This variability can be explained by differences in the population included in the studies (all acute PE vs. symptomatic PE vs. survivors, with or without risk factors for VTE) and how CTEPH is diagnosed (by right heart catheterization or echo).

Almost half the patients in whom CTEPH will be diagnosed present with an acute event on top of preexisting chronic disease. Many patients diagnosed with

CTEPH that allegedly developed following an acute PE were found in retrospect to have CTEPH and were misclassified at the time of the alleged acute event. Several radiological features present on CT-pulmonary angiography are suggestive of the presence of CTEPH rather than acute PE. Good quality CTPA images and experienced pulmonary radiologists are needed to correctly diagnose these patients.

4 Screening for CTEPH

In light of the low likelihood of developing CTEPH following an acute episode, routine screening of all patients following acute PE is not recommended. As a rule, evaluation for the presence of CTEPH should be performed three months after acute PE. Screening with echocardiography is indicated in patients with persistent or new onset symptoms of dyspnea. There may be a role for cardio-pulmonary exercise testing (CPET) to clarify the cause of dyspnea and rule out CTEPH in patients with dyspnea post- acute PE. Follow-up ventilation-perfusion scan does not seem useful as a screening tool for CTEPH post-PE as persistent defects are seen in up to 30–50% of cases and their physiological significance is unclear [11].

Several risk factors for the development of CTEPH have been identified, including post- splenectomy, the presence of infected intravascular line (ventriculo-atrial shunts, pacemaker), thyroid replacement therapy, lupus anticoagulant/antiphospholipid antibodies, malignancy, chronic inflammatory conditions, such as osteomyelitis and inflammatory bowel disease and essential thrombocythemia [6]. It seems logical to screen patients in these high-risk groups for CTEPH following acute PE, but to date no definite recommendations to this effect have been published.

5 Diagnosis

The median age of patients diagnosed with CTEPH is 63 years and men and women are equally affected [1]. Initial clinical features are generally non-specific, such as dyspnea, exercise intolerance, fatigue and chest pain, and there is a median lag time of 14–24 months between symptom onset and diagnosis. Delay in diagnosis is associated with worsening disease. Patients may present with clinical features suggestive of acute PE or with syncope, hemoptysis or signs of right heart failure [1]. Findings on physical examination are similar to those seen in pulmonary hypertension in general, including accentuation of the sound of pulmonic closure (P_2) with or without fixed splitting of the second sound, right ventricular heave, systolic murmur of tricuspid regurgitation, a right sided third heart sound (S_3) and signs of right heart failure.

Routine laboratory tests are not particularly helpful early in the evaluation process. Electrocardiography may show signs of right atrial or ventricular abnormalities. Chest radiography is usually unrevealing but may demonstrate enlargement of the central pulmonary arteries and right cardiac chambers [12]. CTEPH is usually accompanied by a reduced transfer factor (diffusion capacity) for carbon monoxide (DLCO) on pulmonary function tests. Reduced DLCO in the presence of normal lung flows and volumes is suggestive of pulmonary vascular disease, but these tests are not specific enough for diagnosis.

A diagnostic algorithm is presented in Fig. 1. More definitive diagnostic tests include the following:

- **Echocardiography**: Transthoracic echocardiography with Doppler imaging is sensitive for the detection of PH and right ventricular dysfunction, but it is not specific for the diagnosis of CTEPH. Common echocardiographic findings include right ventricular dilatation, hypertrophy, and hypokinesia, right atrial enlargement, right ventricular pressure overload as suggested by interventricular septal deviation toward the left ventricle during systole, and tricuspid regurgitation. Echocardiography cannot be used to reliably differentiate between acute and chronic PE.
- **Ventilation-perfusion radionuclide scan** is the recommended test of choice to diagnose CTEPH and is the best test available at present for exclusion of chronic thromboembolic disease. A normal V/Q scan effectively excludes CTEPH with a sensitivity of 90–100% and a specificity of 94–100% [13, 14]. In a study of confirmed cases of CTEPH, V/Q scan was found to be superior to CTPA with a sensitivity of 97.4% versus 51%. Single photon emission computed tomography (SPECT) is more sensitive than planar VQ. This modality is superior to planar imaging and has been recommended as the methodology of choice to exclude

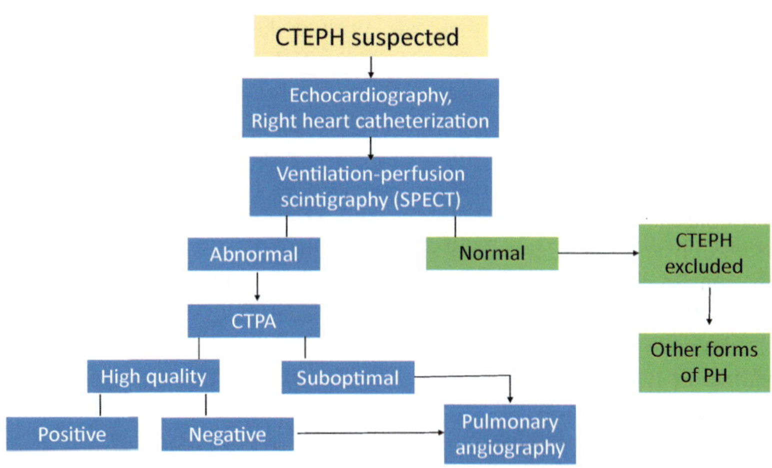

Fig. 1 Algorithm for the diagnosis of CTEPH (adapted from Delcroix). Evidence of pulmonary hypertension on echocardiography and right heart catheterization and an abnormal V/Q scan are adequate to diagnose CTEPH. Subsequent imaging confirms the diagnosis and is required for treatment decisions

CTEPD [15], although interpretation and use may be limited by physician experience.

- **Computerized tomography pulmonary angiography (CTPA)**: Pulmonary vascular imaging is usually performed to evaluate the extent of disease and allow for decisions regarding patient management. CTPA cannot exclude peripheral small vessel CTEPH, but has a high sensitivity and specificity in detecting chronic thromboembolic lesions at the main/lobar (89–100% and 95–100%, respectively) and segmental levels (84–100% and 92–99%, respectively). CTPA can also be valuable by revealing bronchial artery collaterals, which correlate with more central disease and enables evaluation of the lung parenchyma and mediastinum [15]. Findings on CTPA that suggest CTEPH include eccentric wall-adherent filling defects, abrupt tapering and truncation, complete occlusion and pouch defects, intimal irregularity, intravascular webs and bands, stenosis, post-stenotic dilatation and vascular tortuosity [16]. There are several newer diagnostic imaging options that are likely to be incorporated in the workup of CTEPH patients [15]:
  - Dual energy CT (DECT) allows for differentiation between CTEPH and PAH and between CTEPH and acute PE. This technique improves the sensitivity of distal disease.
  - Coned beam CT is more sensitive and accurate than selective angiography in evaluating sub-segmental vascular disease.
- **Right heart catheterization**: This remains the gold standard for diagnosis and evaluation of all forms of pulmonary hypertension, including CTEPH and is required to confirm the diagnosis. Vasoreactivity testing is not routinely recommended in patients with CTEPH. However, there is data to suggest that reduction in pulmonary-artery pressure after administration of a vasodilator, such as inhaled nitric oxide, may be indicative of increased long-term survival among patients with CTEPH who undergo PEA [17]. Of note, many patients with CTEPH may present with elevated wedge pressures but normal LVEDP. Non-invasive methods of measuring hemodynamics, including MRI, are promising but certainly not established enough to replace conventional RHC. The diagnostic significance of an exercise-induced increase in pulmonary pressure in patients with normal resting pressure has long been the subject of debate in pulmonary hypertension patients in general. Although not incorporated in guidelines, a steep rise in pulmonary pressure (>3 mmHg L^{-1} min^{-1}) relative to cardiac output (mPAP/CO) is indicative of reduced pulmonary vascular compliance.
- **Selective digital subtraction pulmonary angiography** (DS-PA) may be used to provide high-resolution imaging of more distal pulmonary vasculature. This can be combined in a single procedure with RHC. Although considered the 'gold standard' for the diagnosis or exclusion of acute PE, a recent ERS expert statement on CTEPH recommends that this is no longer necessary as high quality CTPA offers similar diagnostic accuracy and is safer to perform [15].

- Cardio-respiratory exercise testing (CPET) is at present not part of the diagnostic algorithm in patients with CTEPH. CPET may be of value in CTEPD and can differentiate between pulmonary vascular disease and deconditioning in dyspneic patients after acute PE. Typical findings in pulmonary vascular disease include: elevated slope of minute ventilation (VE)/carbon dioxide output (VCO_2); elevated ventilatory equivalents for oxygen (EQO_2) and carbon dioxide ($EQCO_2$); low and decreasing end-tidal carbon dioxide tension ($PETCO_2$), elevated alveolar–arterial oxygen tension gradient ($PA–aO_2$) and elevated arterial–end-tidal carbon dioxide gradient ($Pa–ETCO_2$) [7].
- MRI. Cardiac MRI can be used for diagnosis and follow-up in patients with CTEPH but is not as yet part of routine management in most centers. This modality is an excellent tool for evaluation of right ventricular function and may be used to monitor improvement in RV function in response to treatment. Contrast enhanced MR pulmonary angiography is of comparable diagnostic yield to CTPA for proximal disease but less sensitive for diagnosing peripheral disease.

Differentiating CTEPH from recurrent PE can be challenging because there is an overlap among risk factors for the two conditions. Additional conditions that can mimic CTEPH and should be considered in differential diagnosis include pulmonary artery sarcomas or other endovascular tumors, pulmonary vasculitis or congenital stenosis, in situ thrombosis associated with IPAH or structural lung disease, extrinsic vascular compression from mediastinal fibrosis, adenopathy, and neoplasm.

6 Treatment of CTEPH

A multidisciplinary team including pulmonary, cardiac, radiology, hematology and surgical specialists is critical for the management of CTEPH patients.

6.1 Anticoagulants

Patients with CTEPH require lifelong anticoagulation therapy. Vitamin-K antagonists (VKAs) are most commonly used in CTEPH. However, there is uncertainty as to whether new oral anticoagulants (NOACs) are an acceptable alternative. The rate of recurrent venous thromboembolism following PEA was higher with NOACs than with VKAs, but the frequency of recurrent VTE and of bleeding seems to be similar in CTEPH patients receiving medical therapy [18]. Patients with antiphospholipid syndrome should receive VKAs.

To date, there is no proof that aggressive treatment of acute pulmonary embolism can prevent CTEPH. In a 3-year follow up of the PEITHO trial, systemic

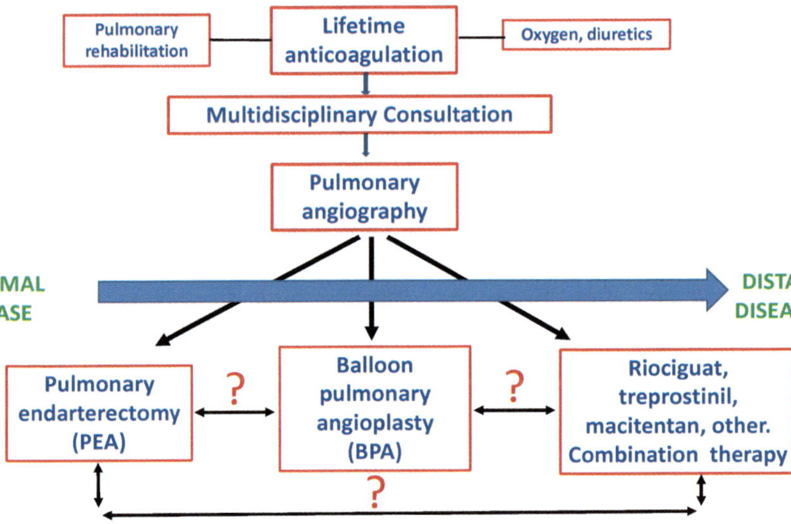

Fig. 2 Algorithm for the treatment of CTEPH. CTPA and pulmonary angiography are of value in determining whether there is proximal pulmonary artery occlusion or narrowing suitable for PEA (up to segmental and even sub-segmental disease), intermediate size arterial disease suitable for BPA or distal disease suitable for medical therapy. Question marks refer to uncertainty regarding the place for sequential or combination of different treatment modalities. The blue arrow shows that the transition from proximal to distal disease is a continuum and there is considerable overlap between patients suitable for different treatment options

thrombolysis did not reduce the risk of CTEPH in patients with intermediate/high-risk (submassive) pulmonary embolism [19].

6.2 *Pulmonary Endarterectomy (PEA)*

Surgical removal of fibrotic organized clots from the segmental and sub-segmental pulmonary arteries is the most effective treatment option for CTEPH. In experienced centers, PEA is associated with a perioperative mortality rate of 3% and a 3-year survival of 89% (vs. 70% for non-operated patients) [20] and 72% 10-yr survival rate. PEA is associated with a significant improvement in functional class [21]. The majority of patients experience substantial relief of symptoms and near normalization of hemodynamics, including reverse right ventricular remodeling, reduction in tricuspid regurgitation, and the return of right ventricular systolic and diastolic function toward normal levels [22]. PEA necessitates a true bilateral endarterectomy through the medial layer of the pulmonary arteries, which is performed under deep hypothermia and circulatory arrest [19]. Operability of patients with CTEPH is determined by multiple factors that are related to the suitability of the patient, the expertise of the surgical team, and available resources. General criteria include preoperative World Health Organization functional class (WHO-FC) II–IV and surgical accessibility of thrombi in the main, lobar or segmental pulmonary arteries. Absolute contraindications for PEA include the presence of significant parenchymal lung disease in areas that would reperfuse with surgery. Risk factors for a less favorable outcome after PEA surgery, though not absolute contraindications, include an absent history of venous thromboembolism (VTE), WHO-FC IV, right heart failure, a PVR >15 Wood units, absence of appreciable lower lobe disease, and significant left heart disease [21].

In addition to the usual complications associated with cardiac surgery, hypoxemia is common after PEA surgery and may result from reperfusion pulmonary edema that develops within the first 72 h of surgery [23]. Residual postoperative PH due to an incomplete endarterectomy or distal small-vessel vasculopathy remains a significant cause of postoperative morbidity and mortality [24].

IVC filter prior to surgery did not influence long-term survival and is no longer recommended [25].

6.3 *Pulmonary Balloon Angioplasty (BPA)*

This technique has become an option for patients with inoperable CTEPH. There are several large cohorts that show that BPA improves functional ability (functional class, 6-min walk, CPET) and well as pulmonary hemodynamics (PVR, CO) and right ventricular function. In a recent cohort [26], 6MWT was improved by 45 m, mPAP reduced by 18% and PVR by 43%. The complication rate reported in large cohorts is 10%, however this has dropped to 5% in more recent large center studies [26]. The most common complications are related to pulmonary vessel injury with hemorrhage. Mortality for the procedure is 3.8%. It is important to take into consideration that most patients require several sessions (median of 3, but up to 12) in order achieve a hemodynamic and clinically significant result. Positive outcomes are heavily dependent on operator experience. BPA resulted in a significant improvement in functional status (WHO class), quality of life, pulmonary pressures (mPAP: 44.7 ± 11.0 vs. 34.4 ± 8.3 mmHg, $p < 0.0001$), and pulmonary vascular resistance: (663 ± 281 vs. 436 ± 196 dyn s cm^{-5}, $p < 0.0001$). Exercise capacity, 6MWD (366 ± 107 vs. 440 ± 94 m, $p < 0.0001$), right ventricular function and NT pro-BNP (442 vs. 202 pg/mL, $p < 0.0001$) were also improved. Long-term outcomes and survival data are not available for this procedure.

6.4 *Medical Therapy*

Standard medical therapy for PH including diuresis for volume overload and supplemental oxygen for hypoxemia are recommended. Several drugs that specifically target the pulmonary vasculature have been evaluated in CTEPH:

- **Riociguat (Adempas)** is a guanylate cyclase stimulator, which increases nitric oxide production in the pulmonary vasculature. This was the first drug to show efficacy in a trial specifically targeting CTEPH patients (the "CHEST-1" trial). Overall, 261 CTEPH patients not suitable for PEA or with persistent/recurrent PH post PEA received riociguat or placebo. The primary endpoint was a change in 6MWD at 16 weeks. There was an improvement of 39 m in the 6MWD ($P < 0.001$) and in pulmonary vascular resistance (246 dyn cm s^{-5} ($P < 0.001$), but no change in time to clinical worsening. The drug has FDA approval for this indication. Long-term treatment with riociguat significantly reduced right heart size and improved RV function in PAH and CTEPH [27]. There is no data on survival benefit for patients treated with riociguat. There are ongoing trials to evaluate riociguat in patients prior to PEA and comparing riociguat to BPA in inoperable patients.
- Treprostinil, administered subcutaneously, led to improvement in clinical and hemodynamic parameters in a 24 week study in 105 patients with inoperable or persistent CTEPH [28].
- Macitentan, a dual endothelin receptor antagonist drug, was found to improve PVR and 6MWT in a 16 week study of 80 patients with inoperable CTEPH [29].
- Bosentan and sildenafil did not show efficacy in small trials with CTEPH patients. Despite the absence of supportive clinical trials or FDA approval, other drugs approved for class I PAH are frequently used for CTEPH, as single agents or in combination, including PDE-5 inhibitors, ERAs and prostanoids.

6.5 *Pulmonary Rehabilitation*

Pulmonary rehabilitation has shown clinical benefit in patients with diverse causes of pulmonary hypertension including CTEPH [30, 31].

6.6 *Pulmonary Artery Denervation*

There is limited data regarding efficacy of pulmonary artery denervation. Denervation lead to greater improvement in 6MWT and PVR at 12 months in patients with persistent PH following PEA as compared to riociguat [32].

6.7 Open Questions Relating to Treatment in CTEPH

There are still several open questions relating to the treatment of patients with CTEPH:

- Which treatment modality is preferable, surgery or BPA, in borderline patients with sub-segmental disease?
- Is BPA preferable to medical therapy in patients with more distal disease? This is being evaluated in ongoing clinical trials. A recent meta- analysis, including 1604 patients from 34 studies found that both treatments resulted in significant improvement in 6MWD (71.0 m with BPA vs. 47.8 m with pulmonary vasodilators), PVR (−3.1 WU vs. −1.6 WU) and mPAP (−14.8 mmHg vs. −4.9 mmHg). The authors conclude that while BPA may offer greater functional and hemodynamic improvements, it is associated with more complications [33].
- Is combination drug therapy preferable to single drug treatment for inoperable CTEPH?
- Should patients receive drug therapy in preparation for PEA or BPA? Using medical therapy as a "bridge to PEA" is more controversial, and is felt to delay timely surgical referral and, therefore, definitive treatment. In the international registry and in a University of California San Diego cohort, 28% and up to 37%, respectively, of the patients were on some form of PH-targeted drug(s) at the time of surgical referral [34]. In both cohorts, the delay between diagnosis and surgery was doubled in the pre-treated patients, without demonstrable clinical benefit. In the international registry, pre-treatment even independently predicted worse outcome (hazard ratio 2.62; $p = 0.0072$) [25].
- Is there a place for BPA or repeat PEA or medical therapy in patients with persistent or recurrent CTEPH following PEA? In some cases, CTEPH patients may remain symptomatic even when therapy (medical or interventional) reduces pulmonary vascular resistance but failed to improve pulmonary vascular compliance. Riociguat has been shown to improve pulmonary arterial compliance in CTEPH patients [35].
- Is there a place for tapering or withdrawing therapy in patients that show improvement post PEA or BPA?
- CTEPD has only recently been given attention and there is little data on how to treat these patients.

7 Evaluating Risk and Prognosis

A number of predictors for risk stratification are used in PAH, such as the REVEAL score and its modifications (REVEAL-2, REVEAL Lite 2) and ESC/ERS predictor. These combine clinical and laboratory measures and can be used to predict clinical deterioration and mortality. These predictors have not been evaluated specifically in patients with CTEPH.

References

1. Galiè N, Humbert M, Vachiery J-L, et al. 2015 ESC/ERS Guidelines for the diagnosis and treatment of pulmonary hypertension. Eur Heart J. 2016;37(1):67–119. https://doi.org/10.1093/eurheartj/ehv317.
2. Simonneau G, Montani D, Celermajer DS, et al. Haemodynamic definitions and updated clinical classification of pulmonary hypertension. Eur Respir J. 2019;53(1):1801913. https://doi.org/10.1183/13993003.01913-2018.
3. Morris TA, Marsh JJ, Chiles PG, Auger WR, Fedullo PF, Woods VL. Fibrin derived from patients with chronic thromboembolic pulmonary hypertension is resistant to lysis. Am J Respir Crit Care Med. 2006. https://doi.org/10.1164/rccm.200506-916OC.
4. Galiè N, Kim NHS. Pulmonary microvascular disease in chronic thromboembolic pulmonary hypertension. Proc Am Thorac Soc. 2006;3(7):571–6. https://doi.org/10.1513/pats.200605-113LR.
5. Fedullo P, Kerr KM, Kim NH, Auger WR. Chronic thromboembolic pulmonary hypertension. Am J Respir Crit Care Med. 2011;183(12):1605–13. https://doi.org/10.1164/rccm.201011-1854CI.
6. Gall H, Hoeper MM, Richter MJ, Cacheris W, Hinzmann B, Mayer E. An epidemiological analysis of the burden of chronic thromboembolic pulmonary hypertension in the USA, Europe and Japan. Eur Respir Rev. 2017. https://doi.org/10.1183/16000617.0121-2016.
7. Held M, Kolb P, Grün M, et al. Functional characterization of patients with chronic thromboembolic disease. Respiration. 2016. https://doi.org/10.1159/000447247.
8. Pengo V, Lensing AWA, Prins MH, et al. Incidence of chronic thromboembolic pulmonary hypertension after pulmonary embolism. N Engl J Med. 2004;350(22):2257–64. https://doi.org/10.1056/NEJMoa032274.
9. Klok FA, van Kralingen KW, van Dijk APJ, Heyning FH, Vliegen HW, Huisman MV. Prospective cardiopulmonary screening program to detect chronic thromboembolic pulmonary hypertension in patients after acute pulmonary embolism. Haematologica. 2010. https://doi.org/10.3324/haematol.2009.018960.
10. Coquoz N, Weilenmann D, Stolz D, et al. Multicentre observational screening survey for the detection of CTEPH following pulmonary embolism. Eur Respir J. 2018. https://doi.org/10.1183/13993003.02505-2017.
11. Boon GJAM, Huisman MV, Klok FA. Why, whom, and how to screen for chronic thromboembolic pulmonary hypertension after acute pulmonary embolism. Semin Thromb Hemost. 2020. https://doi.org/10.1055/s-0040-1718925.
12. Woodruff WW, Hoeck BE, Chitwood WR, Lyerly HK, Sabiston DC, Chen JT. Radiographic findings in pulmonary hypertension from unresolved embolism. Am J Roentgenol. 1985. https://doi.org/10.2214/ajr.144.4.681.
13. Kan Y, Yuan L, Meeks JK, Li C, Liu W, Yang J. The accuracy of V/Q SPECT in the diagnosis of pulmonary embolism: a meta-analysis. Acta Radiol. 2015. https://doi.org/10.1177/0284185114533682.
14. Hess S, Frary EC, Gerke O, Madsen PH. State-of-the-art imaging in pulmonary embolism: ventilation/perfusion single-photon emission computed tomography versus computed tomography angiography—controversies, results, and recommendations from a systematic review. Semin Thromb Hemost. 2016. https://doi.org/10.1055/s-0036-1593376.
15. Delcroix M, Torbicki A, Gopalan D, et al. Early View Task force report ERS statement on chronic thromboembolic pulmonary hypertension. Eur Respir J. 2020.

16. Konstantinides SV, Meyer G, Bueno H, et al. 2019 ESC Guidelines for the diagnosis and management of acute pulmonary embolism developed in collaboration with the European respiratory society (ERS). Eur Heart J. 2020. https://doi.org/10.1093/eurheartj/ehz405
17. Skoro-Sajer N, Hack N, Sadushi-Koliçi R, et al. Pulmonary vascular reactivity and prognosis in patients with chronic thromboembolic pulmonary hypertension a pilot study. Circulation. 2009. https://doi.org/10.1161/CIRCULATIONAHA.108.794610.
18. Humbert M, Simonneau G, Pittrow D, et al. Safety of riociguat in patients with pulmonary arterial hypertension and chronic thromboembolic pulmonary hypertension with concomitant novel oral anticoagulants or vitamin K antagonist use: data from the EXPERT registry. In: C104. Latest clinical investigations in acute and chronic thromboembolism disorders of the pulmonary circulation. American Thoracic Society; 2020. p. A6043.
19. Madani MM, Auger WR, Pretorius V, et al. Pulmonary endarterectomy: recent changes in a single institution's experience of more than 2,700 patients. Ann Thorac Surg. 2012. https://doi.org/10.1016/j.athoracsur.2012.04.004.
20. Delcroix M, Lang I, Pepke-Zaba J, et al. Long-term outcome of patients with chronic thromboembolic pulmonary hypertension: results from an international prospective registry. Circulation. 2016. https://doi.org/10.1161/CIRCULATIONAHA.115.016522.
21. Kim NH, Delcroix M, Jais X, et al. Chronic thromboembolic pulmonary hypertension. Eur Respir J. 2019. https://doi.org/10.1183/13993003.01915-2018.
22. Jenkins D, Mayer E, Screaton N, Madani M. State-of-the-art chronic thromboembolic pulmonary hypertension diagnosis and management. Eur Respir Rev. 2012. https://doi.org/10.1183/09059180.00009211.
23. Levinson RM, Shure D, Moser KM. Reperfusion pulmonary edema after pulmonary artery thromboendarterectomy. Am Rev Respir Dis. 1986. https://doi.org/10.1164/arrd.1986.134.6.1241.
24. Dorfmüller P, Günther S, Ghigna MR, et al. Microvascular disease in chronic thromboembolic pulmonary hypertension: a role for pulmonary veins and systemic vasculature. Eur Respir J. 2014. https://doi.org/10.1183/09031936.00169113.
25. Anand V, Frantz RP, DuBrock H, et al. Balloon pulmonary angioplasty for chronic thromboembolic pulmonary hypertension: initial single-center experience. Mayo Clin Proc Innov Qual Outcomes. 2019;3(3):311–8. https://doi.org/10.1016/j.mayocpiqo.2019.06.006.
26. Brenot P, Jaïs X, Taniguchi Y, et al. French experience of balloon pulmonary angioplasty for chronic thromboembolic pulmonary hypertension. Eur Respir J. 2019;53(5):1802095. https://doi.org/10.1183/13993003.02095-2018.
27. Marra AM, Egenlauf B, Ehlken N, et al. Change of right heart size and function by long-term therapy with riociguat in patients with pulmonary arterial hypertension and chronic thromboembolic pulmonary hypertension. Int J Cardiol. 2015.
28. Sadushi-Kolici R, Jansa P, Kopec G, et al. Subcutaneous treprostinil for the treatment of severe non-operable chronic thromboembolic pulmonary hypertension (CTREPH): a double-blind, phase 3, randomised controlled trial. Lancet Respir Med. 2019;7(3):239–48. https://doi.org/10.1016/S2213-2600(18)30367-9.
29. Ghofrani H-A, Simonneau G, D'Armini AM, et al. Macitentan for the treatment of inoperable chronic thromboembolic pulmonary hypertension (MERIT-1): results from the multicentre, phase 2, randomised, double-blind, placebo-controlled study. Lancet Respir Med. 2017.
30. Mereles D, Ehlken N, Kreuscher S, et al. Exercise and respiratory training improve exercise capacity and quality of life in patients with severe chronic pulmonary hypertension. Circulation. 2006. https://doi.org/10.1161/CIRCULATIONAHA.106.618397.
31. Ehlken N, Lichtblau M, Klose H, et al. Exercise training improves peak oxygen consumption and haemodynamics in patients with severe pulmonary arterial hypertension and inoperable chronic thrombo-embolic pulmonary hypertension: a prospective, randomized, controlled trial. Eur Heart J. 2016.
32. Romanov A, Cherniavskiy A, Novikova N, et al. Pulmonary artery denervation for patients with residual pulmonary hypertension after pulmonary endarterectomy. J Am Coll Cardiol. 2020. https://doi.org/10.1016/j.jacc.2020.06.064.

33. Kalra R, Duval S, Thenappan T, et al. Comparison of balloon pulmonary angioplasty and pulmonary vasodilators for inoperable chronic thromboembolic pulmonary hypertension: a systematic review and meta-analysis. Sci Rep. 2020;10(1):8870. https://doi.org/10.1038/s41598-020-65697-4.
34. Pepke-Zaba J, Delcroix M, Lang I, et al. Chronic Thromboembolic Pulmonary Hypertension (CTEPH). Circulation. 2011;124(18):1973–81. https://doi.org/10.1161/CIRCULATIONAHA.110.015008.
35. Thenappan T, Al-Naamani N, Ghio S, et al. Effect of riociguat on pulmonary arterial compliance in the PATENT and CHEST studies. Pulm Circ. 2020. https://doi.org/10.1177/2045894020963836.

Pulmonary Thromboembolism in COVID-19

Kateryna Yevdokimova and Hooman D. Poor

1 Introduction

Coronavirus disease 2019 (COVID-19) is a clinical syndrome caused by the novel coronavirus, severe acute respiratory syndrome coronavirus 2 (SARS-CoV-2). This virus was first discovered after a series of outbreaks of pneumonia of unknown cause in December 2019 were traced to a seafood market in Wuhan, China [1]. The highly virulent pathogen spread through the population and in March 2020, the World Health Organization declared COVID-19 a global pandemic. By May there were greater than five million confirmed cases worldwide, and by December 2020 that number had exponentially increased to greater than 70 million cases with over 1.6 million deaths [2].

SARS-CoV-2 is part of the Coronoviridae family: enveloped, single-stranded RNA viruses with mammalian and avian hosts. Its mRNA genome codes for several proteins including membrane spike (S) protein which binds to the ACE2 enzyme on the plasma membrane of type 2 pneumocytes and intestinal epithelial cells [3] (Fig. 1). Primarily spread by respiratory droplet as well as aerosolization, it has been found to have both symptomatic and asymptomatic transmission. Up to 80% of cases are asymptomatic, but for those who become symptomatic, usually with fever, cough, fatigue, there is an average incubation time of four to five days [4]. For some patients, particularly those over 60-years-old and with comorbid conditions, the disease worsens after about a week, culminating in sepsis, acute respiratory distress syndrome (ARDS), and multiorgan failure. Patients with severe pneumonia requiring ICU admission have an unfavorable prognosis, with mortality rates up to 50% [5, 6]. Compared to influenza, COVID-19 is associated with higher rates of ICU admission, mechanical ventilation, and mortality [7]. Unlike influenza,

K. Yevdokimova · H. D. Poor (✉)
Division of Pulmonary, Critical Care, and Sleep Medicine, Icahn School of Medicine at Mount Sinai, New York, NY, USA
e-mail: hooman.poor@mountsinai.org

E. Herzog (ed.), *Pulmonary Embolism*,
https://doi.org/10.1007/978-3-030-87090-4_18

the global population has had no immunity related to prior exposure, and the rapid spread of COVID-19 among vulnerable populations caused many healthcare systems to become overwhelmed. Within a month of the onset of the pandemic, cities experiencing a COVID-19 outbreak had overcrowded emergency rooms, ICUs past capacity, and shortages of life saving equipment such as ventilators and dialysis machines. This situation was further exacerbated by understaffed units despite redeployment of healthcare workers and insufficient personal protective equipment, resulting in infections among hospital staff. In such difficult circumstances many hospitals adopted "crisis standard of care" with double-rooming in ICUs and pop-up units in the lobby and even outdoor tents [8].

Among all this chaos, an astonishingly high rate of thromboembolic events was noted in COVID-19 patients. These events included not only deep vein thrombosis (DVT) and pulmonary emboli (PE), but also splenic and renal artery infarcts and strokes, often in patients lacking classic risk factors for venous thromboembolism (VTE). At the same time, many patients with COVID-19 presented with severe hypoxemia in the setting of normal lung compliance, a combination not typically seen in ARDS and potentially explained by pulmonary thrombosis. Additionally, small autopsy series of COVID-19 patients demonstrated a high incidence of both pulmonary macro- and microthrombi despite the use of prophylactic anticoagulation. Given the high mortality and morbidity associated with severe COVID-19, and the concern that aspects of the disease may be driven by thrombosis, many hospital systems instituted aggressive anticoagulation protocols above standard VTE

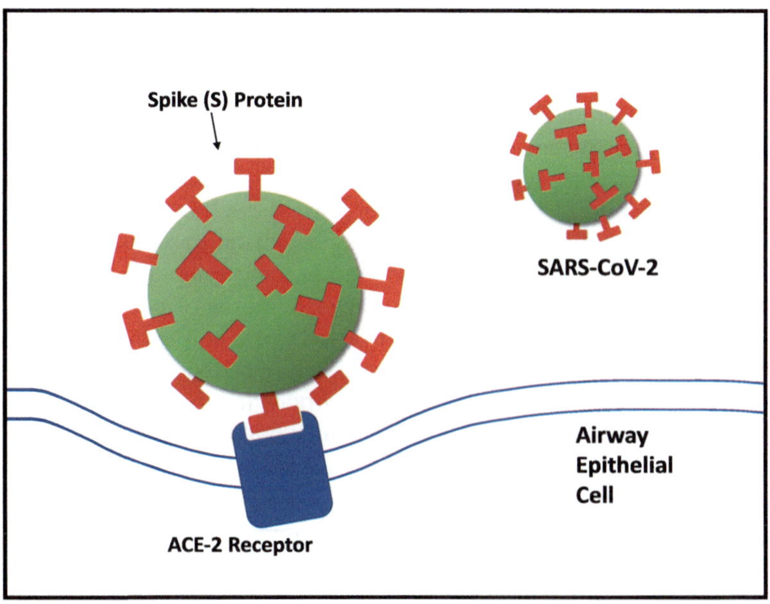

Fig. 1 Interaction between the SARS-CoV-2 virus spike protein and the ACE2 enzyme on the plasma membrane of airway epithelial cells

prophylaxis, despite the absence of randomized clinical trials supporting such practices. This chapter will explore the epidemiology, pathophysiology, diagnosis, and treatment of PE in COVID-19.

1.1 Epidemiology

Accurate assessments of the incidence of VTE in COVID-19 remains elusive, with VTE rates ranging from 4.8 to 85% [9]. The significant variability in the reported incidence is likely a consequence of multiple factors, including assessment setting (e.g. ICU vs. non-ICU), type of events counted (e.g. symptomatic vs. asymptomatic), testing strategies (e.g. clinical suspicion vs. systematic screening), and degree of thromboprophylaxis. In a study of 3334 COVID-19 patients in NYC, thrombosis, which included PE, DVT, stroke, and MI, occurred in 16% [10]. Notably, ICU patients had a higher rate of thrombotic events (29%), compared to ward patients (11%). A study of 184 COVID-19 patients in the ICU had a 30% VTE rate, of which 81% were PE [11]. A metanalysis of 48 studies and over 18,000 COVID-19 patients showed a pooled incidence of VTE of 17%, with high variance based on location: 7.1% for patients in the wards and 27.9% for patients in the ICU [9]. Overall, rates of thrombosis are higher than expected in other causes of sepsis. Compared to non-COVID-19 admissions to the same ICU in 2019, one hospital in France noted the rate of PE was two to three times higher in patients with COVID-19 in 2020 [12]. These statistics likely underestimate the true incidence as many studies did not routinely screen patients and gold standard testing was often deferred to limit transport of critically ill patients and limit exposure to health care professionals.

2 Hypercoagulable State

Sepsis and infection have been linked to coagulopathy long before the COVID-19 pandemic. Virchow's triad of hypercoagulability, stasis, and endothelial injury are particularly evident in sepsis as patients are immobilized and infection causes cellular and endothelial injury that activates the coagulation cascade. Many innate pathways that are triggered to fight infection also cause coagulopathy because this limits pathogen invasion.

This inflammatory state is likely responsible for hypercoagulability associated with SARS-COV2. In COVID, initial laboratory values reveal abnormal inflammatory and coagulation markers with elevated CRP, ESR, fibrinogen, and D-dimer [13] . D-dimer is a degradation product of fibrinolysis, and while a multitude of inflammatory processes can influence D-dimer levels, to some extent its elevation likely reflects intravascular thrombosis in COVID-19 patients. Higher D-dimers have been shown to correlate with increased mortality [13]. The biochemical

Table 1 Alterations of hematologic parameters in COVID-19 coagulopathy and DIC

Hematologic parameter	COVID-19 coagulopathy	DIC
D-dimer	↑	↑
Platelets	↔	↓
PT, aPTT	↔	↑
Fibrinogen	↑	↓
Thrombin	↑	↑
Factor VIII, factor V	↑	↓

aPTT = activated partial thromboplastin time; DIC = disseminated intravascular coagulation; PT = prothrombin time

coagulation phenotype in COVID-19 is distinct from disseminated intravascular coagulopathy (DIC). DIC is a consumptive coagulopathy, characterized by low platelet counts, decreased plasma levels of clotting factors, and prolongation of prothrombin time. In contrast, neither platelet nor clotting factor consumption are common features in COVID-19, suggesting a different mechanism of coagulopathy in COVID-19. Table 1 summarizes and compares the main coagulation parameters of DIC and COVID-19 coagulopathy.

Early autopsy reports have shown diffuse neutrophil extracellular traps (NETs), tangles of DNA released from neutrophils that propagate intravascular thrombosis [14]. Additionally, the binding of alveolar epithelial ACE2 receptor to the S protein of SARS-COV2 upregulates tissue factor, activating a prothrombotic cascade [15]. In addition to the inflammation related to sepsis, the severe hypoxemia seen in many patients also drives inflammation, vasoconstriction, and thrombosis. Hypoxia also triggers upregulation of PAI-1 which suppresses fibrinolysis and possibly causes fibrosis [16]. The micro- and macrothrombi triggered by proinflammatory cytokines and the overall hyperinflammatory response both cause endothelial injury, which further propagates the vicious cycle.

3 Endothelial Injury

In bacterial sepsis, tissue injury caused by cell necrosis or bacterial endotoxin also directly activates the intrinsic blood coagulation pathway [17, 18]. In COVID-19, the virus binds to the ACE-2 receptor, causing the host cell to undergo pyroptosis, a form of programmed cell death driven by infection and inflammation. This process releases damage-associated molecular patterns (DAMPs), which trigger cytokine and chemokine release from nearby epithelial cells, including IL-6. These proteins then attract more immune cells causing a pro-inflammatory cycle. Tissue factor is upregulated on platelets, immune, and endothelial cells which activates the intrinsic and extrinsic pathways which end in production of thrombin and fibrin, which further activates platelets and promotes clot formation and stabilization [16].

The virus also directly causes endotheliitis as SARS-COV2 elements and accumulated inflammatory cells were found in endothelial cells of COVID-19 patients [19]. The widespread endothelial injury was associated with increased microthrombi burden, likely due to overexpression of tissue factor on damaged endothelium. This overall pro-inflammatory, pro-thrombotic state, also termed immunothrombosis, leads to a combination of macrothrombi and microthrombi, both of which play a significant role in the COVID-19 syndrome pathogenesis.

4 Microthrombosis

Microthrombi, while present in many pro-inflammatory states, seem to be particularly prevalent in COVID-19. Pathological analysis showed micro- and macrothrombi in all lung samples of 11 COVID-19 patients in the setting of diffuse alveolar damage and endothelial injury [20]. In an autopsy study comparing seven COVID-19 patients to seven influenza-ARDS and 10 healthy lung controls, the prevalence of alveolar capillary microthrombi was nine times higher in COVID-19 patients compared to patients with ARDS due to influenza [19].

Many critically ill patients with COVID-19 have profound hypoxemia without a significant decrease in lung compliance, a feature that is atypical in classical ARDS [21]. Furthermore, COVID-19 patients have more aerated lung on CT compared to PaO_2/FiO_2-matched-ARDS patients [22]. Pulmonary thrombosis, particularly microthrombi, may explain the disconnect between gas exchange and lung compliance in patients with COVID-19.

Pulmonary emboli increase pulmonary vascular resistance (PVR) and pulmonary artery pressure (PAP), with higher thrombotic burden correlating with higher PVR and PAP. With sufficiently elevated RV afterload, pulmonary emboli can induce right ventricular (RV) dilation and dysfunction. Somewhat strikingly, patients with COVID-19 requiring mechanical ventilation have invasive hemodynamic profiles that are characterized by low, not high, PVR [23]. It is possible that the hemodynamic effect of pulmonary thrombosis is mitigated by a primary pulmonary vasodilatory process in some patients with COVID-19. Dual-energy computed tomographic imaging has demonstrated pulmonary vessel dilation in COVID-19 pneumonia [24]. One study reported that 83% of mechanically ventilated patients with COVID-19 had a positive bubble study as assessed by contrast-enhanced transcranial Doppler, likely indicative of abnormal pulmonary capillary dilation and/or pulmonary arteriovenous malformations. Additionally, the degree of transpulmonary bubble transit correlated with PaO_2/FiO_2 ratio, suggesting that these pulmonary vascular dilations may be a significant cause of hypoxemia in COVID-19 ARDS [25]. While pulmonary macro- and microthrombi increase PVR, pulmonary vasodilation decreases PVR; when both processes occur simultaneously, each can "cancel out" the hemodynamic effect of the other. The coexistence of both obliterative and vasodilatory processes in the pulmonary vasculature is reminiscent of what can occur in chronic liver disease, specifically portopulmonary hypertension (obliterative) and hepatopulmonary syndrome (vasodilatory). Ultimately, in COVID-19 ARDS, the obliterative processes may dominate, leading to severe RV failure and cardiogenic shock.

5 Diagnosis

Diagnosing PE in COVID-19 can be challenging because many clinical signs, such as dyspnea, tachycardia, chest pain, and hypoxemia are shared by both PE and COVID-19 pneumonia. While clinical probability scores, such as the Wells and Geneva scores, are helpful in raising clinical suspicion of PE in patients, they have not been validated in patients with COVID-19, and likely underestimate the probability of PE in COVID-19.

D-dimer, in conjunction with clinical probability assessment, has great utility in ruling out PE in patients with low or intermediate probability of PE, though its utility in COVID-19 is unclear. Elevated D-dimer has been associated with poor prognosis [13, 26]; however, as an acute phase reactant, it is not specific for PE. While D-dimer levels in COVID-19 correlate with rates of thrombosis, it is not clear whether a particular D-dimer value "rules in" or "rules out" PE. Computed tomography pulmonary angiography (CTPA) is the gold standard for PE but its use may be limited in critically ill patients with COVID-19 who are not stable enough for transfer, and for patients with renal failure, a common complication in severe COVID-19. Ventilation-perfusion scanning can be used for patients in whom CTPA is contraindicated or inconclusive. Scans performed on patients with abnormal chest radiographs, as is often the case in patients with COVID-19 pneumonia, are more likely to result in false positives because the images rarely appear as normal or low probability of PE in such patients. Compression ultrasonography can be performed to assess for DVT when chest imaging is contraindicated or indeterminate; however, the absence of DVT does not imply the absence of pulmonary thrombosis, especially since in situ pulmonary thrombosis is a potential mechanism in COVID-19. Echocardiography can raise suspicion for the diagnosis of PE with the presence of clot in the right side of the heart or new right heart strain. While it has limited diagnostic value, echocardiography is most useful for risk stratification of confirmed PE.

6 Treatment

Considering that PE is one of the most common preventable causes of hospital death, thromboprophylaxis is a crucial component in the care of hospitalized patients, and COVID-19 is no exception. However, standard doses of prophylactic anticoagulation are likely insufficient for the prevention of VTE in COVID-19 patients. One study in ICU patients using standard prophylactic anticoagulation noted a 47% incidence of VTE [27]. In addition to its antithrombotic properties, heparin also has anti-inflammatory properties, with some evidence it can inhibit neutrophil chemotaxis, decrease adherence of leukocytes to endothelium, and decrease vascular permeability [28]. With these anti-immunothrombosis properties, heparin is an important part of COVID-19 therapy, though the optimal dosing strategy has not yet been determined. Some hospitals have increased VTE prophylaxis to an "intermediate dose," equivalent to enoxaparin 40 mg twice a day [11]. Some institutions have even gone so far as using therapeutic anticoagulation for prophylaxis. In over 4000 COVID-19 patients at a New York hospital with an aggressive anticoagulation protocol, therapeutic anticoagulation, after controlling for relevant clinical factors, was associated with a 14% reduction in the hazard of mortality compared with prophylactic anticoagulation, though the finding was not statistically significant ($p = 0.08$). As expected, bleeding rates were higher in patients receiving therapeutic anticoagulation [29]. Currently, a large NIH multi-platform randomized controlled trial incorporating three global networks (REMAP-CAP, ATTACC, and ACTIV-4A) is examining the benefit of therapeutic versus prophylactic anticoagulation in patients hospitalized with COVID-19. Enrollment was recently paused for patients requiring ICU level of care at enrollment as interim pooled analysis demonstrated futility in full dose anticoagulation to reduce the need for organ support or mortality. Additionally, it was reported that full dose anticoagulation was superior to usual care prophylactic dose anticoagulation in reducing the need for organ support and mortality in moderately ill hospitalized COVID-19 patients. The full results and official publication of these studies are anxiously awaited, as they will undoubtedly help establish the optimal anticoagulation dosing strategies for patients with COVID-19.

Treatment of confirmed PE in COVID-19 patients is currently the same as for confirmed PE in non-COVID-19 patients. Risk stratification is the central tool to identify patients at increased risk for early death who may benefit from reperfusion therapy (i.e. thrombolysis, embolectomy) and/or mechanical circulatory support [30] (Fig. 2). While thrombolysis is established in the use of high risk or high-intermediate risk PE, it may also be potentially useful in COVID-19 patients who have evidence of pulmonary thrombosis despite anticoagulation. Given the potential pathophysiologic role of pulmonary microthrombosis, thrombolysis has been used in small case series of COVID-19 ARDS. In one case study, four ICU patients already on therapeutic anticoagulation with evidence of increased dead space ventilation, near normal compliance, and presence of shock received tPA; within hours of the infusion, these patients had significant improvement in oxygenation and/or vasopressor requirement [31]. Another case study of 12 patients showed significant improvement in PaO_2:FiO_2 ratio in 24 h after infusion [32]. Randomized clinical trials investigating the efficacy of thrombolysis for COVID-19 ARDS are underway.

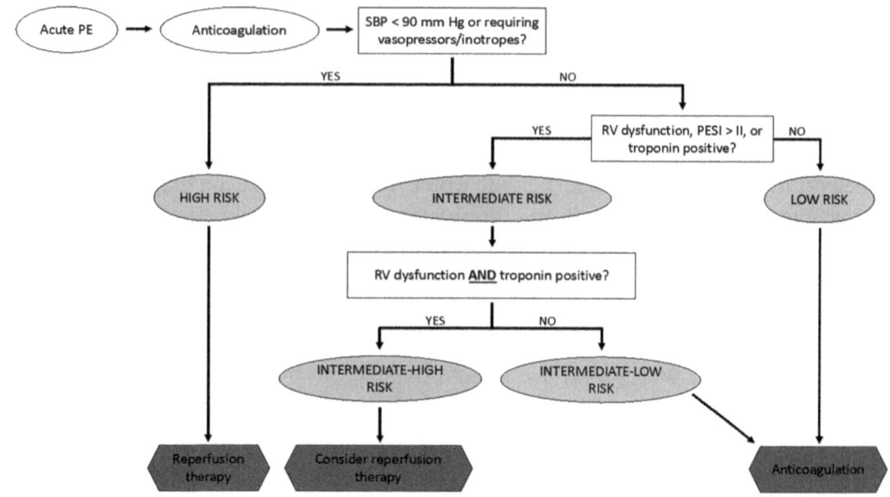

Fig. 2 Risk stratification algorithm and treatment strategy, adapted from the European Society of Cardiology Guidelines [30]. Reperfusion therapy includes thrombolysis and embolectomy. PE = pulmonary embolism; PESI = pulmonary embolism severity index; RV = right ventricle; SBP = systolic blood pressure

7 Conclusion

COVID-19 is associated with significantly elevated rates of VTE. Thrombosis, inflammation, and pulmonary vascular endothelial dysfunction play a significant role in COVID-19 respiratory failure. Optimal treatment strategies with anticoagulation and thrombolysis are being investigated.

References

1. Zhu N, et al. A novel coronavirus from patients with pneumonia in China, 2019. N Engl J Med. 2020;382(8):727–33.
2. WHO. WHO Coronavirus Disease Weekly Report: December 2020. 2020. http://covid19.who.int.
3. Oberfeld B, Achanta A, Carpenter K, Chen P, Gilette NM, Langat P, Said JT, Schiff AE, Zhou AS, Barczak AK. Snapshot: COVID-19. Cell. 2020;181(4):954.
4. Day M. Covid-19: four fifths of cases are asymptomatic, China figures indicate. BMJ. 2020;369:m1375.
5. Amit M, et al. Clinical course and outcomes of severe Covid-19: a national scale study. J Clin Med. 2020;9(7):2282.
6. Bhatraju PK, et al. Covid-19 in critically ill patients in the Seattle region—case series. N Engl J Med. 2020;382(21):2012–22.

7. Xie Y, et al. Comparative evaluation of clinical manifestations and risk of death in patients admitted to hospital with covid-19 and seasonal influenza: cohort study. BMJ. 2020:m4677.
8. Mareiniss DP. The impending storm: COVID-19, pandemics and our overwhelmed emergency departments. Am J Emerg Med. 2020;38(6):1293–4.
9. Jiménez D, et al. Incidence of VTE and bleeding among hospitalized patients with coronavirus disease 2019. Chest. 2020.
10. Bilaloglu S, et al. Thrombosis in hospitalized patients With COVID-19 in a New York City health system. JAMA. 2020;324(8):799.
11. Klok FA, et al. Incidence of thrombotic complications in critically ill ICU patients with COVID-19. Thromb Res. 2020;191:145–7.
12. Poissy J, et al. Pulmonary embolism in patients with COVID-19. Circulation. 2020;142(2):184–6.
13. Zhou F, et al. Clinical course and risk factors for mortality of adult inpatients with COVID-19 in Wuhan, China: a retrospective cohort study. The Lancet. 2020;395(10229):1054–62.
14. Barnes BJ, et al. Targeting potential drivers of COVID-19: neutrophil extracellular traps. J Exp Med. 2020;217(6).
15. He L, et al. Expression of elevated levels of pro-inflammatory cytokines in SARS-CoV-infected ACE2$^+$ cells in SARS patients: relation to the acute lung injury and pathogenesis of SARS. J Pathol. 2006;210(3):288–97.
16. Price LC, et al. Thrombosis and COVID-19 pneumonia: the clot thickens! Eur Respir J. 2020;56(1):2001608.
17. Esmon CT, Xu J, Lupu F. Innate immunity and coagulation. J Thromb Haemost. 2011;9:182–8.
18. Gailani D, Renné T. The intrinsic pathway of coagulation: a target for treating thromboembolic disease? J Thromb Haemost. 2007;5(6):1106–12.
19. Ackermann M, et al. Pulmonary vascular endothelialitis, thrombosis, and angiogenesis in Covid-19. N Engl J Med. 2020;383(2):120–8.
20. Lax SF, et al. Pulmonary arterial thrombosis in COVID-19 with fatal outcome. Ann Intern Med. 2020;173(5):350–61.
21. Laverdure F, et al. Impact of initial respiratory compliance in ventilated patients with acute respiratory distress syndrome related to COVID-19. Crit Care. 2020;24(1):412.
22. Chiumello D, et al. Physiological and quantitative CT-scan characterization of COVID-19 and typical ARDS: a matched cohort study. Intensive Care Med. 2020;46(12):2187–96.
23. Caravita S, et al. Haemodynamic characteristics of COVID-19 patients with acute respiratory distress syndrome requiring mechanical ventilation. An invasive assessment using right heart catheterization. Eur J Heart Fail. 2020.
24. Lang M, Som A, Mendoza DP, Flores EJ, Reid N, Carey D, et al. Hypoxaemia related to COVID-19: vascular and perfusion abnormalities on dual-energy CT. Lancet Infect Dis. 2020:30367–4.
25. Reynolds AS, et al. Pulmonary vascular dilatation detected by automated transcranial Doppler in COVID-19 pneumonia. Am J Respir Crit Care Med. 2020;202(7):1037–9.
26. Connors JM, Levy JH. COVID-19 and its implications for thrombosis and anticoagulation. Blood. 2020;135(23):2033–40.
27. Middeldorp S, et al. Incidence of venous thromboembolism in hospitalized patients with COVID-19. J Thromb Haemost. 2020;18(8):1995–2002.
28. Li X, Ma X. The role of heparin in sepsis: much more than just an anticoagulant. Br J Haematol. 2017;179(3):389–98.
29. Nadkarni GN, et al. Anticoagulation, bleeding, mortality, and pathology in hospitalized patients with COVID-19. J Am Coll Cardiol. 2020;76(16):1815–26.

30. Konstantinides SV, et al. 2019 ESC Guidelines for the diagnosis and management of acute pulmonary embolism developed in collaboration with the European Respiratory Society (ERS). Eur Heart J. 2020;41(4):543–603.
31. Poor HD, et al. COVID-19 critical illness pathophysiology driven by diffuse pulmonary thrombi and pulmonary endothelial dysfunction responsive to thrombolysis. Clin Transl Med. 2020;10(2).
32. Arachchillage DJ, et al. Thrombolysis restores perfusion in COVID-19 hypoxia. Br J Haematol. 2020.

Travel Related Venous Thromboembolism

Oren Yagel, Momen Abbasi, David Leibowitz, and Eyal Herzog

1 Introduction

In 2019 more than 4.53 billion people traveled by airplane worldwide. The number of passengers has almost doubled in the past decade and presumably will continue to grow in the future.

Figure 1, adapted from the "International Civil Aviation Organization", demonstrates the marked increase in passenger numbers over the past decade with a decline in 2020 secondary to the COVID 19 pandemic [1].

Venous thromboembolism (VTE), the combined syndrome of deep vein thrombosis (DVT) and pulmonary emboli (PE), is currently the third most frequent acute cardiovascular syndrome globally following myocardial infarction and stroke [2]. According to the 2020 AHA statistical update for heart disease there were a total of 1,220,000 VTE events annually in the US, of which 370,000 were cases of PE [3].

PE is associated with substantial mortality and therefore preventive strategies should be applied for individuals with elevated risk for VTE.

Even though travel related VTE is relatively uncommon, given the expected increase in passenger traffic, a substantial increase in the frequency of this clinical syndrome can be expected to occur.

The link between air travel and the development of deep vein thrombosis (DVT) and subsequent pulmonary embolism (PE) was first suggested in 1954 by a report describing a patient with a DVT after a 14-hour flight [4].

O. Yagel · D. Leibowitz · E. Herzog (✉)
Department of Cardiology, Heart Institute, Hadassah Hebrew University Medical Center, Jerusalem, Israel

M. Abbasi
Department of Internal Medicine, Hadassah Hebrew University Medical Center, Jerusalem, Israel

E. Herzog (ed.), *Pulmonary Embolism*,
https://doi.org/10.1007/978-3-030-87090-4_19

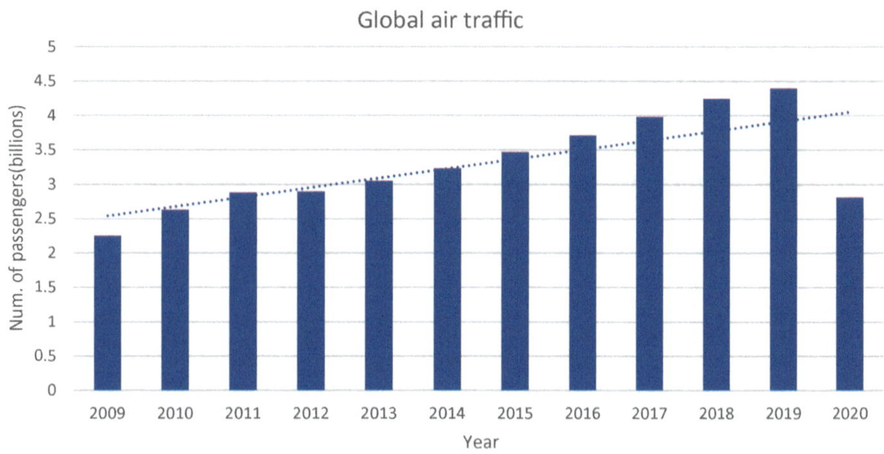

Fig. 1 Number of air passengers per year

In 1998 the term "economy class syndrome" was coined to describe the relation between long distance air travel and venous thrombosis [5], with a description of 6 patients who developed VTE after long haul flights.

In this chapter we discuss the current literature regarding travel related VTE and summarize our recommendations for VTE prevention in this setting.

2 Incidence

Venous thromboembolism (VTE) is currently the third most frequent acute cardiovascular syndrome globally following myocardial infarction and stroke [2].

The prevalence of VTE in the global adult population is approximately 1:1000 adults per year [6].

According to the 2020 AHA statistical update for heart disease there were a total of 1,220,000 VTE events annually in the US, of which 370,000 were cases of PE [3].

VTE secondary to travel is the minority of these cases. Several studies have demonstrated that the risk for VTE is elevated by two to four fold after travel [7–9].

There is no formal international surveillance for VTE related to air travel. The data of VTE incidence is based on past studies [10] with several limitations: part of the studies [8, 11] are based on medical records and not on imaging or precise diagnostic tests, and different studies [12, 13] define flight related VTE with differing time frames after flights.

The overall incidence of pulmonary embolism is 0.39 per one million passengers; for flights up to 8 hours the incidence was 0.25 per one million, while, for flights longer than 8 hours, this increased to 1.65 per one million passengers [13].

3 Pathogenesis

Several mechanisms have been proposed to explain the elevated risk for VTE during long travel and especially during long haul flights.

1. **Immobilization**
   The pathogenesis is based on Virchow's classic triad described in 1856, postulating that stasis, changes in the vessel wall, and changes in the blood composition lead to thrombosis. Immobilization is a leading risk factor for VTE and is a fundamental part of any assessment of patient with suspected VTE. The relationship between immobilization during air travel and VTE is not well established. Most of the studies describing a relationship between immobilization and VTE examined patients during illness or after trauma in patient with other risk factors, and the relationship between immobilization to VTE in healthy people is unclear. Case reports describing VTE in healthy persons after prolonged immobilization such as traffic jams [14], sitting in bomb shelters [15], prolonged prayer [16], and sitting for long periods at a computer [17] have been published, however case control studies are lacking.
2. **Hypobaric hypoxia**
   The cabin pressure in commercial flights is equivalent to a height of 6000–8000 ft above sea level. The oxygen saturation (SpO_2) of hemoglobin measured by pulse oximetry is expected to be between 85 and 95% in this range of cabin altitudes. In normal, healthy individuals, the change in SaO_2 during air travel occurs on the flat portion of the oxyhemoglobin dissociation curve, so that large changes in PaO_2 will produce relatively modest changes in SaO_2 [18].
   The decreased air pressure and relative hypoxia (hypobaric hypoxia) in the cabin reduce fibrinolytic activity and lead to release of vein wall relaxing factors, that may enhance venous stasis.
   The results of hypobaric chamber studies in healthy volunteers failed to demonstrate any association between hypobaric hypoxia and prothrombotic alterations in the hemostatic system [19].
3. **Cramped conditions**
   "The economy class syndrome" was coined to describe the relationship between sitting for long hours in a cramped position leading to stasis and the development of VTE [5]. Venous stasis provoked by the seated position maintained for long periods of time with little space between the rows to enable regular movement of feet and lower limbs, especially in economy class, can trigger the coagulation cascade during a flight and lead to VTE [20].
   Pressure on the calves from the seat, likely prevalent in shorter individuals can exacerbate venous stasis, and the calf veins appear to be the most common site of thrombosis in patients with travel associated VTE [20].
   The BEST (Business class versus Economy class Syndrome as a cause of Thrombosis [21] study is a large prospective study comparing the incidence of VTE in economy class and business class passengers. It did not find higher rates of VTE in economy class travelers. It did find in part of the travelers in both

groups elevation in D-dimer that was higher in travelers with factor V Leiden mutation.

4. **Hypovolemia**
   Low relative air humidity inside the airplane during a flight can cause dehydration.
   Low volume state was considered in the past as a risk factor for VTE, based on the fact that dehydration or alcohol induced dehydration (via its diuretic effect) elevate blood viscosity and upregulate coagulation. Currently, there is no clear evidence for an association between dehydration and travel-associated VTE [22].
5. **Passenger seat location**
   Another aspect of air travel which may be related to immobilization is seat position. The MEGA (Multiple Environmental and Genetic Assessment of risk factors for venous thrombosis study) trial [7] was a large case control study that assessed the effect of several flight related behaviors on the incidence of venous thrombosis and found a two fold increase in the VTE incidence in window seating compared to aisle seating particularly in obese passengers [22].

The risk of VTE for passengers sitting in window seats was higher in overweight participants with BMI 25–30 kg/m^2, and was highest in the obese population with BMI above 30 [7] kg/m^2.

4 Risk Factors

Travel related VTE is multi-factorial. The risk factors are divided to two major groups:

(1) Travel related factors including factors related to the flight length and the conditions during travel.
(2) Patient related factors which are similar to general risk factors of hyper-coagulable state predisposing to VTE.

Table 1 outlines the risk factors for VTE. Risk stratification in each patient should include the patient related risk factors and the travel related risk factors for tailoring the right recommendations for VTE prevention. Of note, prior VTE is probably the most important risk factor that puts the patient in high-risk category for VTE.

5 Guidelines

Multiple societies from around the globe have published recommendations for travel related VTE.

Table 1 Risk factors for VTE

Travel related risk factors	Patient related risk factors
Travel duration—more than 4 hours	Prior VTE
Way of commute	Obesity
Immobility during flight	Malignancy
Hypoxic hypobaria	Thrombophilia
	OCP use or estrogen containing drugs
	Pregnancy
	Recent immobilization
	Elderly patients
	Height (>185 cm or <165 cm)

The British writing group [23] performed an analysis of published data based on 5 prospective studies [10, 21, 24, 25] that investigated the incidence of travel related VTE.

A study by Scurr from 2001 [24] demonstrated reduced symptomless DVT in patients using elastic stockings. The elastic stocking exerted pressure on the leg, especially at the ankle area. The combination of the stockings and muscle activity elevates the blood flow from superficial veins to deep veins and increases blood flow and velocity in the deep vein system, which reduces the stasis and the potential risk for clot formation. Several studies assessed the relation between compression stocking and VTE prevention. A Cochrane review evaluated 11 randomized studies, with almost 3000 patients who had long flights (>5 hours), found evidence of a reduction in the number of asymptomatic DVTs and reduction in superficial venous thrombosis [26].

Two other studies [8, 10] emphasize the relation between flight duration and known risk factors and elevated risk for VTE.

All 5 studies focused on travel over 8 hours. The incidence of DVT or PE was 16/2901 (0.5%) and the incidence of symptomatic VTE was 10/2901 (0.3%).

They concluded with the following recommendations:

(1) There is no evidence for an association between dehydration and travel-associated VTE.
(2) Maintaining mobility is a reasonable precaution for all travelers on journeys over 3 hours, with indirect evidence that maintaining mobility may prevent VTE
(3) Global use of compression stockings and anticoagulants for long distance travel is not indicated, but patients at very high risk undertaking journeys of over 3 hours should wear well fitted below knee compression hosiery.

Table 2 summarizes the British writing group recommendations.

The CDC traveler health guide [27] issued in 2020 based its recommendations on guidelines from 2012 of American College of Chest Physicians. Their focus is

Table 2 British writing group recommendations

Duration of travel	<3 hours	3–8 hours	>8 hours
Risk group			
Low	None	None	None
Intermediate	None	None or stockings	Stockings
High	None	Stockings	Stockings ± anticoagulant
Risk group	*Examples of risk factors for VTE*		
Low	None		
Intermediate	All others e.g. Up to 6 weeks post-partum Previous unprovoked VTE no longer on anticoagulants Previous travel-related VTE Combinations of risk factors		
High	Major surgery in previous 4 weeks Active cancer undergoing chemo-radiotherapy in the previous 6 months, awaiting surgery or chemo-radiotherapy or in palliative phase		

on the following preventive measures for long-distance travelers: calf muscle exercises, frequent ambulation and aisle seating when feasible. For patients with risk factors, they recommend using Graduated Compression Stockings (GCS), for high-risk patients' prophylactic anticoagulation should be considered. Regarding hydration and alcohol drinking they concludes that maintaining hydration is reasonable and unlikely to cause harm, but it cannot be recommended specifically to prevent travel-related VTE.

The Thrombosis Canada [28] published their recommendations in 2019. They summarize that even though there are no good studies assessing the efficacy of preventive measurements they recommend the following preventive measures: walking every 1–2 hours, exercising and stretching legs regularly, wearing loose fitting clothing, minimizing baggage in the space under the seat, staying hydrated and avoiding alcohol while traveling. Graduated compression stockings (20–30 mmHg) should be used only in patients with risk factors. They also recommend that a short course of prophylactic-dose anticoagulation may be considered in select patients who are at very high risk of VTE.

Our team recommends the following:

General measures:

- Frequent ambulation—mostly in long haul flights (more the 4 hours), every 1–2 hours.
- Seat exercise—foot pumps to increase blood flow in the calf, ankle circles, knee-to-chest stretches to prevent stasis.
- Avoid sitting prolonged periods with bent knees (Fig. 2)
- Selecting an aisle seat (Fig. 3)
- Use of graduated compression stockings

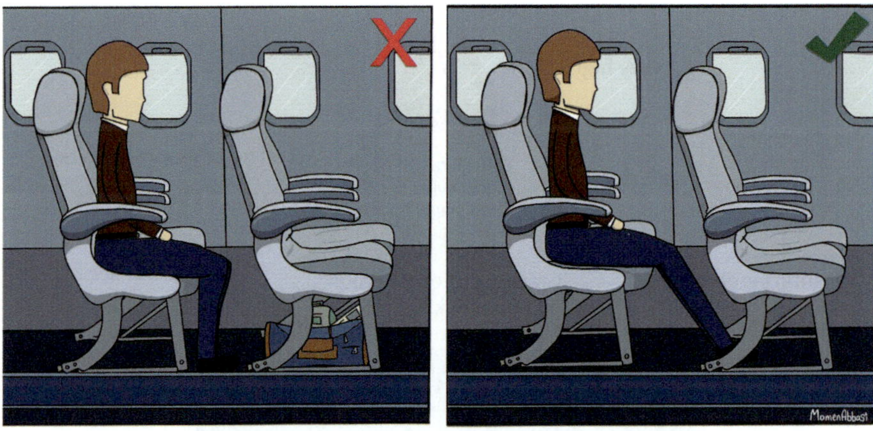

Fig. 2 Recommendation to avoid sitting prolonged periods with bent knees during flight

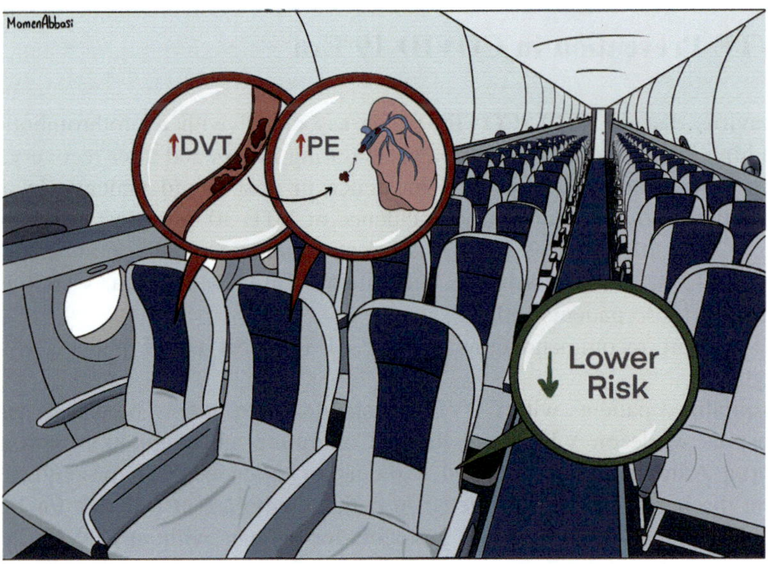

Fig. 3 Recommendation for selecting an aisle seat during flight

Figure 4 demonstrate the relation between the risk for VTE and our recommendations for management.

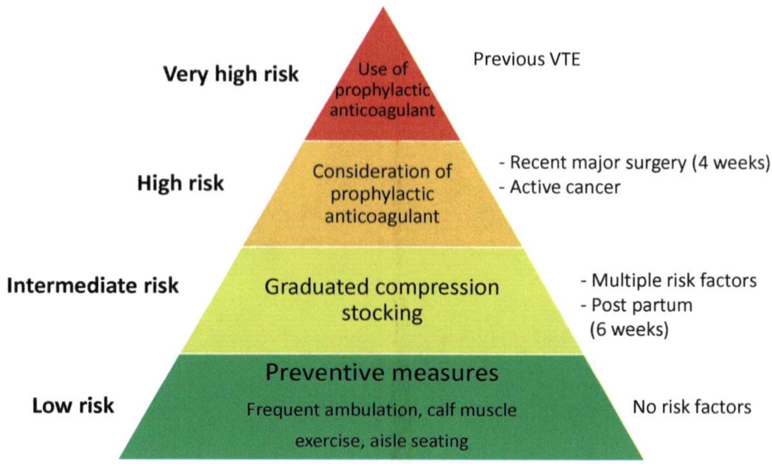

Fig. 4 Relation between the risk for VTE and our recommendations for management

6 VTE Prevention in COVID 19 Era

Coronavirus disease 2019 (COVID-19) is associated with a prothrombotic state with a high incidence of thrombotic events during illness and after recovery. There are few studies that assessed VTE incidence in post Covid patients. In a small retrospective study, the cumulative incidence of VTE 30 days post hospitalization due to COVID 19 was 0.6% [29]. Another study showed similar numbers (0.48%) in the first 42 days after discharge, but compared to pre-covid era, VTE was more prevalent in those patients [30].

The current recommendations from NIH for post covid patients for VTE prophylaxis:

Hospitalized patients with COVID-19 should not routinely be discharged from the hospital while on VTE prophylaxis. Continuing anticoagulation with a Food and Drug Administration-approved regimen for extended VTE prophylaxis after hospital discharge can be considered in patients who are at low risk for bleeding and high risk for VTE, as per the protocols for patients without COVID-19.

There are no studies or recommendations for out-patients post COVID for general VTE prophylaxis and travel related VTE prophylaxis. As noted above, there is no routine treatment of post COVID patients with prophylactic anti-coagulation. As for patients that intend to travel short time after diagnosis unfortunately, there is currently no data. It may be reasonable to recommend for patients who are at high risk for VTE to use non-pharmacological prophylactic measures to prevent VTE. For patients with very high risk including known thrombophilia, patients who had severe illness with reduced mobility prior to the travel, and patients with multiple risk factors, pharmacological prophylaxis should be considered.

References

1. Effects of Novel Coronavirus (COVID-19) on Civil Aviation, from "international civil aviation organization"
2. Raskob GE, Angchaisuksiri P, Blanco AN, Buller H, Gallus A, Hunt BJ, Hylek EM, Kakkar A, Konstantinides SV, McCumber M, Ozaki Y, Wendelboe A, Weitz JI. Thrombosis: a major contributor to global disease burden. Arterioscler Thromb Vasc Biol. 2014;34:23632371.
3. Heart Disease and Stroke Statistics—2020 Update: A Report From the American Heart Association, Salim S. Virani, et al, On behalf of the American Heart Association Council on Epidemiology and Prevention Statistics Committee and Stroke Statistics Subcommittee
4. Homans J. Thrombosis of the deep leg veins due to prolonged sitting. N Engl J Med. 1954;250:148–9.
5. Cruickshank J, Gorlin R, Jennett B. Air travel and thrombotic episodes: the economy class syndrome. Lancet. 1988;2:497–8.
6. Benjamin EJ, Virani SS Callaway CW, et al. American Heart Association Council on Epidemiology and Prevention Statistics Committee and Stroke Statistics Subcommittee. Heart disease and stroke statistics-2018 update: a report from the American Heart Association [published correction appears in Circulation. 2018;137(12):e493]
7. Cannegieter SC, Doggen CJ, van Houwelingen HC, Rosendaal FR. Travel-related venous thrombosis: results from a large population-based case control study (MEGA study). PLoS Med 2006; 3:e307.
8. Kelman CW, Kortt MA, Becker NG, et al. Deep vein thrombosis and air travel: record linkage study. BMJ. 2003;327(7423):1072.
9. Chandra D, Parisini E, Mozaffarian D. Meta-analysis: travel and risk for venous thromboembolism. Ann Intern Med. 2009;151(3):180–90. https://doi.org/10.7326/0003-4819-151-3-200908040-00129 Epub 2009 Jul 6.
10. Schwarz T, Siegert G, Oettler W, Halbritter K, Beyer J, Frommhold R, Gehrisch S, Lenz F, Kuhlisch E, Schroeder HE, Schellong SM. Venous thrombosis after long-haul flights. Arch Intern Med. 2003 Dec 8–22;163(22):2759–64.
11. Philbrick JT, Shumate R, Siadaty MS, et al. Air travel and venous thromboembolism: a systematic review. J Gen Intern Med. 2007;22:107–14.
12. Martinelli I, Taioli E, Battaglioli T, et al. Risk of venous thromboembolism after air travel: interaction with thrombophilia and oral contraceptives. Arch Intern Med. 2003;16:2771–4.
13. Pérez-Rodríguez E, Jiménez D, Díaz G, et al. Incidence of air travel-related pulmonary embolism at the Madrid-Barajas airport. Arch Intern Med. 2003;163(22):2766–70.
14. Eschwege V, Robert A. Strikes in French public transport and resistance to activated protein C. Lancet. 1996;347:206.
15. Simpson K. Shelter deaths from pulmonary embolism. Lancet. 1940;236:744.
16. Eom M, Lim SC, Kim YS. Three cases of pulmonary thromboembolism and extensive prayer (invocation) activity as a new possible risk factor. Am J Forensic Med Pathol. 2009;30:191–4.
17. Beasley R, Raymond N, Hill S, Nowitz M, Hughes R. eThrombosis: the 21st century variant of venous thromboembolism associated with immobility. Eur Respir J. 2003;21:374–6.
18. Mohr LC. Hypoxia during air travel in adults with pulmonary disease. Am J Med Sci. 2008;335(1):71–9.
19. Toff WD, Jones CI, Ford I, et al. Effect of hypobaric hypoxia, simulating conditions during long-haul air travel, on coagulation, fibrinolysis, platelet function, and endothelial activation. JAMA. 2006;295(19):2251–61.
20. Marques MA, Panico MDB, Porto CLL, Milhomens ALM, Vieira JM. Venous thromboembolism prophylaxis on flights. J Vasc Bras. 2018;17(3):215–9.
21. Jacobson B, Münster M, Smith A, Burnand K, Carter A, Abdool-Carrim A, Marcos E, Becker P, Rogers T, Roux D, Calvert-Evers J, Nel M, Brackin R, Veller M. The BEST study

—a prospective study to compare business class versus economy class air travel as a cause of thrombosis. S Afr Med J. 2003;93:522–8.
22. Schreijer AJM, Cannegieter SC, Doggen CJM, Rosendaal FR. The effect of flight-related behaviour on the risk of venous thrombosis after air travel. Br J Haematol. 2009;144:425–9.
23. Watson HG, Baglin TP. Guidelines on travel-related venous thrombosis. Br J Haematol. 2011;152:31–4.
24. Scurr JH, Machin SJ, Bailey-King S, Mackie IJ, McDonald S, Smith PD. Frequency and prevention of symptomless deep-vein thrombosis in long-haul flights: a randomised trial. Lancet. 2001;357:1485–9.
25. Hughes RJ, Hopkins RJ, Hill S, Weatherall M, Van de WN, Nowitz M, Milne D, Ayling J, Wilsher M, Beasley R. Frequency of venous thromboembolism in low to moderate risk long distance air travellers: the New Zealand Air Traveller's Thrombosis (NZATT) study. Lancet. 2003;362:2039–44.
26. Clarke MJ, Broderick C, Hopewell S, Juszczak E, Eisinga A. Compression stockings for preventing deep vein thrombosis in airline passengers. Cochrane Database Syst Rev. 2016;9 (9):CD004002.
27. CDC's Yellow Book (Health Information for International Travel) 2020, chapter 8, Travel by Air, Land & Sea Deep Vein Thrombosis & Pulmonary Embolism
28. Thrombosis Canada - AIR TRAVEL-RELATED THROMBOSIS 2018
29. Patell R, Bogue T, Koshy A, Bindal P, Merrill M, Aird WC, Bauer KA, Zwicker JI. Postdischarge thrombosis and hemorrhage in patients with COVID-19. Blood. 2020;136 (11):1342–6. https://doi.org/10.1182/blood.2020007938.
30. Roberts LN, Whyte MB, Georgiou L, et al. Post-discharge venous thromboembolism following hospital admission with COVID-19. Blood. 2020 August 3

Illustrative Cases of Multimodality Imaging in the Diagnosis and Management of Pulmonary Embolism

Eldad Rahamim, Dotan Cohen, Gabby Elbaz-Greener, David Planer, and Eyal Herzog

1 Introduction

The diagnosis and management of pulmonary embolism (PE) is based on multimodality diagnostic and imaging tests including, but not limited to, electrocardiography, echocardiography, compression ultrasonography, computerized tomography (CT), magnetic resonance imaging (MRI), lung scintigraphy and pulmonary angiography. We recommend to risk stratify patients with pulmonary embolism based on their clinical presentation, their right ventricle (RV) function and their level of cardiac biomarkers into four categories: high risk PE, intermediate high risk PE, intermediate low risk PE and, low risk PE, as described in our pathway for the diagnosis and management of pulmonary embolism [1]. In this chapter we describe four patients who presented to our healthcare system with PE. Each of these patients presents one of these categories.

2 Illustrative Case of Low-Risk Pulmonary Embolism

A 62-year-old female presented to the emergency department with chest pain of three days duration, radiating to her left arm and accompanied by shortness of breath. The patient had a past medical history of ischemic heart disease with a coronary artery bypass grafting surgery two weeks prior to her admission. She also had uncontrolled diabetes mellitus, hypertension, and dyslipidemia.

E. Rahamim (✉) · G. Elbaz-Greener · D. Planer · E. Herzog
Department of Cardiology, Hadassah Medical Center, Hebrew University of Jerusalem, Jerusalem, Israel

D. Cohen
Department of Radiology, Hadassah Medical Center, Hebrew University of Jerusalem, Jerusalem, Israel

E. Herzog (ed.), *Pulmonary Embolism*,
https://doi.org/10.1007/978-3-030-87090-4_20

Upon presentation to the hospital, the patient's vital signs were blood pressure of 130/70 mmHg, heart rate of 87 beats per minute, respiratory rate of 20 breaths per minute, blood oxygen saturation of 99% in room air, and a temperature of 37.1 °C. On physical examination her lung auscultation was clear, her cardiac examination showed regular heart sounds with a 2/6 systolic murmur, intensified with inhalation. There were no physical findings of deep vein thrombosis.

As per our pathway for the diagnosis and treatment of patients with PE, this patient is hemodynamically stable hence the first step in her assessment is the evaluation of the clinical probability of her having PE (Fig. 1 Step 1).

Her laboratory tests showed Di-dimer 3800 ng/mL (Fig. 1 Step 2), high sensitive Troponin T (hsTnT) of 13 ng/L, and C-reactive protein 260 mg/L. ECG showed left axis deviation with no ischemic changes (Fig. 2). Doppler evaluation of the lower limbs excluded deep vein thrombosis. CT angiography of the chest (Fig. 1 Step 4) revealed a bilateral pulmonary embolism, central in the right lung and subsegments on the left lower lobe (Fig. 3a–e). Transthoracic echocardiography (Fig. 1 Step 5) showed normal left ventricular systolic function and did not demonstrate right heart strain (Figs. 4, 5 and 6).

The patient was stratified as a low-risk pulmonary embolism with an sPESI score of 0 (Fig. 1 Steps 5–6). She was admitted to the hospital with an infected surgical site which had prevented her discharge home. She initially received anticoagulation with subcutaneous Enoxaparin sodium 1 mg/kg bid until her laboratory workup excluded antiphospholipid antibodies (as outlined in our pathway). She was then switched to Apixaban 10 mg twice a day for a total of 7 days treatment. Her Apixaban dose was then lowered to 5 mg bid which she was recommended to take for 6 months. She was discharged home and continued follow-up through the outpatient coagulation clinics with an excellent outcome.

3 Illustrative Case of Intermediate Low Risk Pulmonary Embolism

A 65-year-old man presented to the emergency department with three days of dyspnea and a nonproductive cough, worsening with exercise. He denied chest pain. The patient had a past medical history of diabetes mellitus, hypertension, dyslipidemia, and past history of smoking.

On examination, his blood pressure was elevated to 180/100 mmHg, temperature was normal, and the oxygen saturation was 91% in room air. ECG showed sinus tachycardia of 100 bpm, new right bundle branch block with inverted T waves in leads V1-V3 (Fig. 7). Laboratory workup showed a D-dimer of 8,000 ng/mL (Fig. 1 Step 2), and hsTnT was negative on the two consecutive tests. Chest

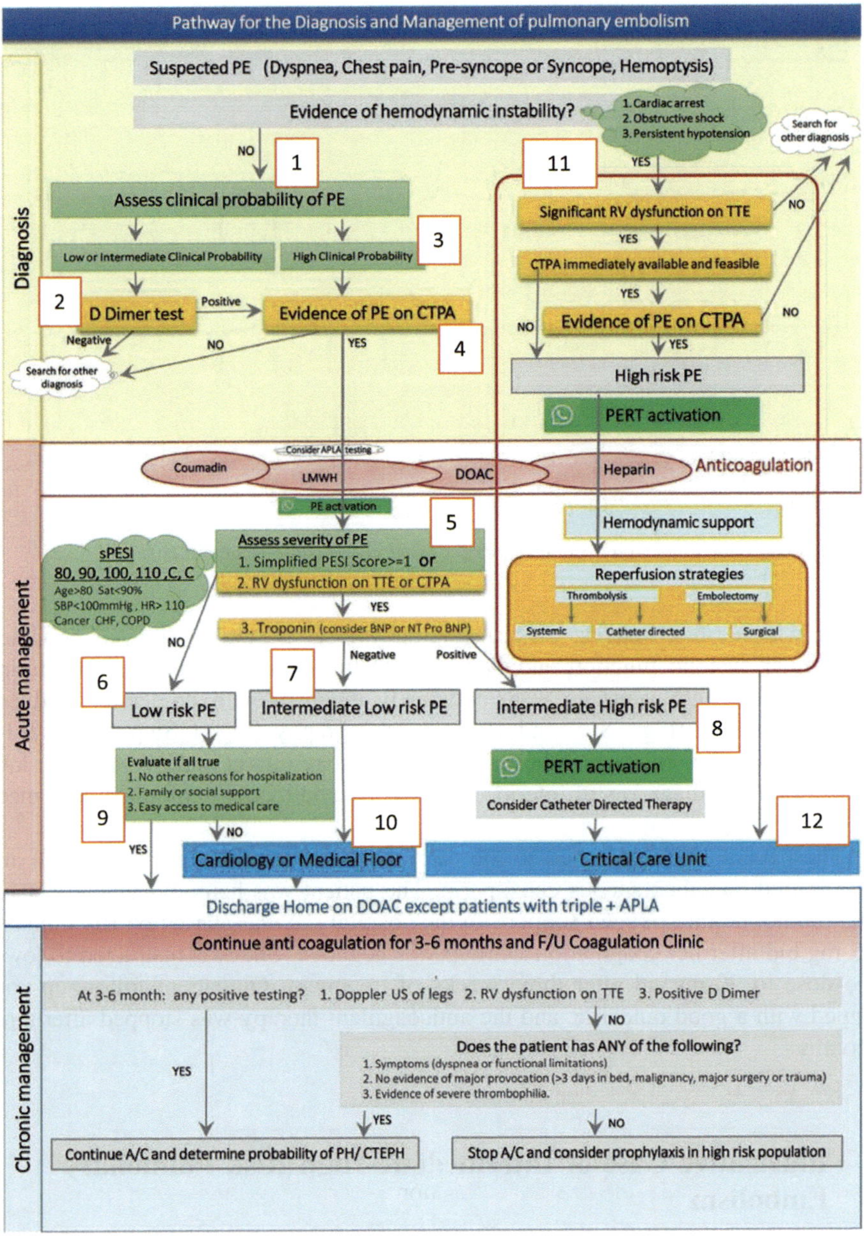

Fig. 1 Pathway for the diagnosis and treatment of pulmonary embolism

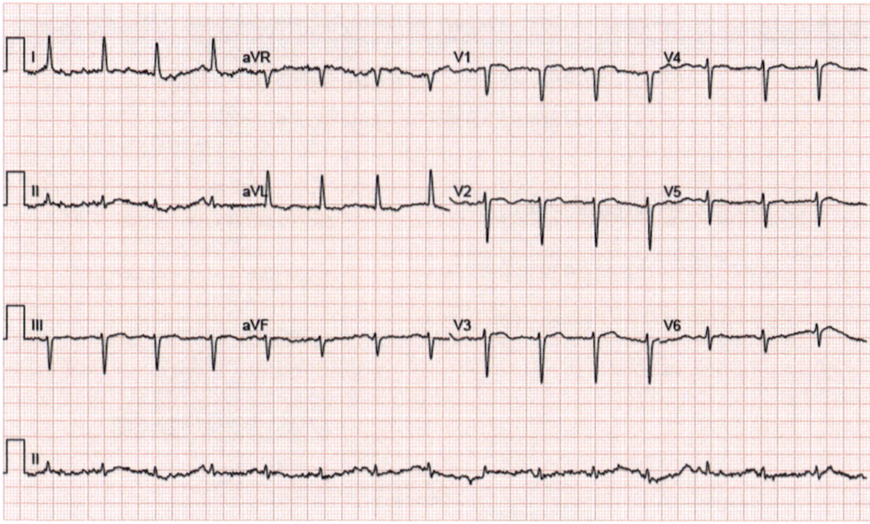

Fig. 2 ECG with sinus tachycardia, left axis deviation, no acute ischemic changes

X-ray was normal; bedside echocardiography (Fig. 1 Step 5) showed good left ventricular systolic function and flattening of the interventricular septum during diastole. The right ventricle was moderately enlarged with moderately reduced systolic function (Figs. 8, 9 and 10). CT angiography (Fig. 1 Step 4) showed a bilateral central pulmonary embolism with pulmonary infarct in the right upper lobe (Fig. 11a–f). A diagnosis of intermediate low-risk pulmonary embolism was made based on our pathway.

The patient was transferred to the cardiology department (Fig. 1 Step 10) and was started on subcutaneous enoxaparin. The patient was hemodynamically stable and did not require oxygen support. In the hospital she was started on Rivaroxaban 15 mg bid after her coagulation workup was negative. She was instructed to lower the dose to 20 mg qd after three weeks of treatment. Outpatient follow-up continued with a good outcome, and the anticoagulant therapy was stopped after three months.

4 Illustrative Case of Intermediate-High Risk Pulmonary Embolism

A 44-year-old female presented to the emergency department with sudden onset of shortness of breath. She denied chest pain, cough or fever, palpitations, or lower limb pain. Her past medical history was significant for lower limb venous insufficiency. She was hospitalized with COVID-19 two months before her current

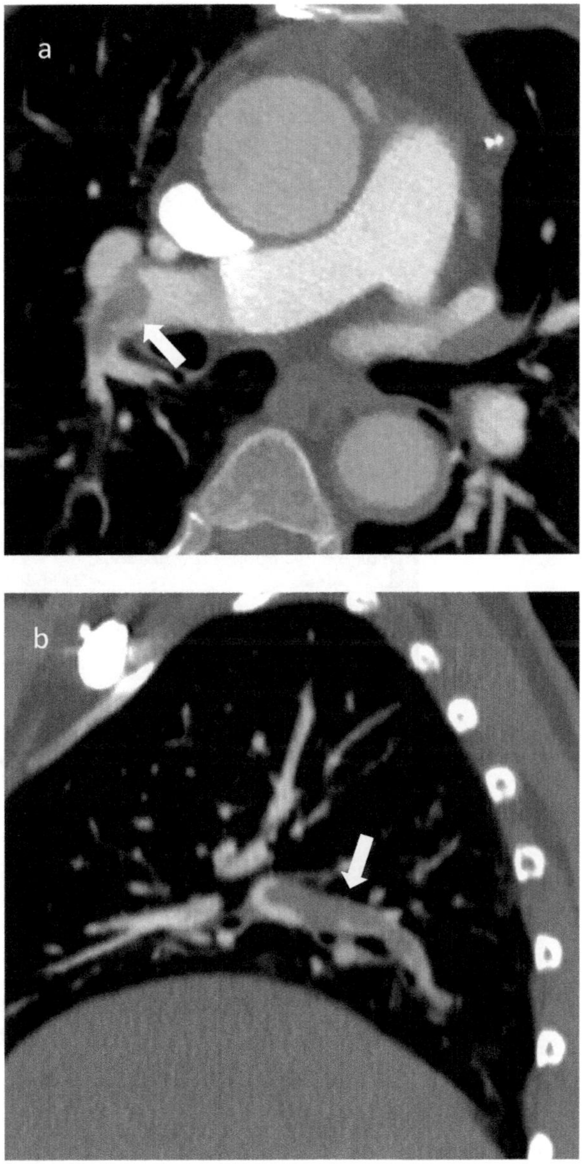

Fig. 3 **a** Axial CTPA image shows a filling defect (arrow) within the right main pulmonary artery extending into the segmental artery to the superior segment of the right lower lobe. **b** Sagittal CTPA image shows filling defects (arrow) within the lobar artery of the right lower lobe extending into a segmental artery. **c** CTPA 4-chamber reconstruction shows no increase in RV:LV diameter ratio (~ 0.7) and normal position of the interventricular septum. **d** Axial CTPA image shows normal diameter of the main pulmonary artery (<29 mm). **e** Axial CTPA image shows no contrast material reflux into the IVC

admission. She was taking oral contraceptives but was not a smoker. Her family history includes venous thromboembolism in her father.

In the emergency department, blood pressure was 132/71 mmHg, heart rate of 122 bpm, temperature of 36.4 °C, and oxygen saturation was 95% in room air. She was tachypneic with respiratory rate of 36 breaths per minute. Heart exam was

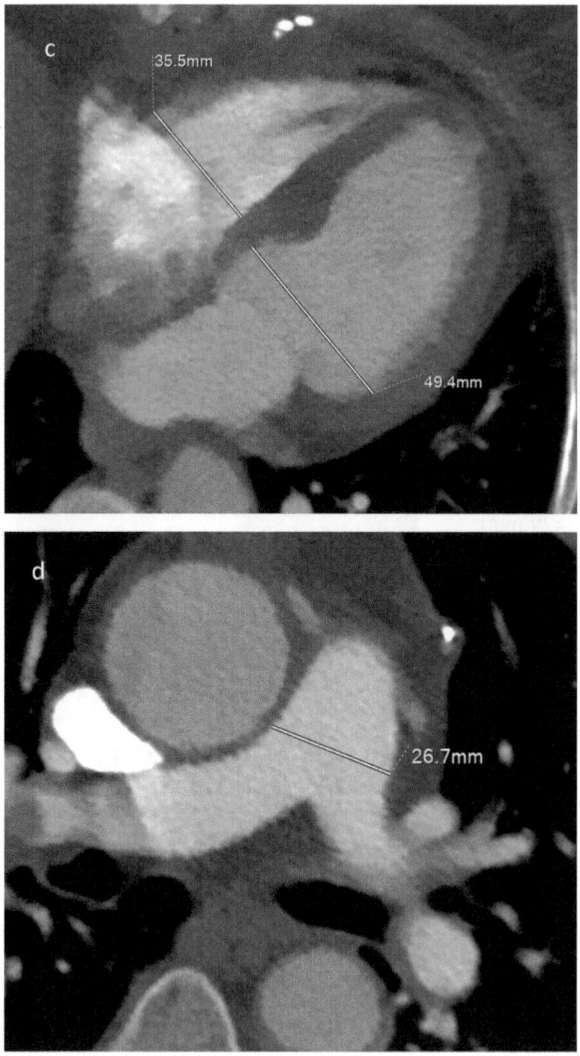

Fig. 3 (continued)

significant for fast and regular heart sounds with a 3/6 systolic murmur intensified with inhalation. lung auscultation was clear, examination of her lower limbs did not show signs of deep vein thrombosis, and she had elevated jugular venous pressure. Lab work revealed significant leukocytosis, d-dimer of 14,000 ng/mL (Fig. 1 Step 2), hsTnT of 1427 ng/L (Fig. 1 Step 5), and lactic acid of 2.4 mmol/L. ECG showed sinus tachycardia with T-wave inversion in leads V1–V3 (Fig. 12).

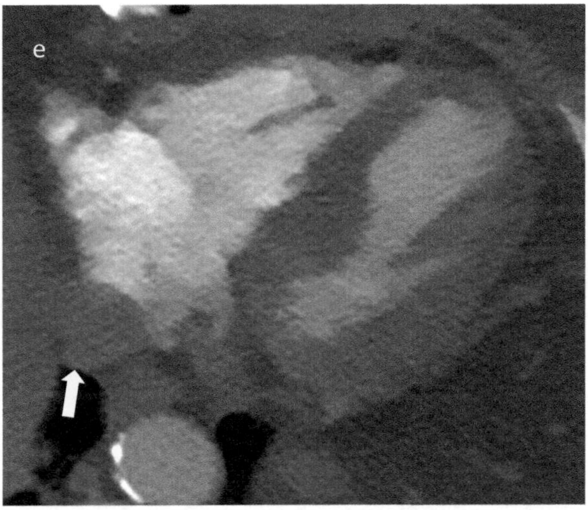

Fig. 3 (continued)

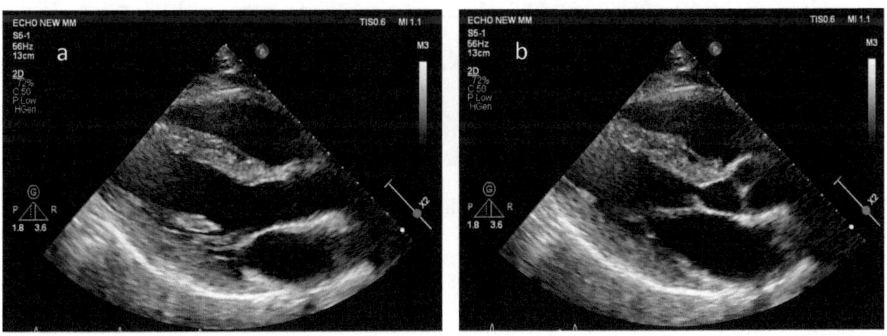

Fig. 4 Parasternal long axis view echocardiography during systole (**a**) and diastole (**b**) showing normal ventricles

CT angiography (Fig. 1 Step 4) showed bilateral central and segmental emboli, most prominent in the left pulmonary artery. The right atrium and ventricle were dilated with flattening of the interventricular septum to the left side. There was reflux of contrast material to the inferior vena cava with no respiratory collapse (Fig. 13a–d). Echocardiography (Fig. 1 Step 5) showed good left ventricular function but severely reduced right ventricular systolic function with a moderately enlarged right ventricle cavity. Free wall akinesis with apical preservation (McConnell's sign) was seen (Figs. 14, 15 and 16). There was severe tricuspid regurgitation and moderate pulmonary hypertension of 57 mmHg.

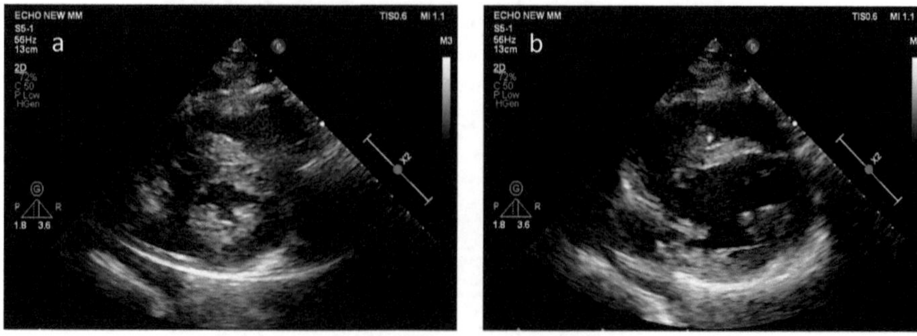

Fig. 5 Parasternal short axis view echocardiography during systole (**a**) and diastole (**b**) showing normal ventricles, with no signs of right ventricular strain

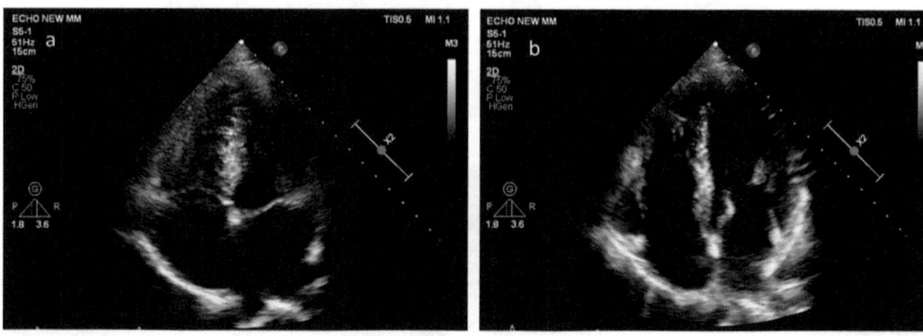

Fig. 6 Four chamber view echocardiography during systole (**a**) and diastole (**b**) showing normal ventricles, negative McConnell sign

With the findings of elevated troponin and reduced right ventricular function, the patient was risk stratified as intermediate high-risk pulmonary embolism. She was given a bolus of 5000 units of unfractionated heparin and was transferred to the cardiac catheterization laboratory. Pulmonary angiography (Fig. 1 Step 8) demonstrated a small embolus in the lobar branch of the right pulmonary artery and a significant embolus with near-total occlusion of the left pulmonary artery (Fig. 17). A catheter directed thrombolysis using pigtail catheter was used to break down the embolus on the left pulmonary artery with immediate clinical improvement. McNamara catheter was inserted beyond the clot with a bolus injection of 3 mg of tPA followed by a continuous infusion of 1 mg per hour drip for the following 12 h. The patient was hemodynamically and respiratory stable and was transferred to the cardiac intensive care unit (Fig. 1 Step 12) for observation.

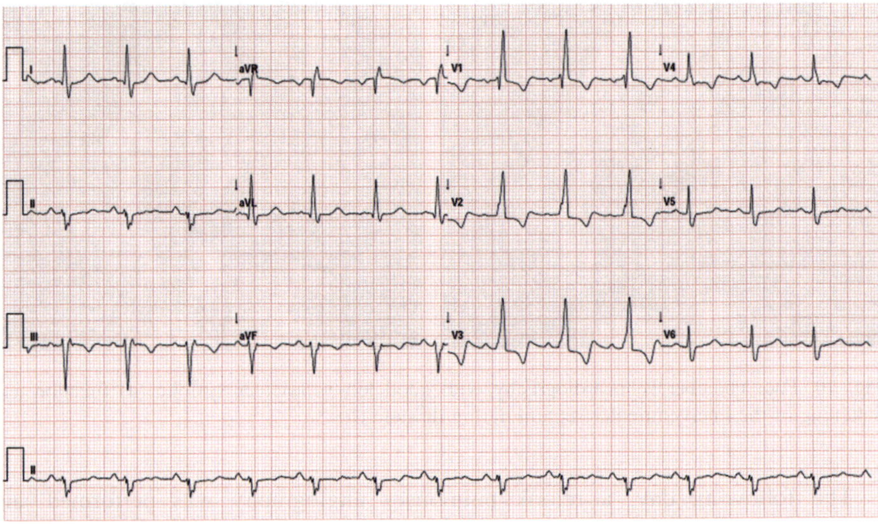

Fig. 7 ECG showing sinus tachycardia of 100 bpm, right bundle branch block with inverted T waves in leads V1–V3

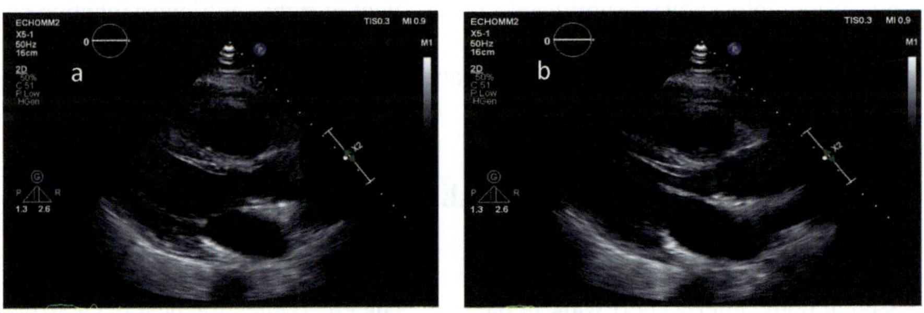

Fig. 8 Parasternal long axis echocardiography with good left ventricular systolic (**a**) function and flattening of the interventricular septum during diastole (**b**)

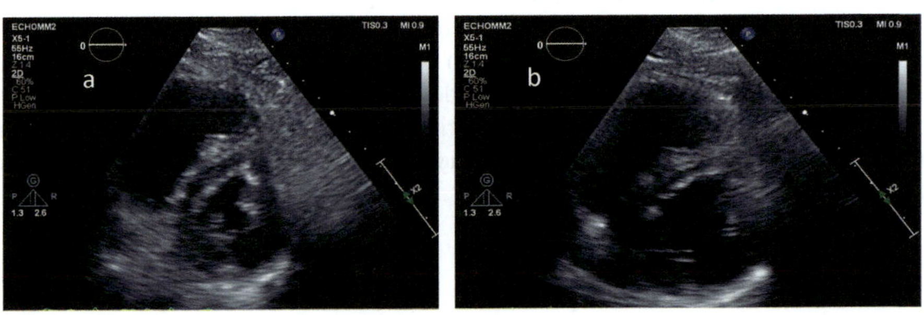

Fig. 9 Parasternal short axis echocardiography with good left ventricular systolic (**a**) function and flattening of the interventricular septum during diastole (**b**)

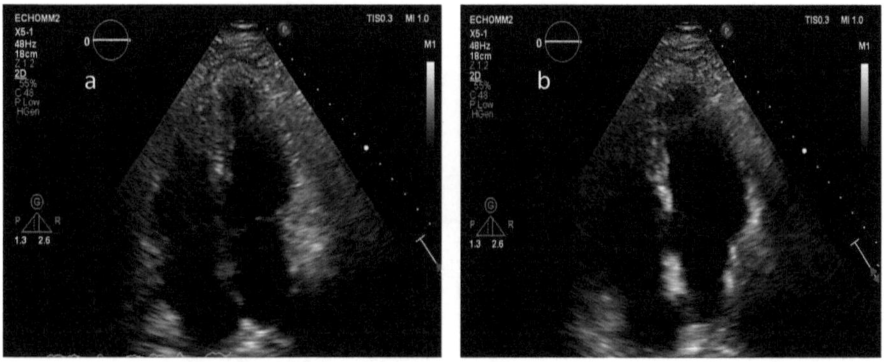

Fig. 10 Four chamber echocardiography with good left ventricular systolic (**a**) function and flattening of the interventricular septum during diastole (**b**)

The following day, a relook pulmonary angiography was performed and excluded the need for further intervention as there was a near normal left pulmonary artery blood flow (Fig. 18). The catheter was removed, and the patient was placed on subcutaneous enoxaparin which was later switched to Apixaban after her blood test was negative for anti-phospholipid antibodies. Repeated transthoracic echocardiography showed significant improvement in right ventricular function and size. The patient was advised to consider alternative forms of contraceptives and was followed up in the coagulation outpatient clinics.

5 Illustrative Case of High Risk Pulmonary Embolism

A 79-year-old female presented to the emergency department with syncope witnessed at home after a short walk in the park. The emergency medical team arrived at the scene and found the patient conscious, but they could not obtain a measurable systolic blood pressure. On arrival to the emergency department, the patient's condition deteriorated. She became bradycardic and hypotensive and eventually progressed to asystolic cardiac arrest (Fig. 1 Step 11).

Cardiopulmonary resuscitation (CPR), including advanced medical therapy with adrenaline, calcium gluconate and sodium bicarbonate was initiated with return of spontaneous circulation (ROSC). Bedside echocardiography showed good left ventricular systolic function but a dilated right ventricle with poor systolic function (Figs. 19 and 20). Soon after, she experienced asystolic cardiac arrest requires a second round of CPR with ROSC.

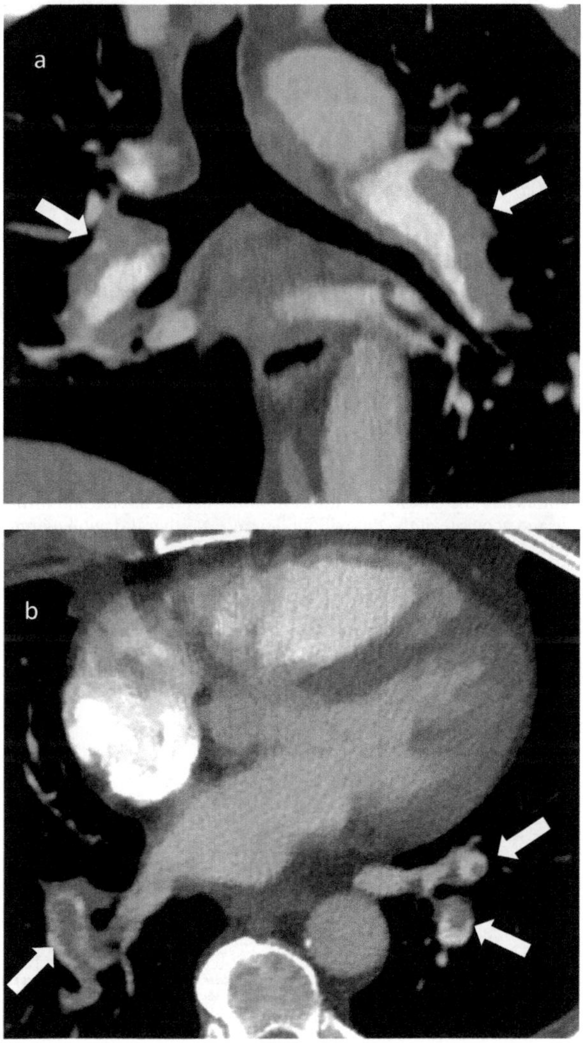

Fig. 11 **a** Coronal CTPA image shows bilateral filling defects (arrows) within the left main pulmonary artery, extending into the lobar artery to the left lower lobe an within lobar arteries to the right upper and right lower lobes. **b** Axial CTPA image shows bilateral filling defects (arrows) within segmental arteries of the left lower lobe and the right lower lobe. **c** Axial CTPA image shows main pulmonary artery dilatation (>29 mm) suggesting pulmonary hypertension. Bilateral pulmonary arteries filling defects are seen as well. **d** CTPA 4-chamber reconstruction shows increased RV:LV diameter ratio of ~1.6 and interventricular septal flattening indicating RV dysfunction. Bilateral pulmonary arteries filling defects are seen as well. **e** Sagittal CTPA image in lung window shows a sub-pleural wedge shaped alveolar opacity (arrow) in the posterior segment of the right upper lobe consistent with pulmonary infarct. **f** Axial CTPA image shows mild contrast material reflux into the IVC

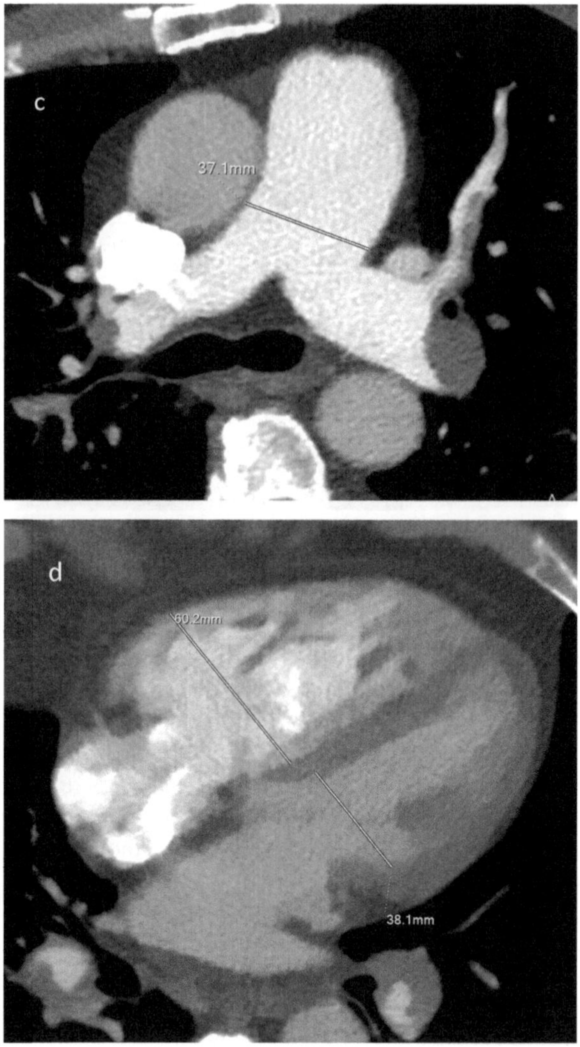

Fig. 11 (continued)

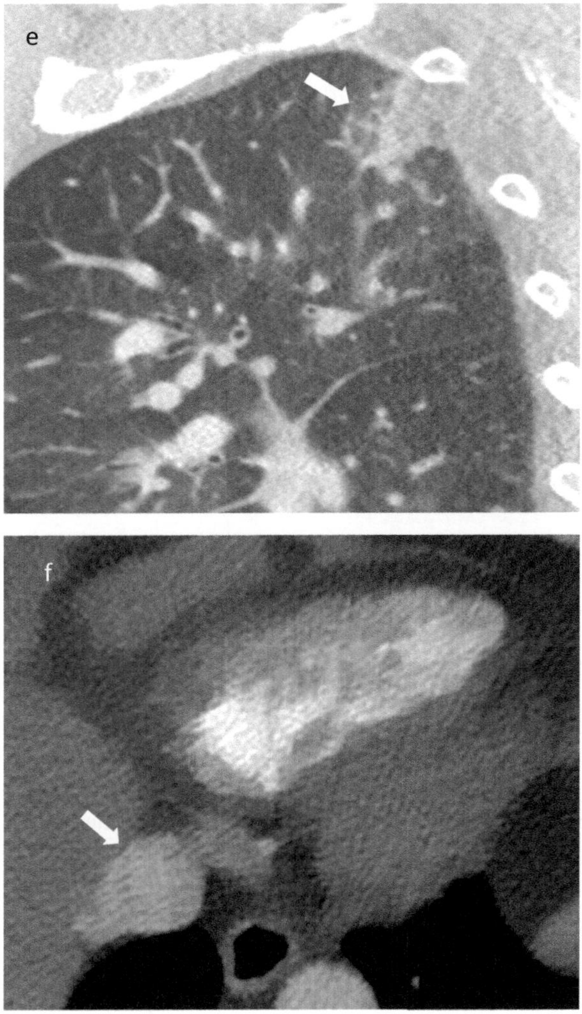

Fig. 11 (continued)

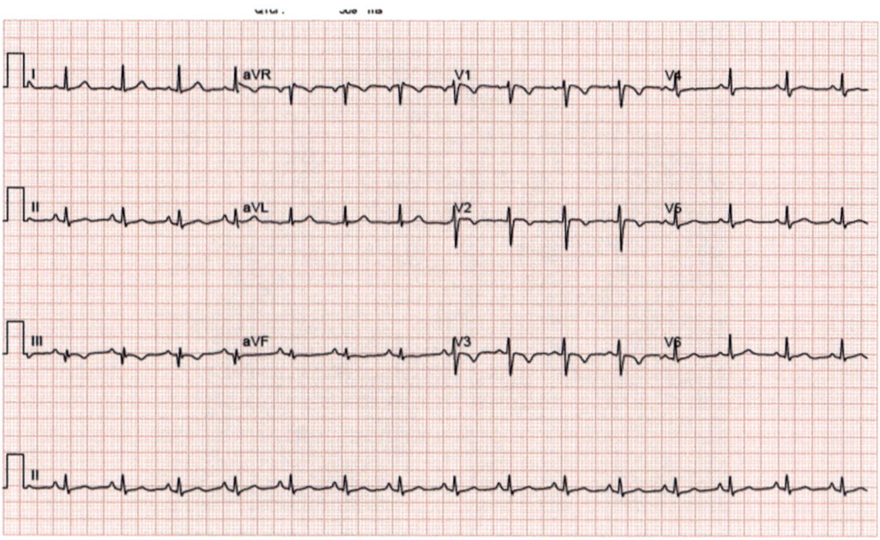

Fig. 12 ECG showed sinus tachycardia with T-wave inversion in leads V1–V3

A femoral central venous line was inserted, and an intravenous drip of noradrenaline and sodium bicarbonate was initiated due to severe metabolic acidosis. The patient was intubated and sedated but was not hemodynamically stable to be transferred to a CT scan. The patient was risk stratified as an "unstable PE" (massive PE). 50 mg of tPA was given over 15 min (0.6 mg/kg). Repeated transthoracic echocardiography showed a mild improvement in right ventricular systolic function. Her blood pressure was 80/30 mmHg on noradrenaline and she was relatively stable to be transferred to the cardiac intensive care unit. Lab work showed severe metabolic acidosis with pH of 6.88, lactic acid of 15.8 mmol/L and d-dimer of 30,000 ng/mL and troponin T of 353 ng/L. ECG showed sinus tachycardia, right axis deviation, S1Q3T3, incomplete RBBB with no other signs of acute ischemia.

On arrival to the cardiac ICU, the patient was started on intravenous unfractionated heparin and intravenous dobutamine. Shortly after her arrival, the patient went into another asystolic cardiac arrest. Additional rounds of CPR failed to restore spontaneous circulation and she was pronounced dead.

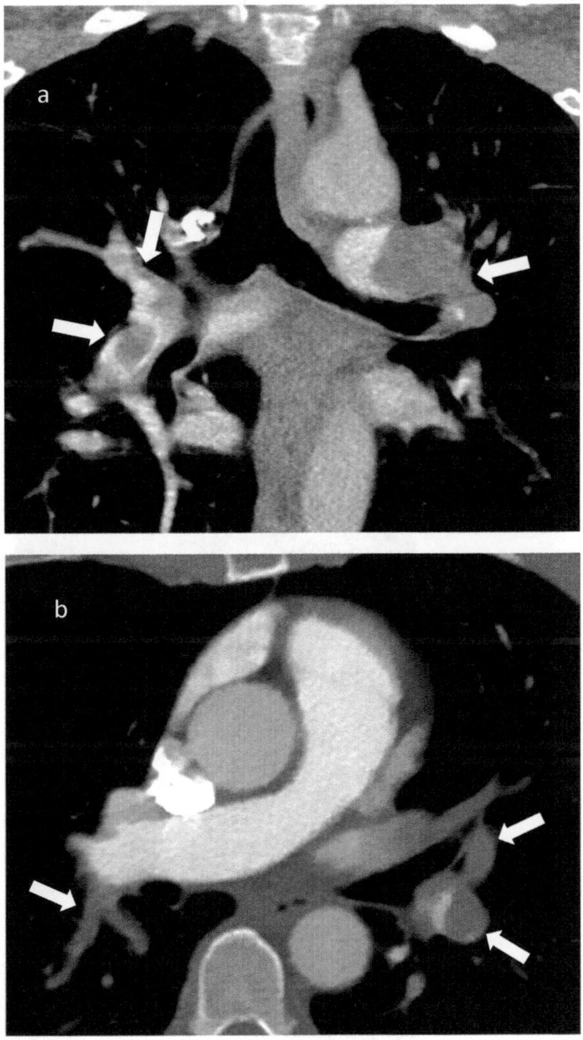

Fig. 13 **a** Coronal CTPA image shows bilateral filling defects (arrows) within the left main pulmonary artery and lobar arteries to the right upper and right lower lobes. **b** Axial CTPA image shows bilateral filling defects (arrows); On the left within the lingula artery and the lobar artery to the left lower lobe and on the right within segmental and subsegmental arteries to the superior segment of the right lower lobe. **c** CTPA 4-chamber reconstruction shows increased RV:LV diameter ratio of 2 and interventricular septal displacement indicating RV dysfunction. **d** Axial CTPA image shows mild contrast material reflux into the IVC and proximal parts of hepatic veins

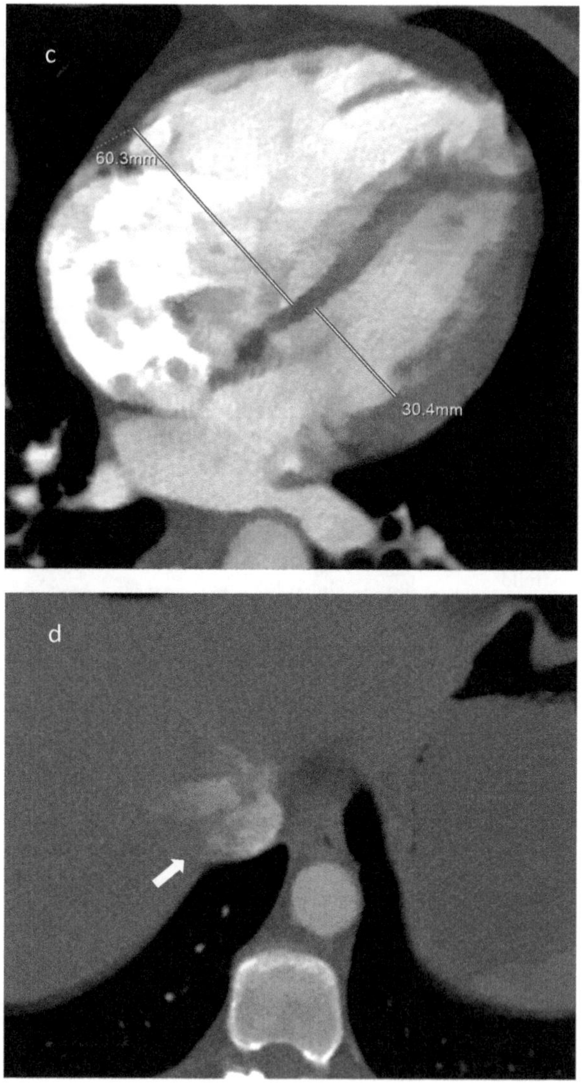

Fig. 13 (continued)

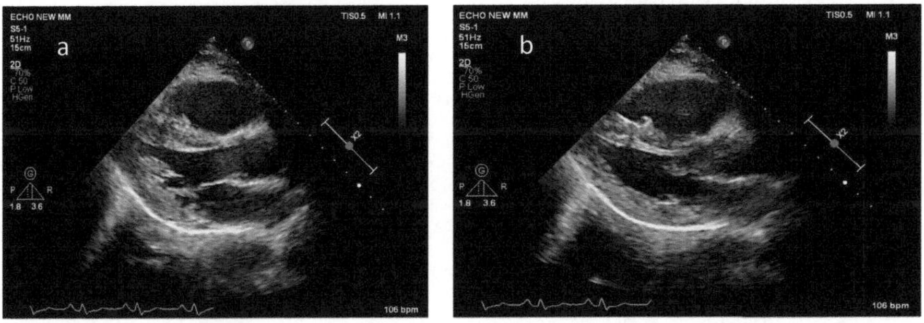

Fig. 14 Parasternal long axis echocardiography with good left ventricular function but severely reduced right ventricular systolic function with a moderately enlarged right ventricle cavity in systole (**a**) and diastole (**b**)

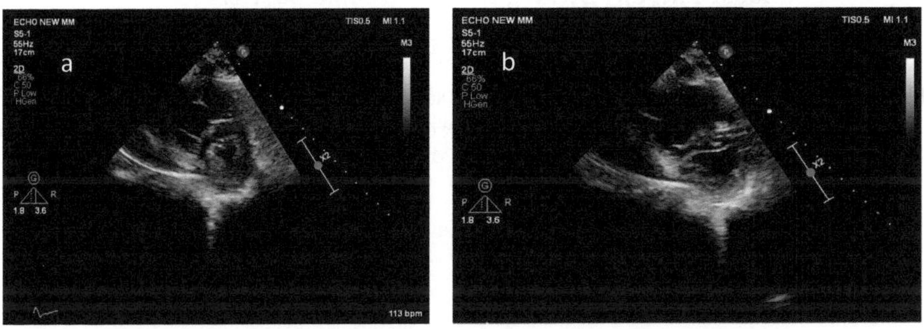

Fig. 15 Parasternal short axis echocardiography with good left ventricular function but severely reduced right ventricular systolic function with a moderately enlarged right ventricle cavity in systole (**a**) and diastole (**b**)

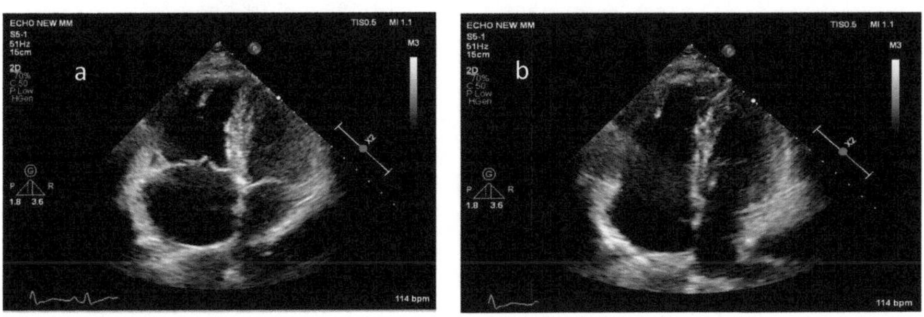

Fig. 16 Four chamber echocardiography with good left ventricular function but severely reduced right ventricular systolic function with a moderately enlarged right ventricle cavity. Free wall akinesis with apical preservation (McConnell's sign) was seen. Systole (**a**) Diastole (**b**)

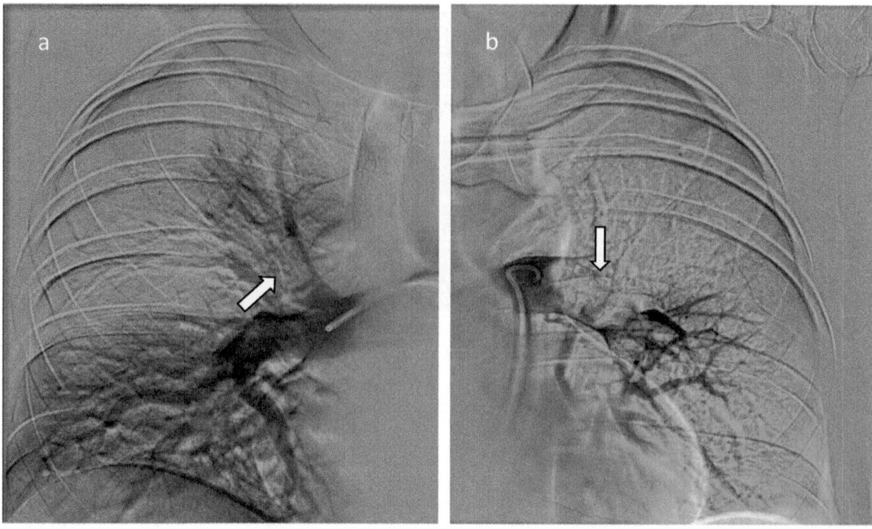

Fig. 17 Pulmonary angiography demonstrated a small embolus in the lobar branch of the right pulmonary artery (**a**) and a significant embolus with near-total occlusion of the left pulmonary artery (**b**)

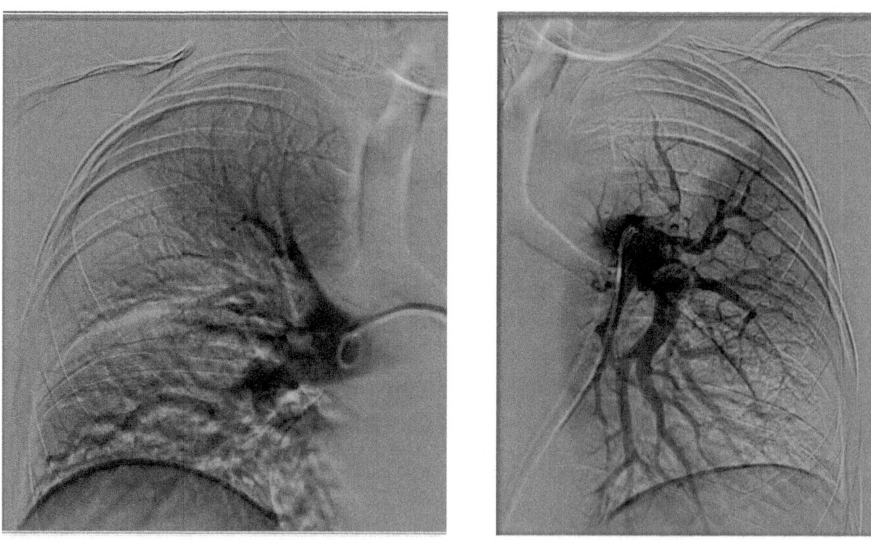

Fig. 18 Relook pulmonary angiography was performed and showed near normal left pulmonary artery blood flow

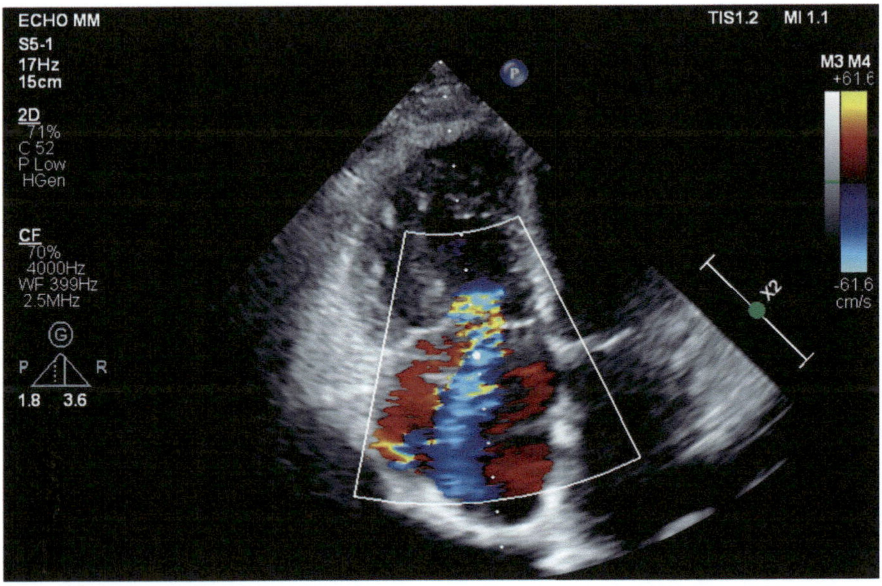

Fig. 19 Apical four chamber echocardiography demonstrating very dilated right ventricle with akinetic base and mid right ventricle and preserved right ventricle apex during systole. There is evidence of very severe wide open tricuspid regurgitation

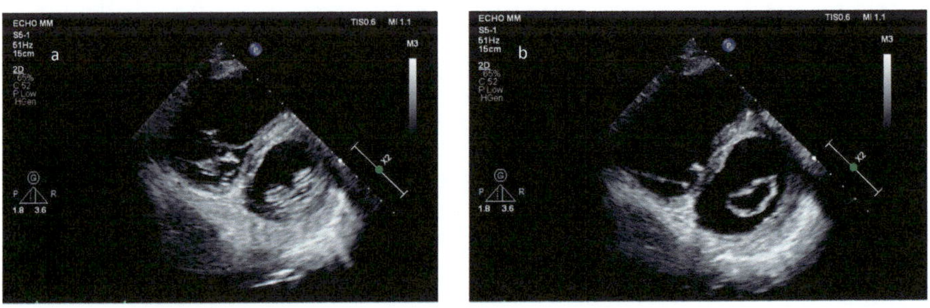

Fig. 20 Parasternal short axis echocardiogram showing enlarged right ventricle during systole (**a**) and D shaped left ventricle during diastole (**b**)

Reference

1. Herzog E, Elbaz-Greener G, Planer D, Koren T, Amir O, Shapiro J, Kalish Y. Pathway for the diagnosis and management of pulmonary embolism. Crit Pathw Cardiol. 2021;20:57–62.

Pulmonary Embolism: Information for the Patient and Family

Saman Setareh-Shenas and Eyal Herzog

1 Pulmonary Embolism: Information for the Patient and Family

1.1 Overview

Pulmonary Embolism (PE) is the consequence of blood clots that obstruct the blood flow in the blood vessels of the lungs. This condition occurs very frequently in the world, in-fact it is the third most common condition affecting the vasculature after heart attack and stroke. The severity of PE varies considerably, it ranges from minor symptoms requiring only at home treatment to requiring hospitalization in the critical care unit and invasive procedures. However, in the past decade we have witnessed notable advancements in novel diagnostic modalities and treatment options.

1.2 Causes

The body naturally utilizes a system to stop a bleed from occurring when there is a breach of blood vessels by creating clots. PE is the result of inappropriate dislodgment of blood clots into blood vessels of the lung, causing a blockage of blood supply to an

S. Setareh-Shenas (✉)
Optum Health, Covina, CA, USA

S. Setareh-Shenas
Division of Cardiology, Smidt Heart Institute, Cedars-Sinai Medical Center, Los Angeles, CA, USA

E. Herzog
Heart Institute, Hadassah Hebrew University Medical Center, Jerusalem, Israel

E. Herzog (ed.), *Pulmonary Embolism*,
https://doi.org/10.1007/978-3-030-87090-4_21

area of the lung and disrupting oxygen delivery. These blood clots most commonly originate from distal blood vessels, such as the deep veins of the legs.

The condition of inappropriate blood clots formation in the deep veins of the legs is known as deep vein thrombosis (DVT). DVTs are usually the results of improper clot formation when there is a sluggish blood flow, for example during long periods of immobility such as a long-distance air travel or trauma. Improper clot formation can also occur in patients where the body's natural mechanism of blood maintenance is more prone to clot formation, a state known as a "hypercoagulable state". Some conditions that are known to cause a hypercoagulable state for example are, cancers, pregnancy, severe infections, and COVID-19.

1.3 Symptoms

The clinical symptoms and presentation of PE varies considerably, depending on the severity of the obstruction, location of the clots, the size of the clots, as well as the presence of comorbidities. Occasionally, some patients may not experience any symptoms and remain asymptomatic. Common symptoms of PE include shortness of breath, chest discomfort, cough, or palpitations (rapid pulse or pounding heart). In addition to the above, symptoms could be accompanied with sudden a faint, lightheadedness, decreased exercise tolerance (shortness of breath during exercise), or leg pain and swelling. In the severe cases of PE, large blood clots could completely block blood flow impairing oxygen delivery via blood circulation and possibly leading to death.

1.4 Diagnosis

If the medical provider has a clinical suspicion for the diagnosis of PE, they will stratify the patient according to the probability of a diagnosis of PE as low, intermediate or high. This classification will allow the clinician efficiently to take appropriate steps to diagnose or rule-out PE.

The patients who are classified as low or intermediate risk will undergo a blood test called D-dimer assay testing, which could assist the clinician with ruling out PE. If the D-dimer assay result is positive, it will then require further testing by imaging modalities, for example computerized tomography (CT) of the pulmonary arteries and the chest, ventilation–perfusion (VQ) scan, or Echocardiography. Other diagnostic tests could be utilized to aid the medical team further with diagnosis and prognosis, for example cardiac biomarkers (e.g., Troponin, brain natriuretic peptide), anti-phospholipid antibody, arterial blood gases, and electrocardiogram (ECG).

Patients who are classified in the high-risk group should initially undergo an imaging study, a CT scan of the pulmonary arteries. This imaging study will require "contrast" or a dye to illustrate the presence of blood clots in the vessels of the lung and their extent. Echocardiography will usually be performed to assess the right ventricle of the heart—which will show specific finding of enlarged and decrease function of the right ventricle in the setting of PE. The result of the imaging studies will aid the clinicians in choosing the appropriate treatment options.

1.5 Treatment

Treatment is based on the risk stratification and severity of the PE. The majority of patients who have been classified as low risk PE, are treated with oral anticoagulation also known as blood thinners. Blood thinners help to dissolve the blood clots and to prevent further clot formation. The treatment with blood thinners is usually for a period of 3–6 months, and during this time patients will be followed in a specialty coagulation clinic if available. Very small group of patients will require lifelong treatment with anti-coagulations.

For the patients who have been classified as intermediate-high to high-risk PE, they will be evaluated by a multidisciplinary group of healthcare providers to identify the appropriate treatment modality. This multidisciplinary group includes Cardiologists, Pulmonologists, Intensivists, Radiologists, and Surgeons. In the intermediate high-risk or in high-risk PE cases that are identified to benefit from early intervention, they can undergo a procedure called catheter-directed therapy. Catheter-directed local thrombolysis is a minimally invasive intervention that delivers a medication called thrombolytics directly to the vessels of the lung to dissolve the blood clots that are obstructing the vessels. Following this procedure patients are closely monitored in a critical care unit. In rare occasions where patients are clinically unstable, they may benefit from systemic thrombolysis rather than catheter-directed local thrombolysis.

2 Summary

Pulmonary Embolism (PE) is a common disorder affecting vasculature of the lungs. PE is the result of obstruction of blood flow by blood clots in lungs vasculature. The severity of PE could vary from those who are asymptomatic to those who will require invasive catheter procedures, and unfortunately fatal for some who are unable to seek time sensitive medical interventions. In the recent years we have witnessed many advancements in effective diagnosis and therapeutics for PE. We are hopeful our diagnostic and treatment pathways will further improve prognosis for patients with PE.

Index

E. Herzog (ed.), *Pulmonary Embolism*,
https://doi.org/10.1007/978-3-030-87090-4

GPSR Compliance

The European Union's (EU) General Product Safety Regulation (GPSR) is a set of rules that requires consumer products to be safe and our obligations to ensure this.

If you have any concerns about our products, you can contact us on ProductSafety@springernature.com

In case Publisher is established outside the EU, the EU authorized representative is:

Springer Nature Customer Service Center GmbH
Europaplatz 3
69115 Heidelberg, Germany

Batch number: 10732090

Printed by Printforce, the Netherlands